Removable Denture Prosthodontics

For Churchill Livingstone

Publisher: Simon Fathers
Project Editor: Clare Wood–Allum
Copy Editor: Rich Cutler
Indexer: J. R. Sampson
Production Controller: Neil Dickson
Sales Promotion Executive: Louise Johnstone

Removable Denture Prosthodontics

Alan A. Grant DDSc MSc FRACDS

Professor of Restorative Dentistry, University of Manchester; Consultant in Restorative Dentistry,
Manchester Central Hospitals and Community Care NHS Trust; External Examiner to the Universities of London and of Wales,
The Institute of Dental Surgery and the Manchester Polytechnic; Former Examiner to Dental Students in the Universities of Baghdad,
Birmingham, Bristol, Dublin, Dundee, Leeds, Liverpool, Malaya, Melbourne, Newcastle and Singapore;
Formerly Visiting Associate Professor of Dental Materials, Northwestern University, Chicago

The late Wesley Johnson BSc MSc LDS

Formerly Senior Lecturer in Restorative Dentistry, University of Manchester; Honorary Consultant in Restorative Dentistry,
Manchester Central Hospitals and Community Care NHS Trust; Honorary Member of the City and Guilds of London Institute;
Formerly Examiner and Assessor to the City and Guilds of London Institute for the Dental Technician's Certificate;
Formerly Visiting Associate Professor of Dental Materials, Northwestern University, Chicago

SECOND EDITION

CHURCHILL LIVINGSTONE
EDINBURGH LONDON MADRID MELBOURNE NEW YORK AND TOKYO 1992

CHURCHILL LIVINGSTONE
Medical Division of Longman Group UK Limited

Distributed in the United States of America by Churchill
Livingstone Inc., 650 Avenue of the Americas, New York, N.Y.
10011, and by associated companies, branches and
representatives throughout the world.

First edition 1983
Second edition 1992

ISBN 0-443-04631-X

British Library Cataloguing in Publication Data
A catalogue record for this book is available from
the British Library.

Library of Congress Cataloging in Publication Data
A catalog record for this book is available from the Library of
Congress.

The
publisher's
policy is to use
**paper manufactured
from sustainable forests**

Published by Longman Singapore Publishers Pte Ltd
Printed in Singapore

Preface

The second edition of this book has been produced in response to continuing requests for an undergraduate text of a basic nature. Several new sections have been included in order that the overall needs of undergraduate courses in prosthodontics in terms of subject coverage might be satisfied. The FDI system of tooth notation has been adopted throughout.

As in the previous edition, the text has been kept to a minimum in the interest of simplicity and to help to control costs, since these are matters of prime concern to undergraduates.

No laboratory procedures have been included, as it is common practice in most undergraduate dental courses for the student to acquire a background in dental technology prior to the commencement of the clinical course.

In common with other clinical disciplines, prosthodontic treatment cannot be learned by rote and then applied as a series of procedures which will be equally appropriate to all patients. The physiological differences and psychological individuality of human beings, as well as their physical form, health status, social circumstances and other innumerable factors which make up the individual, must all be considered. They point to the impossibility of a single approach being successfully applied to all patients. The main thrust of this work has therefore concentrated on principles. Detailed description has been included only where existing works differ in some respect from a suggested approach. Further reading lists have been included in the hope that they will be consulted for three main reasons: first, as a means of expanding the content of the relevant chapter; second, to introduce the student gently to some of the controversies which exist in the clinical field; third, to initiate or strengthen the habit of consulting the literature, for it is here that the quality of professional life is nurtured.

Given the fundamental nature of this book, which is directed towards undergraduate dental students, it is hoped that it may also be of value to the various dental auxiliary groups where it may contribute to their understanding more readily than do more advanced texts.

It is with deep regret that the recent death of my co-author, Mr Wesley Johnson, has now to be recorded. Wesley Johnson will be remembered by generations of dentists as a distinguished contributor to the study of prosthodontics, to which he devoted the greater part of his professional life.

Manchester, 1992   A.A.G.

Acknowledgements

The line drawings have been produced by Annemarie Grant to whom we are deeply indebted for her skills and forbearance. All the typing was carried out by Mrs Janet Lear and our gratitude for her patience through the tedious drafting process and in producing the manuscript is gratefully recorded. Mrs Lear has also been a tower of strength in proof reading. We are grateful to Professor R. Yemm, who provided the basis for Figures 5.2 and 5.3, and to Dr J. R. Heath for Figure 31.1. The following photographs were produced by the Department of Medical Illustration, Manchester Royal Infirmary: 29.1, 29.2, 30.1a, 30.1b, 30.6, 30.7, 31.1, 32.2a, 32.2b, 34.1, 34.2, 34.6a, 34.6b, 34.7, 34.12, 34.14, 34.15, 35.1, 39.2, 39.3, 40.1a, 40.1b, 40.2, 40.4, 41.1, 41.2, 41.3a, 41.3b, 41.3c.

Finally, we acknowledge the support of Heather and Anne over the period of rewriting and revision of the book, and record our deep appreciation of the support they have given.

A.A.G.
W.J.

Contents

PART I

Basic aspects

1. Essential anatomy and physiology of the masticatory system

INTRODUCTION

A knowledge of the anatomy and physiology of the masticatory system is essential to the treatment of patients requiring prosthodontic service. It must be appreciated that the provision of removable dentures represents an attempt to replace lost vital tissues and, to this end, harmony of the appliance with the biological environment in which it is placed is of fundamental importance. This can only be achieved where the structure, function and functional interdependence of the related tissues is appreciated.

In this chapter it is intended to consider only those aspects of the anatomy and physiology of oral structures which are of direct importance in removable denture treatment. Further details of related tissues and their functions may be obtained from the current literature.

ANATOMY

The anatomical features relevant to the provision of a removable denture service may be considered as follows:

1. Extra-oral surface anatomy
2. Intra-oral surface anatomy
3. Structures influencing the periphery of dentures
4. Deeper anatomy.

Extra-oral surface anatomy

Figure 1.1 illustrates those structures which will be referred to in the descriptions of clinical procedures in later chapters.

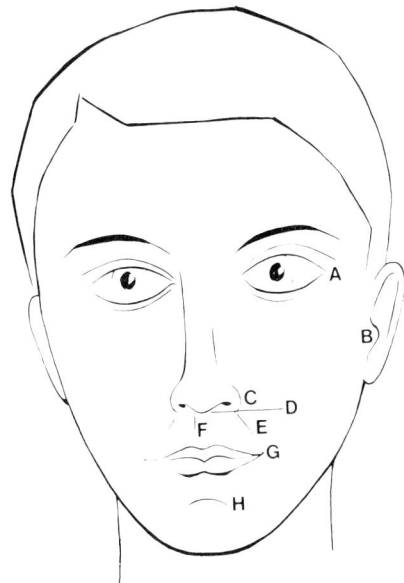

Fig. 1.1 Important landmarks on the face A, outer canthus; B, tragus; C, ala; D, columella; E, nasolabial groove; F, philtrum; G, angle of mouth; H, labiomental groove.

It has been observed that the nasolabial angle, i.e. the angle formed between the columella and the upper lip in the sagittal plane, is, on the average, approximately 90°. However, where proclination of the upper anterior teeth is present, an acute nasolabial angle is often found. In distinction, where the teeth are retroclined, the angle tends to be obtuse (Fig. 1.2).

As with all generalisations relating to human anatomy, the above may be considered useful guidelines only. The value of observations of this nature in the restoration of lost natural tissue is inestimable.

3

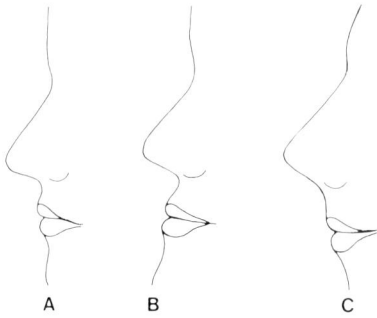

Fig. 1.2   The nasolabial angle in the sagittal plane. A, right angle; B, acute angle; C, obtuse angle.

Intra-oral surface anatomy

Figure 1.3 is a diagrammatic representation of the surface features of the dentate mouth and the edentulous mouth.

With the loss of natural teeth, the alveolar ridge resorbs and becomes the residual alveolar ridge. Resorption is initially rapid following tooth loss and then continues, sometimes intermittently, through the lifetime of the patient.

The aetiology of alveolar ridge resorption

There is a wide variation between individuals in the rate at which alveolar ridge resorption following tooth loss occurs. Some patients may show little change in ridge form over a period of years, while others may suffer gross change over a similar interval of time.

The rate of loss of alveolar bone is generally greatest in the months immediately following tooth loss. Mandibular bone loss occurs at a more rapid rate than does that of the maxilla.

The aetiology of alveolar resorption has not been fully explained, and many factors have been implicated. Some authorities regard resorption to be an atrophic change, while others consider it in the terms of a disease process.

Factors which have been implicated in alveolar ridge resorption include:

1. Anatomical factors
2. Metabolic factors
3. Biomechanical factors.

1. Anatomical factors. These relate to the quantity and quality of bone present. Large, dense ridges might be expected to change at a different rate to small ridges having widely spaced trabeculae. Atwood has suggested that these anatomical factors might be considered to have a direct relationship to ridge resorption.

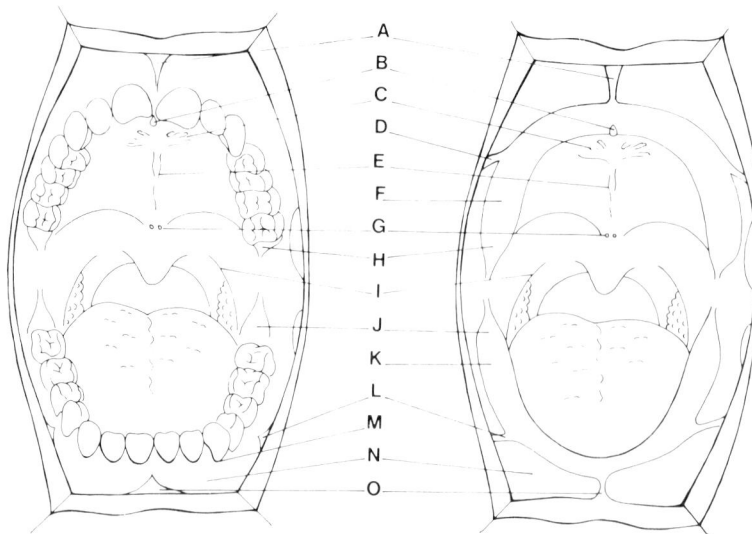

Fig. 1.3   Some surface features of the dentate mouth (left) and the edentulous mouth (right). A, labial frenum (upper); B, incisive papilla; C, rugae; D, buccal frenum (upper); E, median raphe; F, residual alveolar ridge (upper); G, fovea palatinae; H, tuberosity; I, palatoglossal arch; J, retromolar pad; K, residual alveolar ridge (lower); L, buccal frenum (lower); M, gingivae; N, vestibule; O, labial frenum (lower).

2. Metabolic factors. Many of the factors which determine the balance between bone formation and bone resorption have been described. These include systemic, nutritional, metabolic, hormonal, circulatory and local traumatic factors.

The presence or otherwise of osteoporosis or other generalised conditions of bone might also be expected to affect the jaws.

3. Biomechanical factors. The amount, frequency of application, duration and direction of applied forces, whether resulting from normal functional activity or paranormal forces (e.g. bruxism) must be considered.

In addition, the damping effect of the structure of bone and its associated tissues are considered to play a part. The term 'damping effect' refers to the absorption of part of the energy of an applied force, as a result of the viscoelastic nature of the tissues. For example, when teeth are present, the periodontal ligament will act in this way as part of the energy of the masticatory force is used as the ligament deforms under load.

In the edentulous situation, the mucoperiosteum covering the alveolar ridge, being viscoelastic in nature, will play a part. Since the bone of the maxillary ridges is cancellous in nature, it is better suited to damping compressive loads than is the mandible, which is also subject to bending forces and has well defined cortical components.

Atwood has suggested that force factors might be considered to have a direct relationship to resorption, while the damping effect may have a more indirect relationship.

Alveolar bone resorption is a progressive condition which is an inevitable consequence of tooth loss. While the exact processes involved are poorly understood, the following are implicated in its aetiology and progression:

1. Anatomical factors
2 Bone turnover factors
3 Systemic factors
4 Biomechanical factors
5 Time.

Patterns of resorption

The height of the residual alveolar ridge is reduced in both the maxilla and mandible, but in other

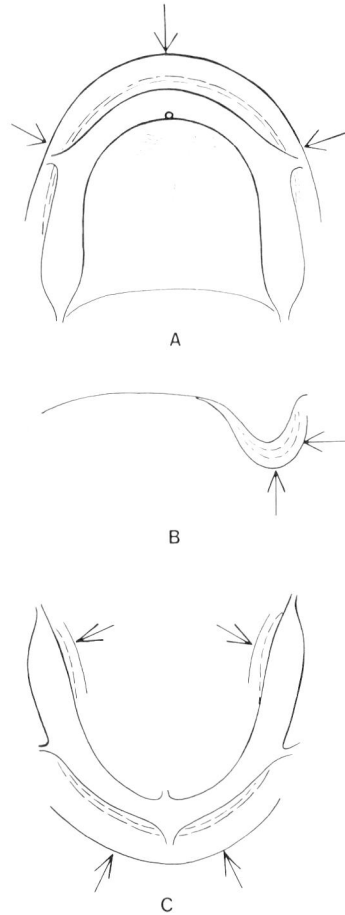

Fig. 1.4 General pattern of bone loss following extractions for the upper and lower arches. **A** Upper residual alveolar ridge and palate in plan view. Rapid resorption of the residual alveolar ridge occurs in the regions indicated by the arrows. **B** Sagittal section of the upper residual alveolar ridge. **C** Lower residual alveolar ridge. Greatest change in the form of the residual alveolar ridge occurs in the regions indicated by the arrows.

aspects the pattern of bone loss in the upper and lower jaws differs.

Resorption of the maxillary ridge occurs mainly labially and buccally (Figs 1.4A and B). In the anterior region, the incisive papilla appears to become more prominent and situated on the 'crest' of the residual alveolar ridge. When the natural incisors are in situ, the midpoint of the incisive papilla is, on the average, 10 ± 1 mm posterior to the labial aspect of the central incisors (Fig. 1.5).

In the edentulous mouth, a thin fibrous band may sometimes be seen passing from the incisive papilla

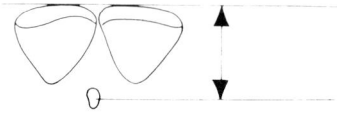

Fig. 1.5 Relation between the incisive papilla and the labial aspect of the central incisors. The average distance as indicated is 10 ± 1 mm.

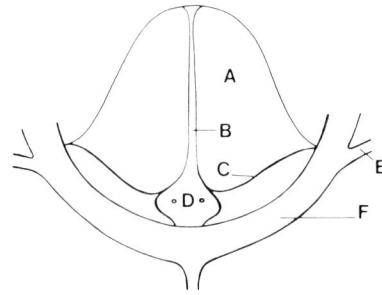

Fig. 1.6 Diagram of some structures visible with the tongue elevated. A, tongue; B, lingual frenum; C, sublingual fold; D, sublingual papillae; E, buccal frenum; F, residual alveolar ridge.

posteriorly along the crest of the residual alveolar ridge. This represents the collapsed palatal gingival margins following extraction of the teeth, and is called the lingual gingival remnant.

Resorption of the lower residual alveolar ridge occurs mainly labially and buccally towards the anterior part of the mouth. In the lower molar regions the residual alveolar ridge tends to retain its width, or, because of the form of the bone in the posterior segments, may even appear to become wider (Fig. 1.4C).

The sulci

The alveolar ridges are defined labially and buccally by a trough of soft tissue called the sulcus. The sulcus is formed by the reflection of the mucosa attached to the tissue overlying the bony ridges into the lips and cheeks. The depth of the sulcus varies in different parts of the mouth.

The lower alveolar ridge also possesses a lingual sulcus, formed by the reflection of the mucosa into the tissues of the floor of the mouth.

Within the sulci are seen frenal attachments (or frenula) which are bands of mucous membrane. A labial frenum occurs in the midline of both the upper and lower jaws. Buccal frenal attachments are present usually, one on each side of both upper and lower buccal sulci in the premolar regions. A lingual frenum is present in the midline of the lower lingual sulcus, formed by the reflection of the mucosa from the lingual aspect of the midline to the underside of the tongue.

Under the ventral surface of the tongue, on both sides of the lingual frenum, is a fold of tissue (sublingual fold) in which many ducts from the sublingual salivary glands are situated. At the frenal end of each sublingual fold is an elevation called the sublingual papilla (Fig. 1.6). The openings of the ducts from all the submandibular, and some of

the sublingual, salivary glands occur via the sublingual papillae.

The palate

The palate consists anteriorly of the hard palate and, posteriorly, the soft palate. Anatomically, the division between hard and soft palates is at the posterior margins of the palatal processes of the palatine bones.

The functional division between hard and soft palates is of more significance in removable denture construction, and this may not coincide with the anatomical division. The functional division is often called the vibrating line and is that palatal line of tissue which just fails to vibrate when the patients says 'aah'. The form of the vibrating line is generally that of a bow, concave posteriorly, whereas the anatomical division between hard and soft palates is that of a double bow, concave posteriorly.

The palate is covered with tissue formed by the periosteum and mucous membrane, which are intimately connected. This tissue is commonly referred to as mucoperiosteum. A linear median raphe is present which may be of variable prominence.

Anterior to the median raphe, the palate shows a number of transverse ridges of soft tissue, known as the palatal rugae. Their functions are obscure, but may be associated with stabilisation of food during mastication.

In many patients, two small depressions occur on either side of the midline in the region of the functional division between hard and soft palates.

These are the fovea palatinae and it is thought that they represent the common ductal openings of some of the palatal salivary glands.

A torus palatinus may be present in the midline of the hard palate. This is a mound of bone usually covered by a layer of thin mucosa. It is a benign structure of variable size and form.

More rarely, the mandible may show a torus mandibularis. This is a benign mound of bone which occurs bilaterally in the lingual aspects of the mandible in the premolar region.

The retromolar pad

The mandibular alveolar ridge terminates distally in an elevated pad of soft tissue called the retromolar pad. This represents the tissue covering the lower anterior part of the ascending ramus of the mandible. Where the last molar tooth has been lost, in some cases a pear-shaped pad is seen just anterior to the retromolar pad. This structure represents the collapsed papilla related to the last molar tooth.

The tissue covering approximately the anterior third of the retromolar pad is fixed. Beyond this, the tissue moves during functional movements of the mouth, due to the presence of muscle tissue.

The mucous membrane

The mucous membrane of the mouth is of the stratified squamous type.

A classification of the oral mucous membrane is as follows:

1. Masticatory — covering the hard palate and most regions of the gingivae.
2. Lining — covering the oral surfaces of the cheeks and lips, the labial and buccal sulci, the floor of the mouth, ventral surface of the tongue and the soft palate.
3. Specialised — covering the dorsal surface of the tongue.

The masticatory mucosa covers immobile tissue and is keratinised, whereas lining mucosa covers mobile tissues and is usually non-keratinised. Specialised mucosa is a mixture of both keratinised and non-keratinised types.

The mucous membrane and submucous tissues which cover the palate and alveolar ridges are of varying thickness and consistency. This tissue may be several millimetres thick and resilient in character, or thin with minimal subepithelial tissue, and wide variation may exist in a single patient.

The mucosa covering the dorsal surface of the tongue is highly specialised, with the anterior two-thirds covered with filiform and fungiform papillae and delineated from the posterior third by the circumvallate papillae.

Smooth mucous membrane covers the lateral borders of the tongue anteriorly. Posteriorly, several parallel vertical folds of tissue called foliate papillae occur and these may be prominent in some patients.

The ventral surface of the tongue is covered with smooth mucosa through which blood vessels may be seen. Some elderly people show a nodular enlargement of the superficial veins of the ventral surface of the tongue and these lingual varicosities, when prominent, are readily visible.

The functions of the oral mucosa are both protective to the underlying structures, and sensory — providing temperature, pressure, taste and, possibly, proprioceptive functions.

Structures influencing the periphery of dentures

The periodontal tissues

The periodontium consists of the investing and supporting tissues of the teeth and includes the gingivae, the periodontal ligament, the cementum and the alveolar bone. The periodontium supports the tooth, provides proprioceptive sensory function and has also a metabolic function.

The most readily observable of these tissues is the gingival tissue, which is that portion of the oral mucous membrane which surrounds the neck of the tooth and covers the alveolar bone crest. The gingival tissues may be divided into three portions:

1. The free (marginal) gingivae. This is the most peripheral portion and comprises a narrow, smooth rim which follows the cervical contours of the tooth. It terminates at the gingival margin on the tooth side and apically at the gingival groove, which demarcates the free and attached gingivae.
2. The attached gingivae. Apically, the attached gingivae merges into the alveolar mucosa at the mucogingival junction, except palatally where no mucogingival junction exists. The attached gingiva

is characterised by a stippled appearance, which results from interconnection of the epithelium — connective tissue interface.

3. The interdental gingivae. This is the tissue located at and within the interproximal space of adjacent teeth. Between posterior teeth which are in contact, the interdental gingiva consists of two elevated portions — the vestibular and lingual papillae — having an apically curved col between them.

Cementum provides a means for attachment of the periodontal fibres. It may become exposed to the mouth as a result of age or periodontal disease. The other periodontal tissues are not visible on examination of the mouth. However, a detailed appreciation of all the periodontal tissues is an essential part of the knowledge required by the prosthodontist and, to this end, a reference text should be consulted. In particular, note should be made of the structure of the periodontal ligament and the arrangement of the fibres, which appear to permit best resistance to forces directed down the long axis of the tooth.

Figure 1.7 is a diagram of a buccolingual section through the gingival tissues, showing their relationship to other periodontal tissues.

The remainder of this section will be considered in respect of complete denture bases, in order that all the peripheral structures are dealt with.

The maxillary denture periphery (Fig. 1.8)

The most anterior part of the periphery of the denture base is grooved by the labial frenum. Further distally, in the region of the lateral incisor, the fibres of the incisivus labii superioris arise from the alveolar border of the maxilla and arch laterally to become part of the muscle tissue comprising a portion of the orbicularis oris muscle. The tissue overlying this muscle limits the denture periphery in the region of the lateral incisor.

In the region of the canine fossa and inferior to the infra-orbital foramen is the origin of the levator anguli oris muscle. This muscle is also inserted into the muscular tissue forming the orbicularis oris muscle.

The buccal frenum limits denture base extension in the premolar region. Distal to this, the zygomatic process of the maxilla — sometimes known as the root of the zygomatic arch — limits extension of the denture base. Further distally, the buccinator muscle arises from the buccal surface of the alveolar process of the maxilla in the region of the upper molar teeth and also from the pterygomandibular raphe. The tissue overlying both these structures influences the denture base extension.

Between the tuberosity of the maxilla and the upper end of the pterygomandibular raphe, a delicate tendinous band bridges the gap between the

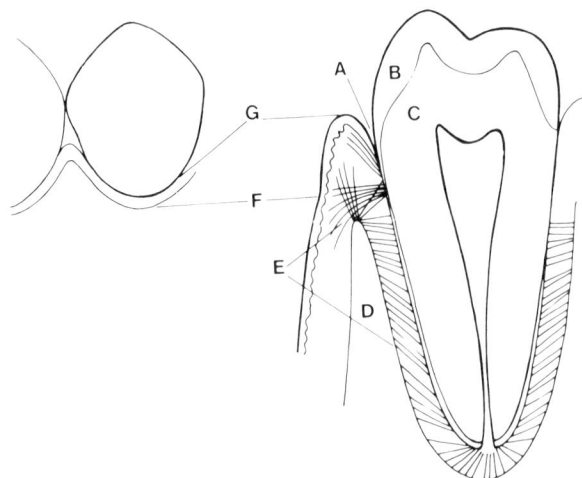

Fig. 1.7 The gingival tissues, showing their relationship to other periodontal tissues. A, gingival crevice; B, enamel; C, dentine; D, bone; E, fibres of the periodontal ligament; F, gingival groove; G, free (marginal) gingivae.

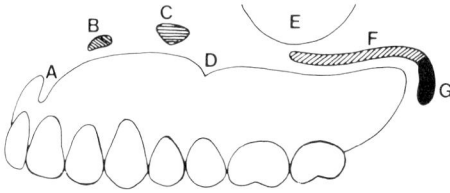

Fig. 1.8 Lateral view of an upper denture showing structures which influence the peripheral form. A, labial frenum; B, incisivus labii superioris muscle; C, levator anguli oris muscle; D, buccal frenum; E, zygomatic process of maxilla; F, buccinator muscle; G, pterygomandibular raphe.

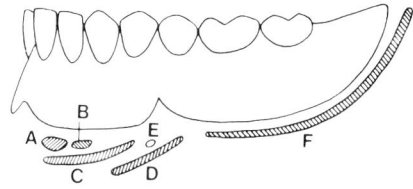

Fig. 1.10 Lateral aspect of a lower complete denture showing the structures which influence the peripheral form. A, mentalis muscle; B, incisivus labii inferioris muscle; C, depressor labii inferioris muscle; D, depressor anguli oris muscle; E, mental foramen; F, buccinator muscle.

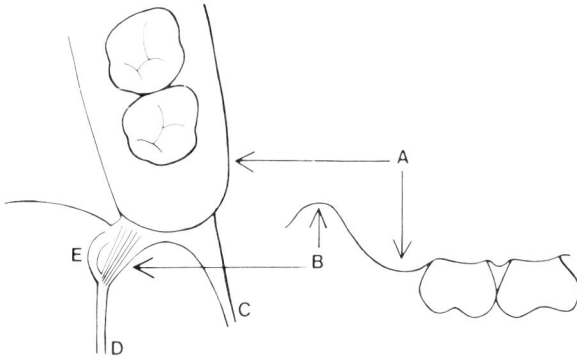

Fig. 1.9 Structures related to the left tuberosity region in plan view (left) and lateral view (right). A, tuberosity; B, hamular notch; C, lateral pterygoid plate; D, medial pterygoid plate; E, pterygoid hamulus.

maxilla and the hamulus of the pterygoid bone. A few fibres of the buccinator muscle arise from this band and form a concavity in the overlying mucous membrane which is known as the hamular notch (Fig. 1.9).

After passing from the buccal sulcus to the posterior aspect of the maxillary tuberosity, the hamular notch limits the extension of the denture base.

The vibrating line lies between the hamular notches and represents the functional division between fixed and movable palatal tissue. It is commonly, but not invariably, just anterior to the fovea palatinae and defines the posterior (anatomical) extension of the fully extended maxillary denture base.

The mandibular denture periphery (Fig. 1.10)

The most anterior part of the labial denture base periphery is usually grooved by the labial frenum.

Lateral to the labial frenum and arising from the incisive fossa of the mandible is the mentalis muscle. The fibres of the mentalis muscle descend to their insertion in the skin of the chin. Further laterally, the periphery is influenced by the tissues overlying the incisivus labii inferioris muscle, which arises at a similar level to the mentalis muscle. The incisivus labii inferioris muscle is inserted into the orbicularis oris muscle.

More distally, the depressor labii inferioris muscle arises between the symphysis menti and the mental foramen and is inserted into the orbicularis oris muscle. Passing further distally, the periphery is influenced by the tissues overlying the depressor anguli oris muscle. It arises from the oblique line of the mandible, below and lateral to the depressor labii inferioris muscle, and up to the medial aspect of the first molar tooth. This muscle is also inserted into the orbicularis oris muscle. A buccal frenum is usually present superior to either the depressor anguli oris or the depressor labii inferioris muscles, and this structure limits the peripheral denture extension in this region.

Lateral to the first molar teeth the tissue overlying the buccinator muscle delineates the buccal sulcus. This muscle is attached to the external oblique ridge of the mandible and the pterygomandibular raphe, and mingles with the superior fibres arising from the maxilla.

Distally, the denture base covers the anterior third of the retromolar pad only, as buccinator fibres are inserted into the posterior two-thirds, and this latter portion therefore moves when buccinator activity occurs.

As the outline of the lower denture proceeds lingually, the attachment of the buccinator muscle to the pterygomandibular raphe, and also the

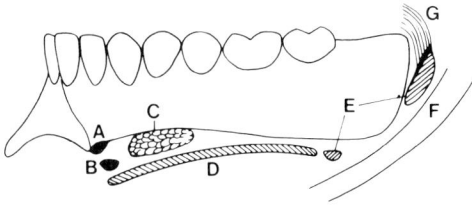

Fig. 1.11 Lingual aspect of a lower complete denture showing structures which influence the peripheral form. A, genioglossus muscle; B, geniohyoid muscle; C, sublingual gland; D, mylohyoid muscle; E, superior pharyngeal constrictor muscle; F, palatoglossal arch; G, buccinator muscle.

superior constrictor muscle of the pharynx, limits possible denture base extension. The forward movement of the palatoglossal arch during actions such as swallowing defines the posterior lingual extension of the denture base (Fig. 1.11).

The lingual extension of the complete lower denture base is mainly influenced by the tissues overlying the mylohyoid muscle, which has as its origin the whole length of the mylohyoid line. It inserts via a midline fibrous raphe to fibres from the opposite side, also to the anterior aspect of the body of the hyoid bone at its inferior border.

More anteriorly, the sublingual salivary gland lies superior to the mylohyoid muscle. In the midline, the tissue overlying the genioglossus muscle at its attachment to the superior genial tubercles delineates the extension of the denture base.

Deeper anatomy

A number of the deeper anatomical structures of the head also influence the shape of removable dentures, especially the surface aspects of the appliance.

Anteriorly, the oral sphincter and the associated orbicularis oris muscle have a strong influence.

Near the angle of the mouth the decussation of the fibres of muscles associated with the orbicularis oris, together with those of the buccinator, form the modiolus (Fig. 1.12). A number of the muscles of facial expression are also inserted into the modiolus. The modiolus is a region of intensive muscular activity and may have a strong influence on denture design in the premolar region. This is further considered in Chapter 3.

The relationship of muscle tissue about the periphery of a lower complete denture, when shown in a plan view, gives an indication of its importance in denture base design (Fig. 1.13).

The temporomandibular joint

The temporomandibular joint is the joint between the cranium and the mandible. The bony elements involved are the articular eminence, glenoid tubercle of the temporal bone and the condyle of the mandible.

The joint is paired and the right and left joints are not independent of each other, as the cranial and

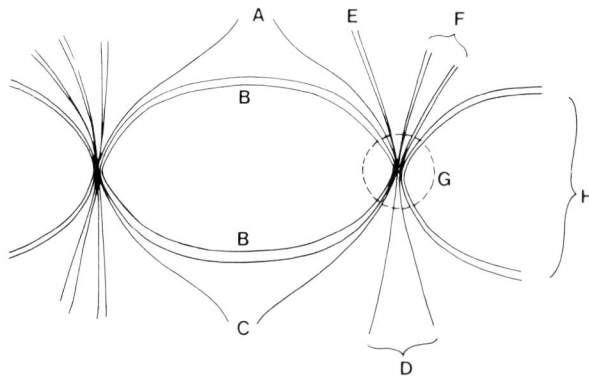

Fig. 1.12 Illustration of the circumoral musculature. A, incisivus labii superioris muscles; B, orbicularis oris muscle; C, incisivus labii inferioris muscles; D, depressor anguli oris and caninus muscles; E, levator anguli oris muscles; F, zygomaticus muscle; G, modiolus; H, buccinator muscle.

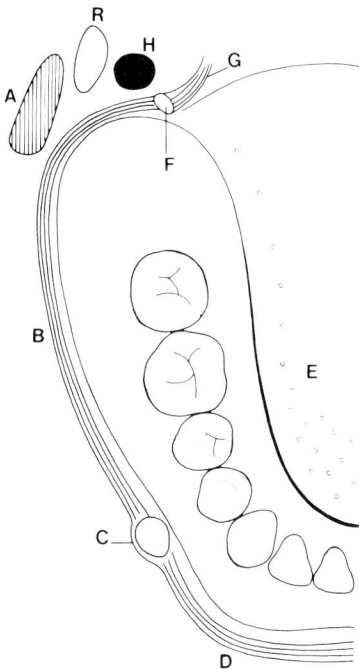

Fig. 1.13 Relationship of muscular tissue to the periphery of the right half of a complete lower denture in plan view. A, masseter muscle; B, buccinator muscle; C, modiolus; D, orbicularis oris muscle; E, tongue; F, pterygomandibular raphe; G, superior constrictor muscle; H, medial pterygoid muscle; R, ramus of mandible.

mandibular elements are, in effect, single bones.

The glenoid fossa is lined with a thin layer of fibrous tissue which is much thicker anteriorly, covering the articular eminence. The slope of the articular eminence varies widely between individuals and may be subject to change during life.

The mandibular condyle is roughly elliptical in form, with the long axis being directed medio-laterally and the short axis anteroposteriorly. The articular surface is covered with a layer of fibrous tissue which is thickest over the convexity of the condyle.

Interposed between the cranial and mandibular elements of the joint is the articular disc or meniscus. The disc is not uniformly thick, having a thin central area and thickened anterior and posterior portions.

Posteriorly, the disc is composed of two layers. The upper lamina of the disc attaches to the squamotympanic fissure and the lower lamina to the posterior surface of the neck of the condyle.

The upper lamina contains loose white fibroelastic tissue. Anteriorly, the disc is attached to the anterior edge of the articular eminence and the articular margin of the condyle (Fig. 1.14).

The capsule of the joint is thin anteriorly and posteriorly, but is strengthened medially and laterally by the capsular ligaments.

The structure of the disc and its attachments are such that a considerable range of movements of the condyle, relative to the temporal bone, can occur. Movement of the disc relative to the roof of the glenoid fossa can take place and also a limited amount of movement between the disc and the condyle.

The lateral poles of the condyles are approximately 1 cm beneath the skin and can be placed in the region of a point some 12 mm anterior to the tragus of the ear on a line extending to the outer canthus of the eye.

A detailed knowledge of the components and relations of the joint is essential to an understanding of the temporomandibular articulation, and reference to the literature should be made. The above description is only intended to serve as a basis for considering the complex and variable nature of possible movements within the joints.

MANDIBULAR MOVEMENTS

In addition to the movements which may occur in the joints themselves, a knowledge of the movements of the mandible is of fundamental importance to an understanding of the functional occlusion of the teeth and dentures.

Mandibular movements are generally represented as the excursions of the mid-incisal point of the mandible.

In order to understand some of the points referred to in considering relations between the jaws, it is necessary first to consider the basic terms used in this field.

Jaw positions and related terminology

There are many positions which the mandible may occupy relative to the maxilla, and also different positions in which the teeth may contact. In order to avoid confusion in the description of jaw and teeth positions which are used throughout this text,

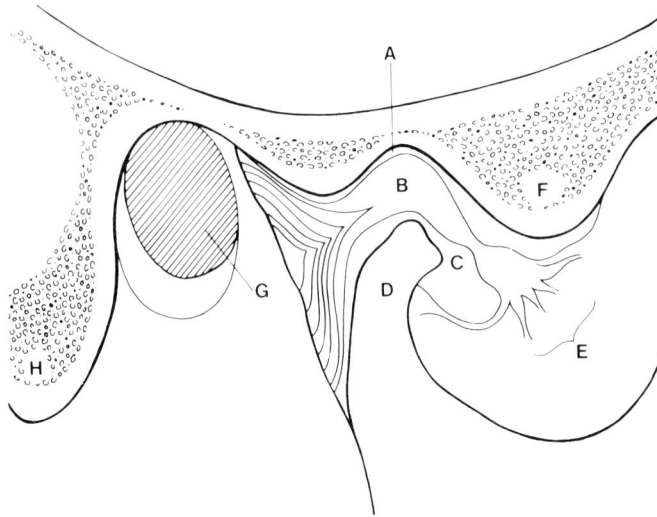

Fig. 1.14 Diagram of an anteroposterior section through the right condyle and glenoid fossa. A, upper joint compartment; B, disc; C, lower joint compartment; D, head of condyle; E, lateral pterygoid muscle; F, articular eminence; G, external auditory meatus; H, mastoid process.

it is important that a standard form of terminology be adopted.

The position of the mandible is usually described relative to the maxilla and is termed a 'jaw relation', which may be defined as 'the positional relationship which the mandible bears to the maxilla', and is usually considered in a vertical or horizontal plane.

When referring to tooth contact, the term 'occlusion' is used and may be defined as 'the contact relationship of the masticatory surfaces of the teeth or their equivalent'.

The rest jaw relation

The rest jaw relation of a person is the relationship of the mandible to the maxilla when the person is seated at ease in an upright position, with the Frankfort plane horizontal and the muscles controlling the mandible in equilibrium. In rest relation, the opposing teeth are not in occlusion and the amount by which they are separated is known as the interocclusal distance or freeway space.

The rest jaw relation is dependent on a balance of muscular forces between the muscles attached to the mandible. The resting posture of the mandible is subject to variations both in short- and long-term periods. Since muscular forces are involved, a change in the posture of the patient will produce a change in the interocclusal distance. For a patient with the trunk erect, if the head is tilted forward, the interocclusal distance becomes smaller and the mandible moves anteriorly. Tilting the head backwards causes the mandible to move postero-inferiorly.

Other factors which affect the rest jaw relation include emotion, physical health, age, proprioception from the teeth, muscles and oral mucosa, and the pattern of tooth loss. Because of the clinical significance of the rest jaw relation it is important that the student becomes familiar with the current literature on this topic.

Measurement of interocclusal distance

The interocclusal distance between individual teeth is rarely measured directly and a convenient clinical method for assessing its magnitude can be obtained from reference points chosen on the midline of the face.

With a patient seated upright as described above, the interocclusal distance has been estimated to average between 2 and 4 mm.

The presence of an adequate interocclusal distance is essential to the success of removable denture treatment. Over- or underestimation of the interocclusal distance may result in the clinical effects described in Chapter 10.

Horizontal relations

Horizontal relations between the jaws and teeth may be considered to exist anteroposteriorly in the sagittal plane and laterally in the coronal plane.

Retruded jaw relation (centric jaw relation). Retruded jaw relation is the unstrained, most retruded relation of the mandible to the maxilla at the established vertical dimension of occlusion. It should be noted that although this is essentially a horizontal jaw relation, reference is made also to the position of the mandible in the vertical plane. When the retruded jaw relation is recorded, the clinician establishes the vertical dimension of the occlusion either by accepting contact of the patient's natural teeth, or by reference to the rest vertical dimension, so that an adequate interocclusal distance will result.

Maximal intercuspal position. This is the relation of opposing occlusal surfaces at which the cusps of the maxillary and mandibular teeth contact with maximum intercuspation. It is dependent upon the presence of tooth contact, whether natural or artificial, in the molar and/or premolar regions of both maxilla and mandible.

A further position to which reference may be made is the muscular position. This is the horizontal contact relation of the teeth determined by the habitual muscle pattern.

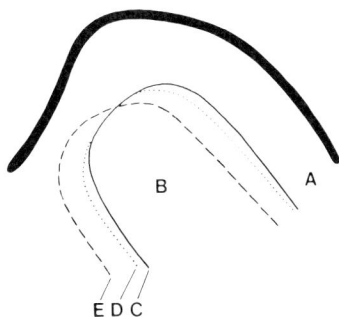

In many dentulous subjects, retruded jaw relation and the maximal intercuspal position do not correspond (Fig. 1.15).

In the treatment of edentulous subjects, however, the teeth are arranged in the maximal intercuspal position and must contact in this position in the mouth when the mandible is in the retruded jaw relation.

Border movements of the mandible

Border movements are the maximum excursive movements of the mandible which can be achieved. These movements are rarely, if ever, performed during normal functional activity such as occurs during mastication and speech. Consequently, most functional movements are intraborder movements.

Recording of border movements in the sagittal plane produces the form of excursion illustrated in Figure 1.16.

Hinge movement (or terminal hinge movement) is considered to be a purely rotational movement of the mandible about an intercondylar axis and occurs over a short distance at the commencement of opening, extending from closure to approximately the rest position of the mandible.

In the coronal plane, the border movement appears as in Figure 1.17.

In the horizontal plane, the border excursions appear as shown in Figure 1.18.

The form of excursion in the horizontal plane,

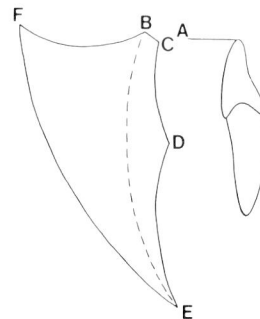

Fig. 1.16 Border movements of the mandible in the sagittal plane. A, represents a pointer attached to the mid-incisal point of the lower incisors; B, teeth in the maximal intercuspal position; C, teeth in retruded jaw relation; D, extent of hinge movement of the mandible; E, maximum opening; F, maximum protrusion. Line EB represents the path of habitual closure from the position of maximum opening.

Fig. 1.15 Illustration of various condyle positions. A, anterior part of fossa; B, condyle; C, maximal intercuspal position; D, retruded jaw relation; E, muscular stimulation.

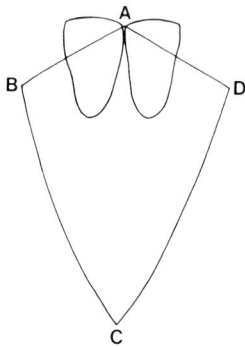

Fig. 1.17   Border movements of the mandible in the coronal plane. A, teeth in retruded jaw relation; B, right lateral excursion of the mandible; C, maximum protrusion; D, left lateral excursion of the mandible.

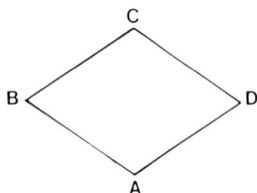

Fig. 1.18   Border movements of the mandible in the horizontal plane. A, teeth in retruded jaw relation; B, left lateral excursion of the mandible; C, maximum protrusion; D, right lateral excursion of the mandible.

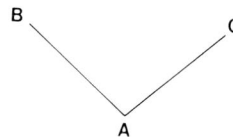

Fig. 1.19   The 'Gothic arch' form. A, retruded jaw relation; B, left lateral excursion of the mandible; C, right lateral excursion of the mandible.

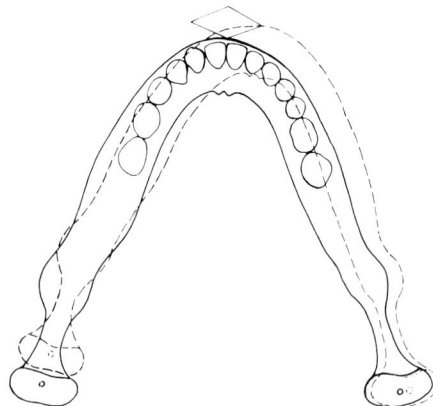

Fig. 1.20   Plan view of the mandible. The position of the mandible following a right lateral excursion is shown by the dashed line. Bennett movement is shown by the lateral movement of right condyle.

from the retruded jaw relation to the extremity of lateral movements, produces a pattern which has been styled a 'Gothic arch' (Fig. 1.19) and has been adapted to a clinical technique. This is considered in Chapter 24.

Bennett movement

A further detail of movements of the mandible which occurs during lateral excursions should be appreciated, especially in relation to restoration of the natural dentition. This is known as the Bennett movement and consists of a bodily lateral translation of the mandible to the side towards which the mandible is moving, and is illustrated in Fig. 1.20. The condylar movement which occurs on the side towards which the mandible moves is of the order of 1–2 mm.

The muscles producing mandibular movement

Primary movements of the mandible result from the contraction of muscles attached to the mandible. The principal muscles involved are designated the muscles of mastication and they are the:

1. Masseter
2. Medial pterygoid
3. Lateral pterygoid and
4. Temporalis muscles.

The digastric, geniohyoid, mylohyoid and platysma muscles are also associated with depression of the mandible.

From a functional point of view, the muscles of mastication may be divided into four groups, as illustrated in Figure 1.21.

In considering the movements of the mandible, it is important to appreciate that various combinations of muscle groups are always involved, and that contraction of similar muscles of the right and left sides does not necessarily occur simultaneously and equally. The nature of the muscle activity which takes place is that of coordinated and reciprocal

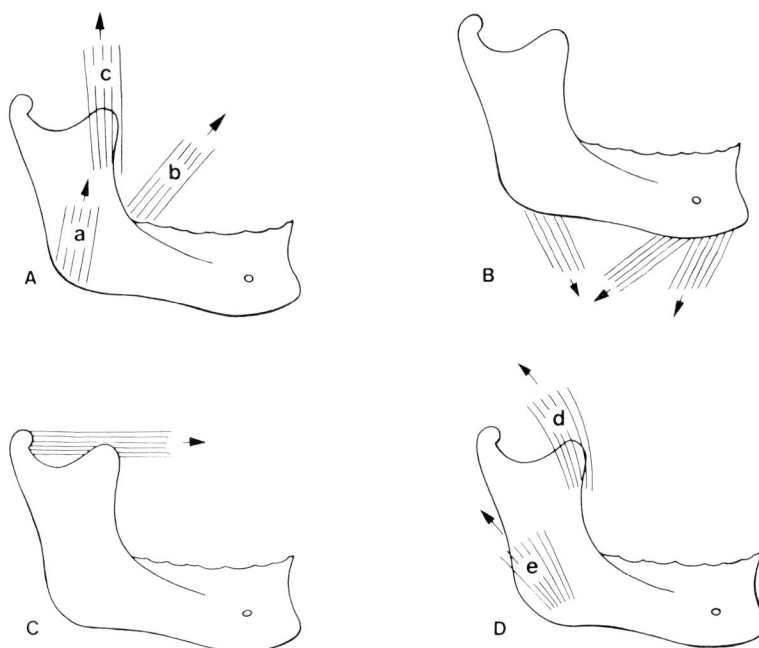

Fig. 1.21 Illustration of the activity of the mandible resulting from contraction of the major muscle groups. **A** Elevators; a, superficial and medial layers of masseter muscle; b, medial pterygoid muscle; c, vertical fibres of temporalis muscle. **B** depressors, including digastric, geniohyoid, platysma and posterior vertical fibres of mylohyoid muscle. **C** Protractors: lateral pterygoid muscles. **D** Retractors; d, horizontal fibres of temporalis muscle; e, deep layers of masseter muscle.

actions of the elevator and depressor muscles. In addition, reflex actions are known to occur during mandibular functional activities.

SALIVA

Saliva is secreted from three large pairs of glands — the parotid, submandibular and sublingual salivary glands — and many others situated in the lips, tongue and palate. Salivary secretion is controlled by the autonomic nervous system.

Many functions have been ascribed to saliva including:

1. Moistening and lubrication —keeping soft tissues pliable and preventing drying.
2. Solvent action — dissolving solids and thus aiding in appreciation of food and taste bud stimulation.
3. Preparation of food for swallowing — altering the consistency and forming a lubricated, plastic mass of food.

4. Digestive function — the presence of, for example, amylase, may help to dissolve starchy food substances.
5. Regulation of water balance — drying of mucous membranes results in a sensation of thirst.
6. Excretory function — many drugs and electrolytes are excreted in saliva.
7. Buffering function — saliva buffers acid in the diet and also acts as a temperature buffer against hot and cold foods.
8. Peripheral seal — saliva acts to form a peripheral seal, necessary for the retention of some removable dentures, and also an oral seal during the suckling process.

From the prosthodontic viewpoint, the formation of a peripheral seal for a denture is an important function. A further effect related to saliva is that of oral galvanism — i.e. the development of an electrical potential difference between dissimilar metals in saliva, which is a good electrolyte.

The amount of saliva secreted each day varies

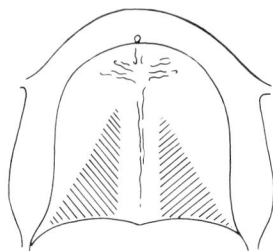

Fig. 1.22   The hatched areas indicate the approximate distribution of the palatine mucous glands.

from individual to individual. In addition, saliva is not an homogeneous fluid but is probably best considered as a suspension of bacteria, food particles, cellular elements and other particulate matter. The composition and physical properties of saliva from an individual may vary widely throughout the day.

The property of viscosity is one which has received considerable attention in considering the retention of dentures and, in general, it has been shown that there is a relationship between viscosity and adhesive capacity. In this respect, the secretions of the palatine mucous glands have been shown to be important in the retention of a complete upper denture (Fig. 1.22).

The role of saliva in denture retention is further considered in Chapter 2.

Variations in flow

The quantity of saliva secreted may be:

1. Diminished (xerostomia)
2. Increased (sialorrhoea).

A temporary decrease in salivary flow may result from an emotional reaction, such as fear. A large number of systemic conditions can also cause xerostomia, and it may also result as an ageing effect as the glands atrophy. Also, and more commonly, it may be a side effect of drug therapy.

Xerostomia may result in a 'burning' sensation of the oral tissues and tongue and cracking of the lips. The oral mucosa becomes dry, smooth and translucent and denture retention is frequently severely diminished. Mucous membranes become susceptible to frictional effects from dentures and are much more friable and readily traumatised.

It is important that an abnormally reduced salivary flow be detected at the examination stage of denture construction, in order that steps may be taken to redress the situation. A possible xerostomia which was previously undetected by a patient may become obvious when a new appliance is provided, with the result that the patient may 'blame' the condition on the treatment provided.

Sialorrhoea, or profuse salivary secretion, is commonly caused by local irritation such as sharp teeth, pathology — e.g. ulcers, or a new denture. It may also result from some diseases of the nervous system. When caused by a 'foreign body', such as a new prosthesis, the effect will be temporary and the rate of flow will return to normal within a few days.

Oral galvanism

Oral galvanism may result in corrosion of metallic restorations in the mouth. Pain resulting from the electrical potentials developed between dissimilar metals in the mouth has also been reported. The presence of metallic and non-metallic ions in the saliva create good conditions for the fluid to act as an electrolyte.

SPEECH

Because of the importance of the oral cavity in the production of intelligible speech, it is necessary to have an understanding of phonetics before attempting to design prostheses for insertion into the mouth.

The sounds of speech are all created by obstructing or shaping the stream of the breath. The shaping and the interruption of the expired air produces the sounds known as vowels and consonants.

The organs involved in varying the contours of the airstream are the lips, the tongue, the teeth, the alveolar ridges, the hard and soft palates and the vocal folds.

Vowel sounds are made by the free and unobstructed passage of air through the various cavity resonators: the larynx, the pharynx, the nasal cavity and the oral cavity. Varying the lip, jaw and tongue positions changes the vowel sounds and makes them different from one another.

To form consonants, the air passage is either closed or narrowed, thus preventing the air passing freely from the mouth. The interruption of the airstream creates the sound. Sounds made when the narrowing or closure of the air passage is created by contact between the teeth, alveolar ridges and palate, and other of the organs of speech, are particularly susceptible to possible difficulties following the loss of teeth and the insertion of a denture.

The tongue is a remarkably adaptable organ and usually requires only a relatively short period of readjustment to changes occurring in the mouth, following tooth extraction or prosthodontic treatment. In respect of the insertion of dentures into the mouth, this statement assumes that the appliance is carefully designed, being well retained and providing adequate tongue space.

Dentures and speech

Vowel sounds

The tip of the tongue lies on the floor of the mouth during the production of the vowel sounds and either contacts, or is very close to, the lingual surfaces of the lower anterior teeth. Any denture having a component which is to be placed in this part of the mouth should not encroach on the space required to accommodate the tongue.

Consonant sounds

As the consonant sounds require contact between various anatomical elements, it is convenient to consider a classification in terms of the parts concerned:

1. Labials — sounds requiring contact between the lips, e.g. 'b', 'p' and 'm'. These sounds may be altered if changes in the occlusal vertical height or forward positioning of the teeth make lip contact difficult.

2. Labiodentals — sounds requiring contact between the lips and teeth, e.g. 'f', 'ph', 'v'. A change in the level of the incisal edge of the upper incisor teeth may affect these sounds.

3. Linguodentals — sounds requiring contact between the tongue tip and the upper incisors, e.g. 'th'. This sound may be affected when the horizon-tal overlap between the upper and lower incisors is excessive, or when an excessive occlusal vertical height has been provided.

4. Linguopalatals — sounds requiring contact between the tongue and the palate. These may be considered as subgroups according to whether the anterior, and/or lateral, portions of the hard palate or the soft palate are involved.

a. Sounds requiring contact between the tongue and hard palate, e.g. 'd', 't', 'l', 'ch', 'j'. A change in palatal contour, such as may be created by reducing the interpremolar width, may produce cramping of the tongue, causing particular problems with sounds requiring the lateral margins of the tongue to contact the lingual surfaces of the upper posterior teeth.

b. Sounds requiring contact between the tongue and soft palate, e.g. 'h', 'g', 'ng'. The thickness and positioning of the posterior border of a denture, or a palatal bar, may cause it to be contacted by the dorsal surface of the tongue in making these sounds, and can result in a feeling of nausea and possibly impair speech.

5. Nasal — Where air cannot escape via the mouth, sounds may emerge via the nose, e.g. lip contact in the production of 'm'. The occlusal vertical height and also the inter-arch width of a denture may be implicated where difficulties with the nasal sounds occur.

Apart from the immediate post-insertion period, speech difficulties arising from removable dentures are not common where the appliance has been carefully designed, provides maximum stability in the mouth, and replaces lost tissue with the minimum of encroachment on tongue activity.

FURTHER READING

Atkinson PJ, Woodhead C 1968 Changes in human mandibular structure with age. Arch Oral Biol 13: 1453
Atwood DA 1971 The reduction of residual ridges. A major oral disease entity. J Prosthet Dent 26: 266
Barker BCW 1971 Dissection of regions of interest to the dentist from a medial approach. Aust Dent J 16: 163
Barrett SC, Haines RW 1962 Structure of the mouth in the mandibular molar region and its relation to the denture. J Prosthet Dent 12: 835
Bates JF, Stafford GD, Harrison A 1975 Masticatory function — a review of the literature. Part 1. the form of the masticatory cycle. J Oral Rehab 2: 281

Chierici G, Lawson L 1973 Clinical speech considerations in prosthodontics: perspectives of the prosthodontist and speech pathologist. J Prosthet Dent 29: 29

Christensen FG 1969 Some anatomical concepts associated with the temporomandibular joint. Parts I and II. An Aust Coll Dent Surg 2: 39

Devlin H, Ferguson MWJ 1991 Alveolar ridge resorption and mandibular atrophy. A review of the role of local and systemic factors. Br Dent J 170: 101

Edgar WM, O'Mullane DM 1990 Saliva and dental health. British Dental Association, London

Jackson RA, Ralph WJ 1980 Continuing changes in the contour of the maxillary residual alveolar ridge. J Oral Rehab 7: 245

Keng SB, Ow R 1983 The relationship of the vibrating line to the fovea palatini and soft palate contour in edentulous patients. Aust Dent J 28: 166

Myer J, Alvares DF, Gerson SJ 1976 The structure and function of the oral mucosa. In: Cohen B, Kramer IRH (eds) Scientific foundations of dentistry. Heinemann, London

Nairn RI 1975 The circumoral musculature: structure and function. Br Dent J 138: 49

Preiskel HW 1972 Lateral translatory movements of the mandible. Critical review of investigations. J Prosthet Dent 28: 46

Rees LA 1954 The structure and function of the mandibular joint. Br Dent J 96: 125

Schroeder HE 1976 Gingival tissue. In: Cohen B, Kramer IRH (eds) Scientific foundations of dentistry. Heinemann, London

Scott JH, Dixon AD 1978 Anatomy for students of dentistry, 4th Edn. Churchill Livingstone, Edinburgh

Tallgren A, Lang SR, Walker CF et al. (1983). Changes in jaw relations, hyoid position, and head posture in complete denture wearers. J Prosthet Dent 50: 148

Tanaka H 1973 Speech patterns of edentulous patients and morphology of the palate in relation to phonetics. J Prosthet Dent 29: 16

Thompson JR 1946 The rest position of the mandible and its significance in dental science. J Am Dent Assoc 33: 151

2. Denture retention

INTRODUCTION

It is fundamental to the success of prosthodontic treatment that appliances placed in the mouth should maintain their planned relationship to the tissues which they contact. In the absence of adequate retention, dentures are unlikely to be functionally effective or physiologically acceptable.

The retention of a denture may be defined as the resistance it possesses to withdrawal from its planned position in the mouth.

Another descriptive term often coupled with that of retention is stability. Stability is a measure of the ability of a denture to remain firm, steady and constant in position when forces are applied to it.

The difference between retention and stability may be illustrated by reference to a simple clinical test applied to dentures to assess, qualitatively, these properties. Retention is generally tested by attempting to remove a denture by means of a force applied in the opposite direction to that in which the appliance was seated in position. Stability may be assessed by observing any movement which occurs by the application of a force in the same direction as that by which the denture was seated in position. A denture may remain in close contact with the underlying tissues (i.e. have good retention) but, by virtue of the displaceability of those tissues, demonstrates appreciable movement when subjected to occlusally directed forces (i.e. it may demonstrate poor stability). Methods of overcoming clinical situations which may lead to instability of a denture are considered in the appropriate sections relating to impression procedures, jaw relationships and tooth arrangements.

FACTORS AFFECTING DENTURE RETENTION

The factors affecting denture retention can be divided into:

1. Physical
2. Mechanical and
3. Physiological forces.

Physical factors

Forces associated with the salivary film

The physical properties of cohesion, surface tension, adhesion and viscosity all play a part in denture retention.

Cohesion. Cohesion refers to the forces of attraction between like molecules. The cohesive forces in a fluid (such as saliva) will act to maintain the integrity of the fluid, whether the fluid is moving or at rest.

Surface tension. The intermolecular forces responsible for cohesion in a fluid act equally on all molecules within the bulk of the fluid. At the surface, one component of these forces is missing, thus resulting in a net attractive force towards the interior of the liquid (Fig. 2.1). This directional energy gives rise to the phenomenon of surface tension, which counteracts forces tending to break the surface of the liquid. It also tends to give the fluid the smallest possible surface area. It should be realised that solids also possess surface tension.

Adhesion. Adhesion refers to the forces of attraction between unlike molecules. For adhesion to be accomplished between a solid and a fluid, wetting of the solid by the fluid must take place, and the degree to which this occurs will depend on their

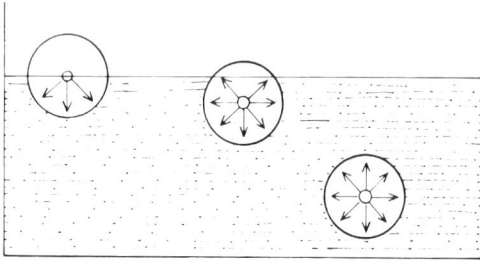

Fig. 2.1 Intermolecular forces within the bulk of a fluid act equally in all directions. At the surface, the net force is directional towards the interior.

relative surface tensions. The wetting characteristics of a fluid may be described in terms of the contact angle formed with the solid surface on which it is placed — a high contact angle indicates poor wetting (Fig. 2.2).

In considering the role of cohesion, wetting characteristics and adhesion in denture retention, the adhesive forces between the saliva and oral mucous membrane present no problems in (physiologically) normal circumstances. This is because saliva effectively wets oral mucous membrane.

The wetting characteristics between saliva and the denture base material will determine the effectiveness of the adhesion of saliva to the denture. Most commonly used non-metallic denture base materials are effectively wetted by saliva.

The cohesive forces within the saliva will complete the mucous membrane–saliva–denture system and, with good adhesion between the saliva and the oral mucous membrane and the denture, these forces will make a significant contribution to denture retention.

Early workers attempted to relate the above factors regarding the relationship between the denture and the underlying tissue as similar to that of two flat parallel plates separated by a fluid film,

which can be represented by the formula

$$F = \frac{2\gamma A}{H},$$

where F is the force required to separate the plates, γ is the surface tension constant of the interposing fluid film, A is the surface area of the plates and H is the distance separating the plates.

It is now appreciated that the above relationship represents an oversimplified account of the problem. In the clinical situation there is considerable variation between patients in respect of, for example, the area covered by the denture base and the direction and magnitude of the displacing forces applied. It also takes no account of the role played by the viscosity of the saliva.

Viscosity. Viscosity is the resistance to flow of a fluid, resulting from intermolecular forces acting within the fluid.

When a fluid is set in motion, the cohesive forces within the fluid act as a form of intermolecular friction to oppose the movement. If a fluid tends to move between parallel plates, the molecules nearest the plates move only slowly because of the adhesive forces acting, while the central molecules move the fastest. The closer the two plates are together, the nearer the flow of fluid approaches the speed of the fluid nearest the plates, so that a thin film of fluid resists flow more readily than a thicker film (Fig. 2.3). In addition, fluids having a high viscosity resist flow more effectively than those of lower viscosity.

Experimental work which has been carried out in respect of denture retention and viscosity of saliva has shown that the retention between glass plates increases with increase in viscosity of an interposed film of saliva. It has also been shown that for a given viscosity value, high retention values result when a denture is subjected to high forces of short duration and, conversely, that small forces acting over an

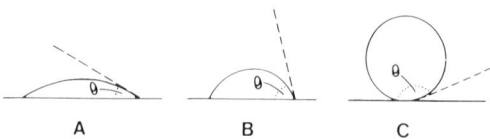

Fig. 2.2 **A** Very small contact angle in a spreading system, e.g. alcohol and clean glass, **B** θ is just less than 90°, e.g. water and acrylic resin; **C** High contact angle in a non-wetting system, e.g. water and wax.

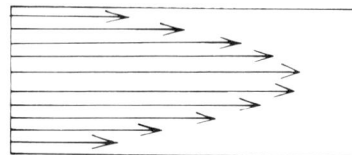

Fig. 2.3 Fluid near the walls of the plates moves slowly while that in the centre moves more rapidly.

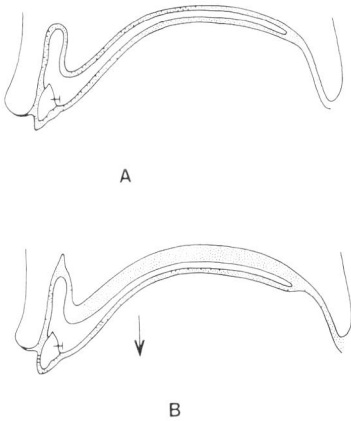

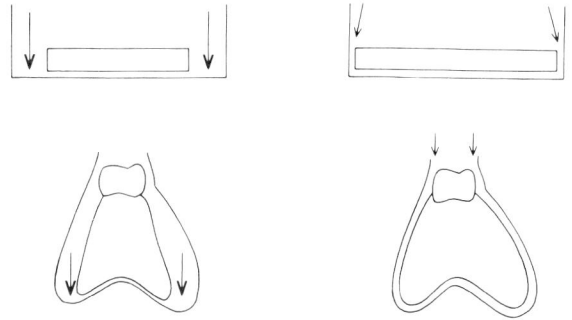

Fig. 2.5   The two diagrams on the left illustrate wide openings and consequent easy displacement of the plate and denture. In the diagrams on the right the plate and denture are shown to fit closely against the sides, and upward displacement is more difficult because more time is required for fluid to pass through the restricted opening.

Fig. 2.4   A downward displacing force causes additional saliva to be drawn under the denture. **A** Denture at rest; **B** Denture subjected to a downward displacing force.

extended period may dislodge a denture. This is because there is little time for flow of saliva to occur when a force is applied suddenly.

When in position in the mouth, a denture is covered over all surfaces by a continuous film of saliva. Should the denture be subject to a force tending to displace it, a reduced pressure will result in the salivary film under the denture, relative to that in the oral cavity. This will cause additional saliva to be drawn under the denture (Fig. 2.4).

The additional saliva will result in loss of retention of the denture, because of the resultant increase in distance between the denture and the mucosa. It is, therefore, essential that the relationship between the periphery of the denture and the surrounding tissue is such that the closest possible adaptation exists. Close adaptation about the periphery will have the effect of delaying the rate of influx of saliva under the denture base (Fig. 2.5). This aspect of close adaptation of the denture base to the tissues is usually referred to as peripheral seal, and is referred to again in the section on physiological forces.

Clearly, the viscosity of the saliva will have a significant effect in the above description, and it should be appreciated that the viscosity of saliva varies markedly between patients and even in a single patient under varying circumstances.

An analysis of factors involved in the separation of two plates in an analogous situation to that of a denture completely surrounded by saliva has produced the following relationship:

$$F = \frac{3\eta A^2}{2h^3} \cdot \frac{\mathrm{d}h}{\mathrm{d}t} \ ,$$

where F is the force required to separate the two plates of surface area A, η is the viscosity of the fluid in which the plates are immersed, h is the distance between the plates and $\mathrm{d}h/\mathrm{d}t$ represents the rate of separation of the plates.

The above formula indicates that increasing the viscosity will increase the force required for separation of the plates and that the greater the area covered, the higher will be the separation force required, especially since this factor is raised to the second power. Low values of h, i.e. the distance between the plates, are very significant as this factor is cubed. The time over which the force producing separation occurs is also taken into account.

As indicated above, the forces derived from cohesion, adhesion and wetting characteristics contribute to denture retention. Thus, in order to obtain the maximum possible benefit for denture retention from the physical forces related to the salivary film, the denture base should:

1. Cover the maximum usable area.
2. Provide for the closest possible adaptation between the denture base and the oral mucous membrane.
3. Provide for accurate peripheral seal.

Gravity

A further force which should be considered in relation to denture retention relates to the weight of the appliance. In the upper jaw, light weight is advantageous as lower gravitational forces will be acting on it. In the lower jaw, however, additional weight may help to keep the denture in place. Care must be exercised in this latter case to ensure that the mass of any appliance is kept within the physiological limits of tolerance for the patient, so that neither muscular fatigue nor accelerated bone resorption occur.

Magnetic forces

Magnetic forces of repulsion have occasionally been used in an attempt to stabilise dentures. The like poles of permanent magnets are contained in opposing dentures, so that the forces of repulsion act to seat the dentures firmly when the dentures are at, or near to, contact. This has not been shown to be effective. More promising is the use of the force of attraction in the overlay denture, where one element of the magnetic system is attached to the remaining root face of the patient, and the other to the denture which fits over the root face.

Vacuum devices

This type of device aims at the production of a reduced pressure in a circumscribed area of the denture base — usually in an upper complete denture. The dangers of older devices such as rubber suction discs — a sucker-like attachment to the tissue side of the palate of an upper denture — are well documented. Their use is now condemned.

Relief areas are sometimes used in upper dentures, in order to compensate for unequal displaceability of the tissues contacted by an overlying denture, and so improve stability. Such areas have the effect of increasing the distance between the denture and the tissue over the area relieved and, as a result, cause a reduction in the retentive forces derived from close contact between the denture and the tissues.

Relief areas may be supplemented by valves which are designed to enable the patient to evacuate the relief area by sucking on the valve. There is no evidence of continuing effectiveness of these valves as the relief area is quickly filled by saliva and tissue, which proliferates into the area.

Mechanical factors

Engagement of undercuts

The use of undercut areas in edentulous regions of the mouth may be possible. This is illustrated in Fig. 2.6.

Springs

Mechanical devices such as springs are used only rarely to assist the retention of complete dentures in such circumstances as post surgical rehabilitation, and are considered to be outside the scope of this text.

Most removable partial dentures depend for their retention on friction or direct mechanical interlocking.

Friction

Friction may be utilised by virtue of contact between parts of a partial denture and the remaining teeth, which may be modified in order to provide for more effective retention. Either naturally present contact points, such as are used in the Every design denture, or tooth and restoration surfaces modified to produce guiding planes, are examples.

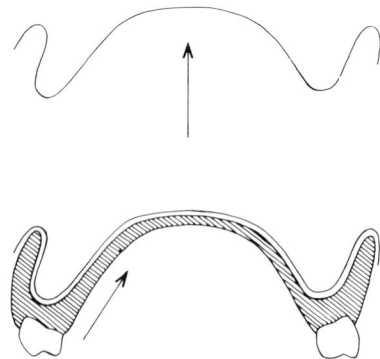

Fig. 2.6   Attempts to insert the denture vertically will fail because of the undercuts present. Inserting the denture from the side allows it to contact the residual ridge and will provide for mechanical resistance to a direct downwards force.

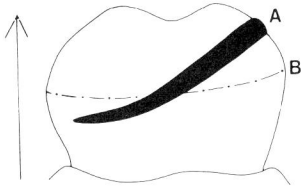

Fig. 2.7 The tip of the clasp arm must deform to allow its withdrawal over the tooth. A, clasp arm; B, survey line (maximum convexity of the tooth with respect to the direction of surveying).

In the majority of circumstances where partial dentures are to be provided, additional retention in the form of:

1. Direct or
2. Indirect retainers

will be required.

Direct retainers

Direct retention is obtained by means of clasps, or by the use of preformed (precision) attachments.

Clasps. Clasps provide resistance to a displacing force because they are so designed that the terminal end rests on an undercut surface. For the denture to be displaced, it is necessary for the clasp arm to be moved over the most bulbous portion of the tooth.

Provided that the force tending to dislodge the denture is less than that required for the clasp arm to be displaced from the undercut, the denture will be retained in position (Fig. 2.7).

Preformed (precision) attachments. These comprise a male component which is usually attached to the saddle (q.v.) of the denture, and a female part which is fabricated into an inlay or crown of an abutment tooth. When assembled in the mouth a dovetailed, ball and socket, or hinged joint is formed, which provides for mechanical retention (Fig. 2.8).

These two types of direct retainer will be considered in more detail in respect of their place in partial denture treatment.

Physiological forces

These relate to the musculature of the oral cavity. In this respect, the buccinator, orbicularis oris and the musculature of the tongue may be regarded as the most important.

Active muscular fixation of dentures may be obtained by careful attention to the form of those surfaces which contact their environmental tissues. The tongue on the lingual surface and the peripherally placed muscles of the lips and cheeks may be considered to act as antagonists, so that in the

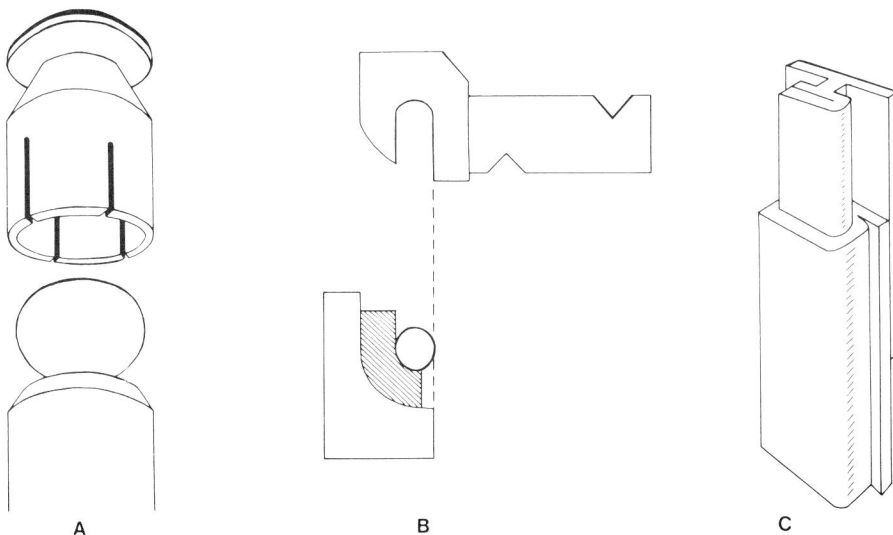

Fig. 2.8 Some types of precision attachment: **A** ball and socket; **B** hinge; **C** dovetailed slot.

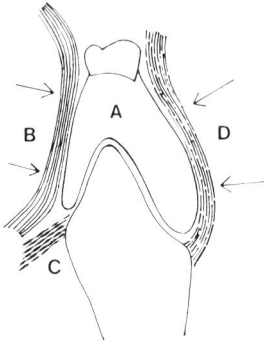

Fig. 2.9 Opposing muscle groups acting to stabilise a lower denture. A, denture; B, tongue; C, mylohyoid muscle; D, buccinator muscle.

event of careful, clinically developed denture form, the simultaneous contraction of the two muscle groups may stabilise the denture and retain it against its foundation (Fig. 2.9).

The accurate approximation of the tongue, cheeks and lips to a denture also acts to impede the flow of saliva about the denture, thus increasing the effective area for retention. When a small displacing force is applied to a denture, the reduced pressure which develops in the salivary film under the denture will cause the soft tissues about the periphery of the denture to move inwards, thus reducing the potential flow of saliva under the denture. Inaccurate extension of a denture may allow increased saliva and even air to enter under a denture and cause loss of retention. Because of the small surface area covered by a complete lower denture relative to the length of border, the potential for saliva and air leaks is high. For the upper denture, there is little or no movable tissue available at the posterior palatal border, so that the breakdown of the film of saliva in this region may occur on only

slight displacement. Consequently, a specially formed addition to the denture is provided to assist in retention in this region. This addition is called the posterior palatal seal or post-dam, and is considered in Chapter 26.

It may be helpful to think in terms of retention derived by accurate denture base extension and approximation to the adjacent tissues as resulting from interfacial seal.

Careful development of the form of the 'polished' surfaces of dentures can be a powerful aid to denture retention. This is well illustrated by the common clinical experience whereby the dentures worn by a patient for many years can be shown to be poorly adapted to the foundation tissues, and yet are regarded by the patient as being a good 'fit'.

In such a situation, muscular fixation has compensated for the loss of retention via physical factors which pertained at the initial insertion of the denture.

Provision for muscular fixation is required in the design of both complete and partial dentures.

FURTHER READING

Avant WE 1971 Factors that influence the retention of removable partial dentures. J Prosthet Dent 25: 265
Barbenel JC 1971 Physical retention of complete dentures. J Prosthet Dent 26: 592
Bates JF 1980 Retention of partial dentures. Br Dent J 149: 171
Brill N 1967 Factors in the mechanism of full denture retention — a discussion of selected papers. Dent Pract 18: 9
Caldwell RC 1956 A method of measuring the adhesion of foodstuffs to tooth surfaces. J Dent Res 38: 188
Clayton JA, Jaslow C 1971 A measurement of clasp forces on teeth. J Prosthet Dent 25: 21
Laird WRE, Grant AA, & Smith GA 1981 The use of magnetic forces in prosthetic dentistry. J Dent 9: 328
Lindstrom RE, Pawelchak J, Heyd A, & Tarbet WJ 1979 Physical–chemical aspects of denture retention and stability. A review of the literature. J Prosthet Dent 42: 371
O'Brien WJ 1980 Base retention. Dent Clin North Am 24: 123

3. Principles related to denture design

INTRODUCTION

The functions to which the oral tissues contribute depend on sensory processes for their control. In the context of removable dentures, the functions related to mastication and speech are of particular interest. In addition, the large number of transient tooth contacts made throughout the day, for instance, in swallowing saliva must also be considered.

It will be helpful to consider briefly some functional aspects of normal occlusion of the natural teeth at this stage.

FUNCTIONAL OCCLUSION

In Chapter 1, the term 'occlusion' was used to define the contact relationship between opposing teeth. During function, the upper and lower dentitions move relative to each other. The dynamic relationships which exist during sliding of the opposing teeth while they are in contact is called articulation.

Balanced occlusion refers to an arrangement of the teeth so that, in any occlusal relationship, as many teeth as possible are in occlusion. When changing from one occlusal relationship to another with a smooth, sliding contact maintained, free from cuspal interference, balanced articulation is said to exist.

The functional occlusion is controlled by a complex neuromuscular mechanism in which various sensory elements play a part.

The features of a functionally optimum occlusion include the following:

1. The teeth should receive occlusal stresses consistent with the physiological requirements of the supporting structures. It has been shown that a tooth must be stimulated to maintain the support provided by the periodontal ligament. Too much or too little stimulation may lead to damage or atrophy of the ligament. The arrangement of the tooth in its socket is such that the periodontium is capable of resisting axial forces better than those directed laterally.

2. The effects of occlusal forces are minimised by firm, interproximal tooth contacts and simultaneous occlusal contacts.

3. Closure into the maximal intercuspal position must be even and free of any premature contacts or cuspal interference.

4. The presence of an acceptable amount of freeway space is essential.

5. During mandibular movements such as in chewing, when occlusal contacts are made other than in the maximal intercuspal position, the teeth usually slide back to that contact relationship before another masticatory cycle commences. Ideally, balanced articulation should exist, but this is rarely achieved with the natural dentition.

RESTORATION OF THE DISRUPTED OCCLUSION

The loss of parts of the dental tissues is accompanied by the loss of some of the exteroceptive and proprioceptive apparatus. This will have a direct effect on the ability of the remaining oral components to function normally. In addition, when attempts to replace the lost tissue by means of a prosthesis have been made, the nervous mechanisms about the mouth may suffer further interference.

On the basis of a knowledge of the functional anatomy and normal occlusion, a number of principles of design for removable prostheses may be defined. These are as follows:

1. The restoration must not interfere with normal physiological processes.

2. The restoration must not prejudice the health of the remaining hard and soft tissues.

3. The restoration must be tolerated in the mouth.

Although the factors listed above are interdependent, they will be considered separately. It should, however, be appreciated that there is considerable overlap between them.

Interference with normal physiological processes

The nervous pathways controlling mandibular movements include voluntary and reflex mechanisms. Only the sensory component of the neuromuscular control mechanism will be considered here, because of its direct relationship to tooth loss.

The sensory nerve endings provide exteroceptive and proprioceptive sense. Exteroceptive sense is that of pressure, temperature, etc., and proprioception is the awareness of position in space.

Proprioceptive elements are located in the tendons, muscles, ligaments (including the periodontal ligaments) and joints of the jaws. Exteroceptive innervation lies in the periodontal ligaments, the epithelial surfaces of the oral cavity, tongue muscles, muscles of mastication and the temporomandibular joints.

Some examples of the way in which removable prostheses may influence sensory mechanisms about the mouth follow and are intended to illustrate the severe interference to normal function which may result.

Premature contact between opposing teeth

In the context of removable dentures, this is a situation which might occur where uneven contact between a natural tooth and part of a denture in the opposing jaw takes place. The proprioceptive nerve endings of the periodontal ligament serve an important function. When a tooth is contacted prematurely, these receptors send impulses through a reflex arc to the muscles of mastication, which contract in a manner which attempts to avoid the premature contact. As pointed out above, the ideal situation exists when the teeth contact simultaneously without interference. This produces simultaneous firing of the periodontal receptors and reinforces the habitual path of closure. If the premature contact cannot be avoided, several consequences may follow:

1. The neuromuscular system attains asynchronous contraction patterns which causes increased muscle tonus and may act as a trigger for bruxism (grinding or forceful clamping together of the teeth and jaws).

2. Pain may develop in the periodontal membrane.

3. Pain may develop in the temporomandibular joint, due to eccentric closure of the jaws in attempting to avoid the pain of premature contact.

4. A general effect on the nervous system may occur, when continual attempts to avoid pain must be made.

Errors in jaw relations

Temporomandibular joint proprioception is thought to play a key role in identifying mandibular position and in control of muscular activities about the jaws. Errors in securing jaw relations in respect of either the vertical or horizontal component might, therefore, be expected to interfere severely with oral function. This type of error is more likely to be associated with patients who have lost several teeth from one or both jaws.

Clasps

As already pointed out, a natural tooth can withstand forces directed along the long axis of the tooth much more effectively than laterally directed forces. Some laterally directed forces are generated during normal mastication and, in addition, where a removable partial denture is present, a clasped tooth will receive stimuli from forces applied to the opposite side of the denture through the denture. Lateral stresses to a tooth contacted by a denture may, therefore, build up to physiologically unacceptable levels.

In addition, the presence of an inaccurately constructed clasp about a tooth can cause a stream of nervous signals to be produced, which may cause interference with the normal controlling mechanism of the masticatory system. This aspect is further considered in the section on surveying, as it is fundamentally important that clasps be accurately constructed, and that any appliance contacting the natural teeth is passive when not in function.

Prejudice to the health of the hard and soft tissues

It is clear that the above examples of possible interference with physiological processes could also be considered in this section. It is, however, intended to consider here two further aspects:

1. Trauma
2. Plaque control.

Trauma

Mention has been made of the effects on the nervous control mechanism of the masticatory apparatus by an inaccurately clasped tooth. Inaccuracy may also result in direct traumatic injury to the periodontal membrane. Similarly, any part of partial or complete dentures which contacts any part of the oral mucous membrane inaccurately may cause traumatic injury. Margins or flanges of dentures which extend excessively onto movable tissues are included in this category, and the trauma produced may result in mild inflammation at one end of the scale, to ulceration of the epithelium and sub-epithelial tissues, or even hyperplasia of the soft tissues where persistent, severe and prolonged damage has occurred.

Dentures which contact the tissues accurately, but where the teeth occlude inaccurately, may also result in trauma to the underlying tissues as a result of the transmission of unplanned forces through the denture. In this context, the diminished sensitivity of the oral mucous membrane on which a denture is placed after tooth extraction, relative to that of the natural tooth, should be borne in mind. The sensitive receptors in the periodontal membrane of the natural tooth provide much better protection to possible tissue overload than does the mucous membrane.

Surfaces of dentures which are not adequately smooth or polished may cause trauma to the cheeks, tongue or mucoperiosteum covering the residual alveolar ridges or palate. In addition, where artificial teeth are not accurately placed in relation to the opposing teeth, trauma in the form of cheek, lip or tongue biting may result.

Plaque control

The presence of a removable denture in the mouth provides an increase in the surface area to which plaque may be retained.

A discussion of plaque formation and the damaging effects of plaque accumulation is beyond the scope of this text. It is, however, important to bear in mind that the presence of plaque accumulations can result in dental caries and periodontal disease. The very fact of a patient seeking removable denture treatment is often an indication that natural teeth have been lost as a result of tooth decay or periodontal disease. Such a patient might be regarded as being particularly at risk in this respect, and particular attention will need to be given to his education in oral hygiene measures.

The design of an appliance to be placed in the mouth must be carried out with an appreciation of the need to minimise plaque retention, coupled with the importance of educating the patient in oral and denture hygiene measures.

A removable partial denture often involves many natural teeth and gingival margins, and covers a large area of the other oral tissues. It is very demanding of good plaque control, as periodontal disease and caries may otherwise occur.

Similarly, complete dentures present large areas for the retention of plaque. In this case, however, no natural teeth or gingival margins are present and the effects of plaque accumulation will be on the soft tissues covered by the denture, and may encourage candidal infection of the mucous membrane.

Details of methods by which the effects of plaque accumulations on removable dentures may be minimised are considered in Chapters 20 and 27.

Tolerance in the mouth

The great majority of patients become accustomed to the wearing of a prosthesis following tooth loss.

This may include even those patients who express strong doubts as to whether they will ever 'get used to' an appliance.

The only somatic mechanism by which a patient can become accustomed to a foreign appliance in the mouth is through readjustment to the changed nervous responses about the oral cavity which result from tooth loss, and the subsequent placement in the mouth of a denture. This requires a carefully designed appliance to facilitate adaptation of the tissues which comprise the denture environment. The space available for removable appliances to be placed in the mouth is a major consideration in this respect, and is discussed below.

Psychological factors can be very powerful in respect of dental treatment, and there are a number of dental conditions which are thought to have psychological involvement. The conditions are best described as psychosomatic processes. The literature includes the following as amongst those in which a psychosomatic component may be present: gagging, temporomandibular joint dysfunction, bad taste, periodontal disease and maxillofacial pain.

Consideration of psychological factors is regarded as an advanced aspect of prosthodontic treatment, and the student is referred to the current literature for further details, beyond those presented in Chapter 4.

The space available for removable dentures

The space available is dependent on the nervous mechanisms discussed above, and also the functional activity of the environmental musculature.

The term used to describe the space which a removable denture may occupy in the mouth is the 'denture space'. It may be described as that space limited by the tongue, cheeks, lips, residual alveolar ridges and any remaining teeth.

A simplified version of the denture space in the edentulous mouth is shown in Figure 3.1 and is based on the concept that:

1. The force developed by the cheek is exactly balanced by that of the tongue and
2. Such a balance of forces is likely to occur at, or near, the crest of the residual alveolar ridge.

While it is possible that this situation may occur during rest, it is unlikely that such a balance of

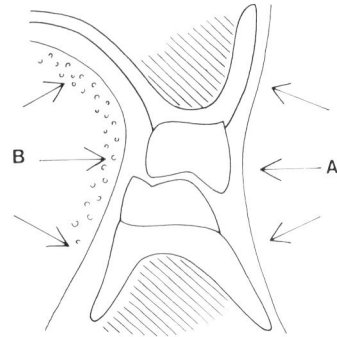

Fig. 3.1 Diagram to illustrate the concept that the force developed by the cheek (A) may balance that developed by the tongue (B).

forces would exist except, perhaps, momentarily during functional activity.

The terms 'neutral zone' and 'zone of equilibrium' have been applied to the concept that equilibrium may exist at any given site in the mouth between the buccally and lingually directed forces generated by muscular activity, during rest and in some functions. It is known that this equilibrium does not exist in the natural dentition and, because of the individuality of the teeth in the natural state, such a balance of forces may have no significance in terms of the stability of the dentition.

If one considers the extreme example of a complete denture, the placement of a denture in a zone of equilibrium would have clear advantages in respect of its retention and stability. The results of the application of a force to an artificial tooth affects the whole denture base to which the tooth is attached. However, a disturbance of equilibrium at one site on a denture does not preclude the possibility that muscular activity in another site might resist displacement of the denture.

In this context, several clinical techniques have been devised in an attempt to define a zone of equilibrium for an individual patient. Such treatment forms are costly in time and resources and, as a consequence, the great majority of removable dentures conform to an 'average' approach to denture design in terms of buccolingual tooth placement. Where only a few natural teeth are missing, a clear guide to tooth placement might be obtained from a study of the position of the remaining teeth.

For complete dentures the 'average' is based, in general, on the assumptions of Figure 3.1 — having due regard to the known patterns of resorption of the residual alveolar bone following tooth loss. The assumptions include the following:

1. The pressures of the cheeks and tongue tend to be balanced in repose, and
2. The polished surfaces of the dentures should be a series of inclines so that forces generated from the muscular environment will help to retain the denture in position.

THE SURVEYOR IN RELATION TO DESIGN PRINCIPLES

Mention has already been made of the biological necessity for ensuring that any part of a removable denture in contact with a natural tooth be passive when not in function.

It is similarly essential from the biological point of view that no part of an appliance meant for insertion and removal from the mouth, without modification, should be fashioned in such a manner as to have rigid portions which enter undercut regions of the mouth.

To avoid the damage which will inevitably result if the above criteria are not met, an instrument called the cast surveyor is used. The cast surveyor is a precision instrument which enables the position of maximum contour of individual teeth and alveolar ridges to be located as one of its functions.

A detailed description of the cast surveyor and its use is included in Chapter 5. Because of its importance in denture design for placement of retaining elements for removable dentures, it is often thought of as having a purely mechanical function. It is, however, important to appreciate the fundamental biological necessity for the use of the surveyor.

FURTHER READING

Bergman B, Hugoson A, Olsson CO 1977 Caries and periodontal status in patients fitted with removable partial dentures. J Clin Periodont 4: 134

Brill N, Tryde G, Schubeler S 1959 The role of exteroceptors in denture retention. J Prosthet Dent 9: 761

Crum RJ, Loiselle RJ 1972 Oral perception and proprioception. A review of the literature and its significance in prosthodontics. J Prosthet Dent 28: 215

Fish SF 1967 Adaptation and habituation to full dentures. Br Dent J 129: 19

Heath RM 1971 A study of the morphology of the denture space. Dent Pract Dent Rec 21: 109

Karlsson S, Hedegård B 1979 A study of the reproducibility of the functional denture space with a dynamic impression technique. J Prosthet Dent 41: 21

Neill DJ, Glaysher JKL 1982 Identifying the denture space. J Oral Rehab 9: 259

Ramfjord SP, Ash MM 1971 Occlusion, 2nd edn. WB Saunders, Philadelphia

Stipho HDK, Murphy WM, Adams D 1978 Effect of oral prostheses on plaque accumulation. Br Dent J 145: 47

The Academy of Denture Prosthetics 1977 Principles, concepts and practices in prosthodontics, 1976. J Prosthet Dent. 37: 204

Watt DM, Durran CM, Adenubi JO 1967 Biometric guides to the design of complete maxillary dentures. Dent Mag Oral Top 84: 109

4. Psychological aspects

INTRODUCTION

In the provision of a removable denture service, the need for an appreciation of the patient from the psychological viewpoint is essential to the success of treatment.

Indeed, the emotional characteristics of both the dentist and the patient, and the relationships which develop between them, may affect the diagnosis and treatment plan adopted by the dentist and also acceptance by the patient of the treatment provided.

Inability to establish empathy with the patient may lead to failure, regardless of the excellence of the treatment provided. Mutual respect and understanding must be developed between the dentist and patient at the earliest moment and be maintained throughout treatment.

Within the practice environment, the state of mind of the patient will depend on many factors. These include the ability and reputation of the dentist, the health of the patient and the atmosphere of confidence, trust and security created by the dentist and his surroundings.

MENTAL ATTITUDE

While it has long been appreciated that people cannot be classified into 'types', it can be helpful to recognise the attitudes of patients seeking removable dentures as an aid to approaching their treatment. Four groups based on those suggested by House may be considered. It must be emphasised that these groupings are suitable largely as an aid to the comparison of patients' attitudes.

Philosophic

Patients having a philosophic attitude trust the dentist and will generally accept without question the advice and treatment plan provided. Even where the conditions in the mouth of the patient present difficulties, these patients are content in the knowledge that the dentist will exercise to the maximum his skill and judgement in their treatment.

Exacting or critical

Patients having a critical attitude often doubt the ability of the dentist to provide satisfactory treatment. They tend to be highly critical of previous dental treatment, and are always ready to provide advice and instruction to the dentist on the way in which treatment should proceed.

It is essential that this attitude be recognised before the commencement of any treatment, and attempts at re-education of the patient be commenced immediately. A careful and sympathetic attitude in dealing with the critical patient is needed, in order that accuracy may be achieved in diagnosis and treatment planning. It must be borne in mind that ill-health may be a factor involved in their outlook.

Hysterical or sceptical

This attitude may have been fostered by previous failures of treatment, resulting in a conviction on the part of the patient that they are a 'hopeless' case and that no form of treatment can ever be successful for them. These patients may make impossible demands in respect of the efficiency or appearance of their dentures. An unfortunate social background (such as bereavement) may be present, and poor health is often a contributing factor.

For this group, the development of confidence in the dentist by the patient is paramount, and must commence as early as possible in the first appointment.

Indifferent

These patients appear unconcerned about their appearance, or the need for replacement of lost natural teeth. Treatment is often sought because of the insistence of relatives and, if early problems with dentures are encountered, they generally do not bother to seek adjustments but prefer, simply, to discard the appliances.

APPLICATION OF PSYCHOLOGY TO THE DENTURE PATIENT

The classification of attitude suggested by House may be considered a useful starting point in patient assessment, but it must be appreciated that there are many factors which influence the individual under treatment. These may be considered as:

1. Intrapersonal factors
2. Interpersonal factors.

The intrapersonal feelings of the patient influence strongly the interpersonal relationships between the dentist and the patient.

Intrapersonal factors

The most important of these are body image and fear and anxiety.

Body image

Body image refers to the unconscious representation possessed by each individual of the image and appearance of the body and associated organs. The retention of this representation of the mental image of the body is important in maintaining a sense of security, and the prospect of change may be interpreted as a threatening action. The adjustment to change takes time, and this has important implications in connection with prosthodontic dentistry because of the distinctive part played by the mouth in body image.

Silverman found that body image was important in denture acceptance, especially for the older patient.

Fear and anxiety

Many people experience some kind of anxiety in the dental surgery, and the reaction which results is highly individual. The role of the dentist in this respect should be an educational one, directed towards helping the patient to manage his anxiety and adjust it to a tolerable level in each situation.

Interpersonal factors

A knowledge of the individual needs of the patient is of basic importance to the success of treatment. By the careful development of his powers of observation and listening ability, the dentist can go a long way towards getting to 'know' the patient before the commencement of treatment.

The dress and posture of the patient, the way he copes with or dramatises symptoms, his handshake, any speech defects, the number of previous dentures and his expectations are all part of the many factors which contribute to the evaluation of the patient.

Good communication is one of the factors of such importance that it cannot be overemphasised in respect of its contribution to a satisfactory dentist–patient relationship. The ability to present information to the patient in respect of the treatment to be undertaken, and interpreting the thoughts of the patient, are abilities which must be acquired and developed.

DEVELOPING RAPPORT WITH THE PATIENT

The first appointment will have a lasting effect on the relationship which develops between the dentist and the patient. Many factors of a general nature will contribute to the patient's concept of the relationship, and the most lasting impressions will be those gained in direct association with the dentist.

A neat, tidy, well-groomed appearance, for example, may provide a non-verbal signal to the patient that any dental treatment is likely to be carefully and competently carried out.

It should be borne in mind that most dental communication takes place within the boundaries of the intimate space (0–45 cm) or personal space (45–130 cm) as described by Hall. Dental treatment takes place within the intimate zone so that some time must be spent in the development of an appropriate relationship before attempting an examination of the mouth. Appropriate conversation is the means by which this can be achieved.

The following are points which may be helpful to remember when meeting a new patient:

1. Greet the patient in a polite, gracious and attentive manner.

2. Remember, and use, the patient's name.

3. Engage the patient in conversation. It is often helpful to be complimentary to the patient.

4. Do not make any derogatory remarks about existing dental work or the condition of the patient's mouth.

The denture patient

The relationship between the dentist and patient is directly related to the degree to which the patient feels satisfied with each appointment.

Patient satisfaction may be increased by the application of the factors considered above, which give rise to the following practice of dealing with the denture patient:

1. Determine the expectations of the patient in respect of dentures and, if it is unlikely that they can be met, explain why.

2. Determine the causes of concern of the patient and do not simply confine the diagnostic visit to gathering objective information about the oral conditions and medical background.

3. Provide full information to the patient concerning the diagnosis and treatment plan.

4. Adopt a friendly attitude rather than a purely business-like one.

5. Spend some time in conversation of a non-dental type. This helps to make it clear to the patient that you have an interest in him as an individual.

Increased satisfaction of the patient with each appointment will result in increased cooperation. The key to increased satisfaction is good communication.

FURTHER READING

Friedman N, Landesman HM, Wixler M 1986 The influences of fear, anxiety, and depression on the patient's adaptive responses to complete dentures I. J Prosthet Dent 58: 687
Friedman N, Landesman HM, Wixler M 1988 The influences of fear, anxiety, and depression on the patient's adaptive responses to complete dentures II. J Prosthet Dent 59: 45
Miller AA 1970 Psychological considerations in dentistry. J Am Dent Assoc 81: 941
Newton AV 1984 The psychosomatic component in prosthodontics. J Prosthet Dent 52: 871
Silverman S, Silverman SI, Silverman B, Garfinkel L 1976 Self-image and its relation to denture acceptance. J Prosthet Dent 35: 131
Smit GL 1978 Psychological considerations in dentistry: a survey of the literature. J Dent Assoc, South Africa 33: 375
Smith M 1976 Measurement of personality traits and their relation to patient satisfaction with complete dentures. J Prosthet Dent 35: 192
Winkler S Davidoff A, Lee MHM 1972 Dentistry for the special patient: the aged, chronically Ill and handicapped. WB Saunders, Philadelphia

5. Examination

INTRODUCTION

In the preceding chapters, some of the factors relating to the provision of prosthodontic treatment have been referred to. Generalisations concerning anatomical and physiological factors have been considered, but it must be appreciated that there is substantial individual variation between patients in respect of these factors, and the way in which they may affect treatment.

Some reference has also been made to psychological factors related to treatment, but no mention has been made of the many other individual and personal factors which affect the approach to, or the outcome of, treatment.

Before treatment is commenced, the operator must undertake a thorough assessment of the patient, who can then be advised on the most appropriate form of treatment. In addition, a careful examination will allow for any possible difficulties to be anticipated, together with the degree of success likely to be achieved.

To do this effectively, an understanding of conditions which might have an effect on the jaws or their movement is required. Skill in recognising general conditions and those disease states confined to the oral cavity is also required. In addition, the effects of drug therapy on denture retention and tolerance must be appreciated.

It is proposed in this chapter to outline an approach to gathering all the information necessary to form a detailed diagnosis and treatment plan for the patient seeking prosthodontic treatment. The information obtained will also enable an assessment of the likely degree of success or outcome of treatment to be made, i.e. a prognosis can be formed.

The procedure by which information gathering is carried out is known as history taking and examination of the patient.

HISTORY TAKING

History taking consists of communicating with the patient in order to obtain essential personal details, including health information.

When properly conducted, the history taking phase of treatment can, in addition to the essential information obtained, provide an opportunity to initiate the development of rapport between the dentist and the patient. Any doubts or fears the patient may have in respect of dental treatment should be elicited as early as possible, as a sympathetic consideration of these may suggest the need to vary the routine approach to information gathering and treatment.

Details which will be required may be considered under the following headings:

1. Personal details
2. Social details
3. Reason for attendance
4. Dental history
5. Medical and surgical history.

Personal details

The name, address and telephone number of the patient must be recorded, so that positive identification may be made and the patient can be contacted as required.

The age of the patient should be determined. For an adult, this is usually best obtained by asking for the date of birth. In general, older patients may have more difficulty in adapting to removable dentures than younger patients. Chronological age of itself is not always a good guide in this context, and an estimation of the physiological age of the patient may be helpful. A 'young' 65 year old can be much more adaptable to change than an 'old' 50 year old. Some pathological conditions, e.g. carcinoma, are known to be age related.

The name and address of the patient's physician should also be recorded, in case it may be necessary to obtain details of any aspect of the health status of the patient.

Where a patient has been referred by a professional colleague, details of this should also be recorded.

Social details

Occupation can provide an indication of the socio-economic class of the patient and may indicate possible difficulties with regular attendance for appointments, e.g. if the patient is a shift worker. Special treatment needs might also be indicated by the patient's occupation, e.g. wind instrument players, who may have special needs in respect of the formation of an embouchure; singers may have special needs concerning the retention of an appliance and the placement of teeth.

Social conditions relating to the patient's personal life may also be significant, e.g. severe emotional disturbance following the death of a spouse, or other stress-inducing circumstances. These can result in apparently excessive reactions to minor trauma, or clenching or grinding of the teeth, or an inability to cope with what would normally be a non-stressful situation.

Reason for attendance

Determining the exact reason for the patient's attendance should be carried out at an early stage in the interview. The patient may never have worn a removable denture before and the reason for presenting might be the absence of some or all of the teeth and a desire for their replacement. If a denture has been worn, or an attempt has been made to wear a denture and a replacement is sought, the reasons for requesting a new denture must be determined so that treatment planning will include

overcoming the present difficulties. If a replacement denture is sought because of fracture of an existing appliance, it is important to determine whether the denture broke during normal use, or if it was dropped and fracture occurred outside the mouth.

Whether or not a denture is present, the attitude and expectations of the patient to removable denture treatment must be determined. The attitude of the patient is often conditioned by knowledge of a third party who has been treated, regardless of whether or not the same type of treatment was required. An enquiry as to why the patient has sought treatment at this particular dental practice may, therefore, be useful in this context.

In questioning patients about difficulties they have experienced with dentures, it must be appreciated that they use their own terminology which must be interpreted by the interviewer. It should also be borne in mind that the length of time a previous denture has been worn will be of significance in relation to the criticism offered. For example, a complaint of looseness of a denture only a few weeks old may have a different basis to that of a denture which is considered to be loose after many years of use.

If the appearance of the denture is said to be unsatisfactory, it is important to know if the patient has initiated the complaint or, as is common with more elderly patients, another member of the family has done so. An exact description of the nature of the complaint should be obtained.

Where looseness is the complaint, it will be important to know the circumstances in which the dentures feel loose. During mastication, a feeling of looseness may be related to faults in tooth positioning or occlusion or the stability or extension of the bases. During speech, a feeling of looseness could result from tongue interference.

If pain is complained of, it will be necessary to determine the character of the pain, whether it is local or general about the mouth or jaws, and if it is present all the time, or is relieved by removal of the dentures.

Clicking noises during speech or eating could result from looseness, or incorrect vertical height estimation.

Retching may result, for example, from stimulation of the soft palate by overextension of an upper denture, or placement of the upper posterior teeth lingually so that they contact the dorsal surface of the tongue. It is important to know whether it is a chronic problem or has just developed.

The above are examples only, and do not represent the whole range of reasons for replacement of denture, or of all the possible bases for the complaints.

At this stage, information in the patient's own words is sought and this phase of history taking merges into the next phase.

Dental history

Where dentures are being worn, questions should be asked concerning their age, how many dentures have been made following the loss of the natural teeth, how long each lasted and why they were replaced. This will give valuable information concerning the tolerance of the patient to dentures. It may also give an indication of the rate at which resorption of the residual alveolar ridges has occurred. Comments on the appearance of the dentures should be encouraged.

If the missing teeth were not extracted by the dental surgeon who is conducting the interview with the patient, information regarding the extractions should be sought. The order in which the teeth were extracted may be significant, in that uncommon masticatory habits may have developed. Where a history of difficult extractions is elicited, the possibility of retained roots in apparently edentulous regions of the jaws should be borne in mind.

Where natural teeth are present in the mouth, it is essential that the oral hygiene habits of the patient are fully explored and also the regularity of attendance for dental treatment. It is known that the success of removable partial denture treatment is strongly dependent on good oral hygiene, and the importance of early motivation of the patient to this end cannot be overemphasised. The denture hygiene habits of the patient must also be determined.

If dentures have never been worn before, it is important to understand exactly what the patient expects. If it is clear that such expectation cannot be met by removable denture treatment, a careful explanation of the limitations of this type of treatment must be given.

Medical and surgical history

The health status of the patient may have a direct bearing on the approach to, or the outcome of, treatment, either as a direct result of a disease process, or of any medication.

A convenient starting point for this part of history taking is to ask whether the patient has ever suffered from a serious illness, or been subjected to a period of hospitalisation. Any current treatment being undertaken should be elicited.

A direct question should be asked concerning any medicine, tablets, capsules or other form of medication being taken. It is possible that a patient may have been consuming tablets as a matter of routine for a prolonged period and come to accept these as part of a daily routine, rather than considering themselves as taking a drug.

It has been shown that this part of history taking can be assisted considerably by allowing the patient to read a list of relevent conditions before history taking commences. An example of a suitable list is shown in Figure 5.1. This is not an exhaustive list of conditions known to influence dental treatment, but it does include many which have direct relevance and it has been shown to act as an effective memory promoter for patients about to undergo dental treatment.

There are many general conditions which have a direct bearing on the treatment of patients seeking removable denture service.

General disorders of the neuromuscular system, such as may occur with Parkinson's disease, can result in poor control of the muscles about the jaws together with excessive salivation. The ability to manage removable dentures in these circumstances is severely diminished. In the diabetic patient, the timing of appointments in relation to dietary control of the condition may be important and, in addition, healing of lesions in the mouth is likely to be slow and the periodontal tissues will require special care where natural teeth are present. The patient suffering from nutritional disturbances, or blood dyscrasias, may show an abnormal response of the oral mucous membrane to denture trauma.

A history of allergy will alert the operator to possible abnormal reactions to materials or drugs which may be used in treatment. The existence of

Before being examined and treated, the following questions should be read carefully.

Your answers are *important* in your own interests.

If you have any disease, condition or complaint not listed below that you think should be taken note of, please inform the person attending to you.

Any matters arising from this questionnaire will be dealt with more fully by the person attending to you, but will in any case be treated in confidence.

HEALTH

1. Are you in good health?
2. Are you under the care of a doctor at the present time?
3. Have you ever had any serious illness or operation at any time?
4. Have you ever been in Hospital, especially within the past year?

ILLNESS

Do you suffer from, or have you had, any of the following:-

RHEUMATIC FEVER
RHEUMATIC HEART DISEASE
CHOREA (St. Vitus Dance)
CONGENITAL HEART DISEASE (Blue baby)
HEART MURMUR or VALVULAR DISEASE OF THE HEART
ANAEMIA
HEART TROUBLE, HEART ATTACK
STROKE, PARALYSIS or THROMBOSIS
TUBERCULOSIS, BRONCHITIS, CHEST PAINS
PERSISTENT COUGH or SHORTNESS OF BREATH

FAINTING SPELLS, BLACKOUTS, FITS
EPILEPSY or LOW BLOOD PRESSURE
ASTHMA, HAY FEVER (Summer colds)
BLOCKED NOSE, ECZEMA or HIVES
  (Urticaria)
DIABETES
JAUNDICE (Yellowing of the skin)
  especially after operation
ARTHRITIS (Rheumatism)
KIDNEY TROUBLE

MEDICINES

1. Are you taking, or have you taken, any of the following medicines, tablets or drugs during the past year?
   (a) Antibiotics (Penicillin, etc.) (b) Tablets for high blood pressure (c) Nerve tablets for depression (d) Insulin or others for Diabetes (e) Anticoagulants (to thin the blood) (f) Cortisone (Steroids) (g) Tranquillisers (sedatives) (h) Digitalis, etc. for the heart.
2. Do you habitually take alcohol?

BAD REACTIONS

1. Are you, or have you been, allergic, sensitive or hypersensitive to any drug, medicine or anything else such as:-
   (a) Local Anaesthetic (b) Penicillin or other antibiotic (c) Sleeping Pills (d) Aspirin or similar pain killing drugs (e) Sticking Plaster (f) Iodine (g) Any other drug (h) Any type of food (i) Ointments.

DENTAL COMPLICATIONS

1. Have you been to the dentist during the past six months?
2. Have you needed treatment for bleeding following dental extractions, operation or injury?
3. Do you bruise easily?
4. Are you employed in any situation which regularly exposes you to X-rays or other ionising radiation?
5. Have you had any bad reactions to any form of dental treatment?
6. Have you or your relatives had any bad reactions to a general anaesthetic (going to sleep for an operation)?

FOR WOMEN

Are you pregnant or taking the contraceptive pill?

FOR PATIENTS OF AFRICAN OR MEDITERRANEAN DESCENT

1. Have you or members of your close family suffered with Sickle Cell Anaemia or Cooley's Anaemia?
2. Have you had a blood test for these diseases?

Fig. 5.1   List of relevant conditions to be read by the patient before history taking commences.

epilepsy in a patient will introduce design considerations such that any appliance provided will not present an additional hazard to the patient. Where an infective condition is suspected, proper protection will need to be provided to the operator and other members of the dental team — nursing staff, receptionists and technicians — as well as to other patients attending the practice.

These few examples given above are intended to underline the need to obtain a full and accurate medical history, and, where any doubt may exist, the patient's own physician should be contacted.

An additional aspect of the patient's health which is important in removable denture treatment relates to drug therapy, which may be either prescribed by a doctor or represent self-medication by the patient.

In either case, drugs being taken must be accurately identified.

Some examples of drug therapy relevant to denture treatment include undue dryness of the oral mucosa, with a resultant predisposition to damage from minor trauma and potential problems with denture retention. This can occur with the use of tricyclic antidepressant drugs and also with antihypertension drugs. Diuretic drugs can cause rapid fluid loss from the tissues, resulting in an apparently altered 'fit' of a soft-tissue-supported denture, causing looseness and local trauma. The prolonged use of phenothiazines, or similar psychotropic drugs, can produce abnormal and unpredictable movements of the oral musculature. The use of non-soluble forms of aspirin can cause ulceration, which may simulate other lesions in the mouth.

CLINICAL EXAMINATION

This will be considered as a series of stages which should be followed as a routine, so that no aspect is overlooked. It is all too easy to examine only that feature of which a patient may complain, and in so doing overlook another condition which might be present.

The clinical examination requires the following to be carried out:

1. Extra-oral examination
2. Intra-oral examination
3. Examination of existing dentures both intra-orally and extra-orally
4. Special tests where indicated.

In addition, the production of study casts will be required for all dentate and some edentulous patients before a final diagnosis can be made.

Extra-oral examination

The overall appearance of the patient should be noted, as this may provide a guide to the importance the patient places on aesthetic values. The symmetry of the face should also be noted, and any abnormal movements about the jaws during speech. It may also be possible to detect abnormal clenching or grinding habits.

The general development of the facial muscula-ture should be observed, as a well-developed musculature may indicate that heavy forces are generated during mastication.

The lips should be observed for their general characteristics such as length, relationship to the teeth, mobility during speech and whether they appear tense and might, therefore, exert strong lingually directed forces against the anterior teeth. Any deep creasing, inflammation or scarring at the angles of the mouth should also be noted, as this might indicate possible vertical dimension loss of the facial height, or the presence of an active or healed angular cheilitis.

The apparent skeletal base relationship should be noted, following observation of the profile, as this information will be useful in assisting the development of correct tooth positions. The nasolabial angle may also be determined by profile observation of the patient.

Temporomandibular joint activity should be observed, and any asymmetry of action during opening and lateral movements of the jaws noted. The presence of any clicking or crepitus or any present or past pain in the region of the joints should be recorded.

Any palpable or tender lymph nodes about the face, jaws or neck should be noted and their cause determined, as these may have a direct relationship to the patient's dental condition and treatment.

The amount of freeway space should be measured and noted on the record card, as this will have a direct influence on decisions relating to the vertical dimension provided during the subsequent treatment procedures.

Intra-oral examination of existing dentures

Any dentures should be examined while in position in the mouth and the extension, retention and stability noted. Methods for testing these properties have been referred to in Chapter 2, and, in addition, careful note should be made of the relationship between the periphery of the denture and the adjacent soft tissues during their manipulation. Where clasped partial dentures are present, the position of clasps and rests and their relationships to tooth surfaces and soft tissues should be noted. Any observable soft or hard tissue lesion related to the in situ dentures should be recorded.

Where no natural teeth are present, the horizontal relationship of the anterior teeth to the lips should be noted, and also the tooth arrangement and their colour. The same procedure should be followed where natural teeth are present, and, additionally, the relationship, form and colour of the artificial teeth and natural teeth should be noted.

The occlusion in the retruded jaw relationship is next observed, and whether balance exists in eccentric contact relationships between the teeth and/or dentures.

Observations made during the above procedures often relate to the difficulties to which the patient may have referred during the history taking stage.

Extra-oral examination of existing dentures

At this stage, the existing dentures are removed from the mouth and carefully examined. Note should be made of the type of base material used, any relief area, and any other elements present. The material and form of the denture teeth should be noted also. Any evidence of chipping of denture teeth may indicate lack of balanced occlusion. Loss of substance from the teeth should be looked at in terms of the length of time the denture has been in use, and also the method used for cleaning the appliance. This is necessary in order to decide whether wear has been excessive, in which case the use of a more abrasion-resistant material may be indicated.

The state of hygiene of the denture will give an indication of the attitude of the patient to oral hygiene, and the degree of care likely to be exercised to the remaining teeth or a replacement denture. Similarly, broken flanges, distorted clasps, etc., may point to lack of adequate education of the patient by previous dentists, or a careless patient.

Where any palatal relief has been provided, this should be noted. The general arch form and arch width of the dentures should be recorded, so that a reduction in tongue space or tissue support may be avoided in a new denture.

The tabulation of information recorded during the extra-oral and intra-oral examination of any existing dentures can often be aided by completing special survey forms. These carry headings covering the individual items which commonly require to be

assessed. An example form that may be used in the examination of complete dentures is given in Figure 5.2, the corresponding form used in the examination of partial dentures being shown in Figure 5.3.

Intra-oral examination

This phase of the clinical examination requires a knowledge of disease states affecting or involving the hard and soft tissues of the mouth.

The mucous membranes

The mucous membranes covering the lips, cheeks, floor of the mouth, tongue, hard and soft palates, tonsillar areas, the jaws and residual alveolar ridges should be carefully examined in turn. Any areas of inflammation or other pathology should be noted and the cause identified, wherever possible. This may involve special tests or referral for diagnosis to a specialist. It will be necessary to institute treatment of any lesions found before undertaking removable denture treatment.

Where natural teeth are present, the gingival condition must be carefully assessed. The standard of oral hygiene must be noted and, by means of a plaque or debris index and a gingival index, the periodontal state should be recorded. This will also necessitate recording the mobility of the teeth and a careful radiographic assessment (see later). The condition at the time of examination must be recorded, to provide a baseline so that the effects of treatment can be determined.

The teeth

The teeth present in the mouth must be charted and the form of the occlusal surfaces noted. Any caries and restorations, and the materials of which they are made, should be noted. The length of the clinical crowns of the teeth and the amount of abrasion present should be noted. Wear facets on the teeth should be observed in relation to the age of the patient, along with the number of teeth which are present. Apparently excessive wear might point to the possibility of parafunctional jaw activity as a cause. Vitality tests may be indicated. The occlusion should be examined with special refer-

COMPLETE DENTURES — ASSESSMENT

Age of Patient:

Patient's Assessment:

Length of Time Edentulous:

Age of Present C/C:

	Incorrect	Alteration proposed
Relationship of C/C:		
Intercuspal Position	☐	
Occlusal Contacts	☐	
Articulation	☐	
OVD/FWS	☐	
Upper Denture		
Labial Fullness	☐	
Incisal Level	☐	
Incisal Plane	☐	
Occlusal Plane	☐	
Mould/Arrangement	☐	
Shade	☐	
Arch Width	☐	
Lower Denture		
Labial Fullness	☐	
Horizontal Overlap	☐	
Vertical Overlap	☐	
Arch Width	☐	
Buccolingual Width	☐	
Cusp Form	☐	

Condition of:

	C/—	—/C
Upper Ridge	—	
Palate	—	
Lower Ridge	—	

Support and Retention

Tissue Adaptation	Incorrect	Alteration Proposed
Depth	Width	

	Depth	Width
Upper	☐	☐
Lower	☐	☐
Extension		
C/— Labial	☐	
Buccal	☐	
Post Border	☐	
Tuberosity	☐	
—/C Labial	☐	
Buccal	☐	
Post Border	☐	
Lingual	☐	
Distolingual	☐	

Fig. 5.2 An example of the type of form which can be used to record information during the extra-oral and intra-oral examination of complete dentures.

PARTIAL DENTURES — ASSESSMENT

Age of Patient:

Length of time wearing P/P:

Age of Present P/P:

Patient's Assessment: P/— —

                        —/P —

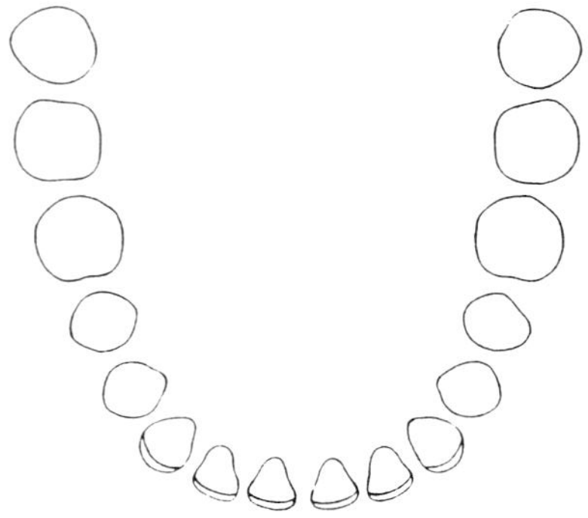

TEETH PRESENT   EXISTING CONS.

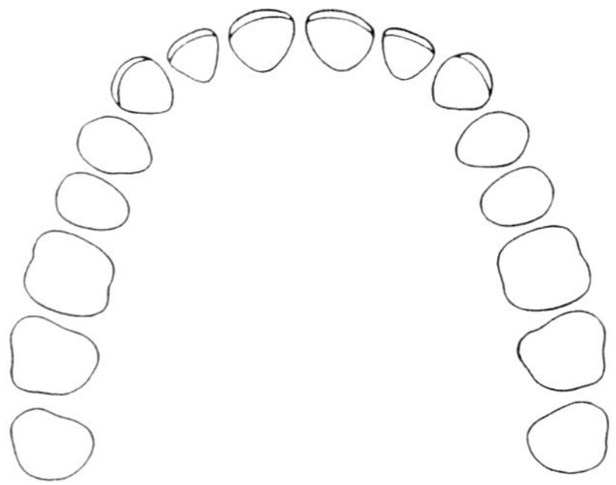

PERIODONTAL CONDITION: ABUTMENT TEETH:
                         OTHERS:

Periodontal Support — Abutment Teeth:
(Radiographic)   — Others:

ORAL HYGIENE: GOOD/FAIR/POOR

Tolerance of previous P/P

REASONS FOR PROVISION OF P/P:
(Delete where inappropriate and list
remainder in order of importance)

Improvement in masticatory efficiency ☐

Improvement in aesthetics and/or speech ☐

Prevention of tilting, drifting and
over eruption of .... ☐

Reduction of load on natural dentition ☐

Prevention of tongue spread and narrowing
of neutral zone ☐

Improvement in occlusion ☐

REASONS AGAINST PROVISION OF P/P:

Inc. risk of caries ☐

High risk of perio
disease ☐

Possible damage to
abutment teeth ☐

TREATMENT REQUIRED
PRIOR TO PROSTHETICS

CONS

PERIO

OHI

PRESENT P/—
(outline)

PRESENT —/P
(outline)

Fig. 5.3   An example of the type of form which can be used to record information during the extra-oral and intra-oral examination of removable partial dentures.

ence to the numbers of teeth in contact on closure of the jaws. Disturbances of normal closure from the rest position to tooth contact should be noted, together with any lack of balance in mandibular excursions. Any mobility of each tooth should be assessed and noted.

The upper jaw

The overall size and form of the maxillary alveolar ridge and residual ridge should be noted. The forward movement of the coronoid processes lateral to the tuberosities should be observed, in case there is limited space available for a denture flange which may be required in this region. The form of the hard palate may provide a possible clue to the retention which might be expected for a denture which does not involve the use of tooth-borne retainers. A flat, horizontal palatal form, with well formed ridges and covered by evenly displaceable mucoperiosteum, will give most favourable conditions where soft tissue support is required. The nature of the mucoperiosteum — whether firm or displaceable — will influence the support and stability which might be expected.

Note should be made of the presence and prominence of the frenae, as these will influence the peripheral form and possibly the positioning of clasps.

The presence of a torus palatinus and/or undercut regions will affect treatment, and note should be made of the position and form of such features.

The mandible

The overall size and form of the mandibular alveolar ridge and residual ridge should be noted. The presence and size of frenae should be noted, as these will have an influence on denture base design, and possibly on clasp placement. In edentulous patients particularly, the prominence of the mylohyoid ridge and the genial tubercles should be noted. The displaceability of the covering mucoperiosteum and its evenness or otherwise, and also the presence of undercuts, should be noted. The presence of a torus mandibularis will influence denture design and should be noted and described.

The tongue

The tongue will have a strong influence on denture design, especially for a lower denture, and note should be made of its size and mobility. Where posterior teeth have been missing for many years, the tongue may tend to spread laterally because of the lack of restriction posterolaterally, and may result in difficulty in the patient adjusting to a denture replacing the missing teeth. A large tongue may also suffer mechanical irritation resulting from friction with a denture.

Saliva

It has been pointed out that the presence of saliva is essential for denture retention, particularly for complete denture wearers, and is also important to the comfort of the patient wearing removable dentures.

Lack of saliva may result in frictional effects, general oral discomfort and trauma. Excessive saliva may tend to cause drooling, and good support of the corners of the mouth will be required. Both of these conditions will require care in the choice of impression materials and in the design of any appliance provided.

SPECIAL TESTS

Radiographic examination

In order to assess further patients presenting for removable denture treatment, a radiographic examination may be required. Where partial denture treatment is being considered, all the teeth which may be directly associated with the denture must be radiographed. In some instances this will involve radiographs of all standing teeth. The amount of bony support available, interproximal caries and any pulpal or periapical pathology may all be disclosed using radiographs.

In edentulous areas, the presence of unerupted teeth, retained roots or other pathological entities may be disclosed. The nature of the residual alveolar bone may provide a valuable indication of possible reactions to denture treatment. where a sound layer of dense cortical bone is present, with a clearly defined pattern of trabeculae in the cancellous bone, good support for a denture might be anticipated. The recommended radiographs for suitable examination of the teeth and jaws include an orthopantomographic-type scan of the jaws, supplemented by intra-oral views of any area which is specifically indicated.

Other special tests

The soft tissue condition in the oral cavity may require bacteriological examination. Biopsy may be indicated in the presence of suspected neoplasia. Blood tests may be indicated where anaemia or other deficiency conditions are thought to exist.

Where suspicion is aroused regarding possible allergy to dental materials, skin sensitivity tests may be indicated.

STUDY CASTS FOR DENTATE MOUTHS

Because of the difficulties involved in close examination of parts of the mouth and in assessing tooth relationships and their contours accurately, study casts are required to provide additional information to assist in planning the treatment to be undertaken.

Study casts are an accurate representation of the teeth, jaws and sulci. They should be fabricated of a durable material such as dental stone. The casts must be mounted on an adjustable articulator. Mounting of the upper cast is accomplished using a face-bow record in order to ensure its correct relationship to the condylar mechanism of the articulator. An accurate record of retruded jaw relation is obtained for attachment of the lower cast to the articulator in its correct relationship to the upper.

Functions of study casts

1. They reveal the surface morphology of the tissues about the jaws, unencumbered by surrounding tissues and the presence of saliva.

2. A detailed study of the occlusion, including the lingual aspects in retruded jaw relation, can be made.

3. The occlusion and its balance in retruded jaw relation and eccentric positions can be examined. A decision to adjust the occlusal surfaces by, for example, judicious grinding or crown modification

using restorative procedures may be reached in order to:

a. Improve tooth contact in retruded jaw relation, or provide freedom of movement and more favourable distribution of occlusal loads in lateral movements.

b. Adjust the level of the occlusal plane of the remaining natural teeth.

4. The need for further extractions might be indicated following examination of the study casts and in the light of the information obtained in the clinical examination. A third molar, for example, could be malpositioned and mitigate against successful denture design, either by virtue of being in contact with the opposing residual alveolar ridge, or by interference with occlusal balance, or perhaps because of a nearly horizontal inclination. Tooth extraction or crown modification will therefore be required.

5. The casts can be surveyed and the pathway by which the denture may be seated into position in the mouth determined. Surveying the casts enables many other decisions relating to partial dentures to be reached. These are considered below.

6. They provide an excellent visual aid for discussion of treatment with the patient.

7. They can be used in the production of special impression trays for subsequent impression procedures and for the production of temporary splints, where a change in the patient's vertical dimension of occlusion is contemplated.

8. They are an essential guide to the technician for subsequent laboratory stages.

SURVEYING

The next step in diagnosis and treatment planning is to survey the study casts. Surveying consists of locating the maximum contour of individual teeth and of the alveolar ridges and residual ridges. The maximum contour is located by means of a vertical plane, which is brought into contact with the cast. If a carbon marker is substituted for the vertical plane, a mark which is called a survey line can be produced on the cast. All parts of the surveyed cast above the survey line are non-undercut areas, and all parts below are called undercut areas, with respect to the direction in which the survey was carried out (Fig. 5.4).

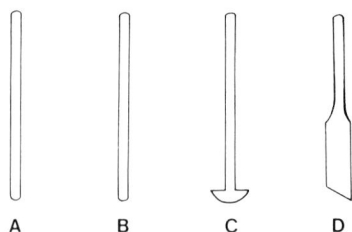

Fig. 5.6   Tools used in the surveyor: **A** analysing rod; **B** carbon marker; **C** undercut gauge; **D** chisel or trimmer.

available in three sizes (0.25, 0.50 and 0.75 mm) and the method of use is shown in Figure 5.7. The use of these gauges is essential to decisions regarding the position in which clasp arms may be placed, the material of which they may be constructed, and their dimensions.

The chisels or trimmers are used in the elimination of unwanted undercuts. Where a cast is to be used in the production of a partial denture, it is essential that unwanted undercuts are eliminated in the same axis as that chosen for insertion and removal of the denture. If the denture is to be produced on a duplicate cast, e.g. such as that used for a cast partial denture base, the undercuts are eliminated using wax prior to the construction of the duplicate cast. Where the denture is to be produced directly on the master cast, unwanted undercuts are eliminated using plaster of Paris. Elimination of unwanted undercuts is essential to ensure that no rigid part of a partial denture can enter an undercut area relative to the paths of insertion and removal. In addition to undercuts about the teeth, the elimination of undercuts related to soft tissues may be required, in order to prevent

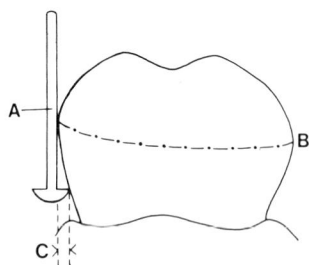

Fig. 5.7   Use of the undercut gauge. A, undercut gauge; B, survey line; C, undercut dimension.

injury to the superficial tissues when such areas are to be included within the denture outline.

Selecting the path of insertion

The selection of the path of insertion for a removable partial denture is fundamental to further detailed planning of the appliance.

Two basic schools of thought may be said to exist in relation to selection of the path of insertion:

1. A vertical path of insertion, where the occlusal plane is horizontal during surveying, should be used. The forces which tend to dislodge a denture during mastication, and which are generated by the adhesion of foodstuffs to opposing occlusal surfaces, are at a maximum at the moment of first separation of the jaws. These forces act at right angles to the occlusal plane, and retention for the denture should be provided to resist these displacing forces. Such an approach would provide for a simple vertical path of insertion and withdrawal for the denture, so that the patient would not have any complicated manoeuvres to learn. Where complex insertion and removal procedures are involved, the possibility of inducing excessive stresses in the periodontium exists.

2. If a vertical path of insertion is used, displacement of the denture is resisted only by clasps. Where the path of insertion is not at right angles to the occlusal plane, rigid portions of the denture will resist displacement in the vertical plane during mastication. Thus, the case should not be surveyed with the occlusal plane horizontal (Fig. 5.8).

The choice between these two approaches is not always so clear-cut as would appear from the above, and there are several other factors which may appear to be in conflict in any given clinical situation:

1. Guiding planes. These are parallel surfaces of teeth and residual ridges, which form a clear pathway along which the denture may be guided to its planned position in the mouth (Fig. 5.9).

Where effective guiding planes are present, part of the retention of the denture may be effected by friction between the denture and the guiding plane, thus reducing the need for reliance on clasps. Where no guiding planes exist, limited modification

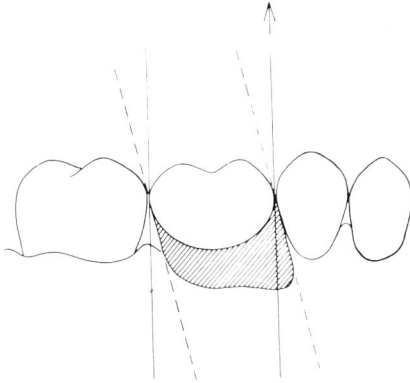

Fig. 5.8 By tilting the cast, rigid portions of the denture can engage undercuts relative to the vertical path of displacement. The solid line represents a vertical direction of survey, and the broken line that of a survey with the cast tilted.

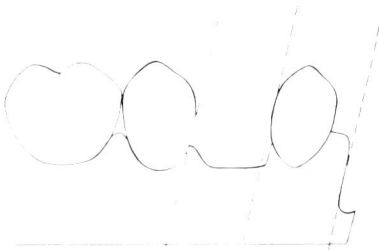

Fig. 5.9 Guiding planes are indicated by the broken lines.

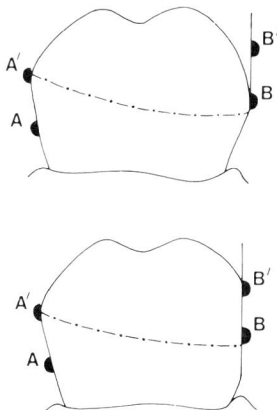

Fig. 5.10 The presence of a guiding plane on a tooth enables the reciprocating arm (B) of the clasp to oppose the action of the retentive arm (A) in all positions of contact of the retentive arm with the tooth. Note how the absence of a guiding plane in the upper diagram results in loss of contact of the reciprocating arm (B′) while the retentive arm (A′) still engages an undercut region of the tooth.

of tooth substance may be undertaken in order to produce them. Guiding planes are also significant in considering effective reciprocation for individual clasps (Fig. 5.10).

2. Retention undercuts. Ideally, undercuts utilised for retention should be equally distributed over the teeth to be clasped.

3. Undercut areas enclosed by the denture. These are in effect dead spaces and should be minimised either by averaging them out in selecting the path of insertion, or by adjusting the form of the abutment teeth.

4. Appearance. When clasps are required about the anterior parts of the mouth, a minimal display of metal must be aimed at.

5. Saddles. Several may be present, each having different characteristics.

Procedure for surveying

The cast to be surveyed is removed from the articulator and firmly attached to the cast table, which is placed on the base of the surveyor.

The occlusal plane of the cast is then oriented with respect to the base of the surveyor, i.e. a degree of tilt is applied to the cast. In the first instance, zero tilt, i.e. with the occlusal plane horizontal, should be adopted. The analysing rod is placed in the surveyor and gently brought into contact with the cast. Guiding planes may be present on the lingual aspect of the remaining teeth; undercuts in regions where retention by means of clasps will be sought should be checked. It may be found necessary to modify the tilt of the cast, in order to even out undercuts and dead spaces. Areas where minor modification of a tooth surface to produce suitable guiding planes are required should be noted. When the final degree of tilt has been decided upon, the analysing rod should be substituted by the carbon marker. All undercut areas should then be recorded, including that part of the cast representing soft tissue.

Where moderate to severe abutment tooth inclination exists, the method of averaging abutment inclination offers a good starting method for tilting the cast. In this approach, the abutment tooth inclinations in the lateral plane are marked on the cast and the average of these taken to provide the degree of lateral tilt for the cast. The antero-

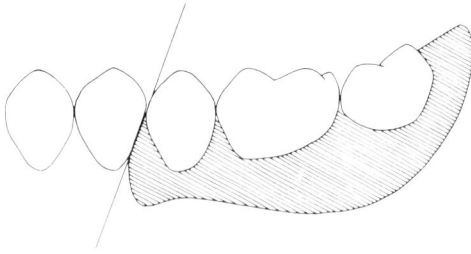

Fig. 5.11   Downwards tilting of the anterior part of the cast enables the distal aspect of 34 to be used as a guiding plane.

posterior tilt is similarly averaged from the mesio-distal inclination of the abutment teeth. The vertical movable post of the surveyor is then made parallel to this average of inclinations of the abutment teeth.

Whatever approach is used, compromises often need to be made to allow for simplicity of insertion consistent with the availability of suitable undercuts, and diminishing dead spaces which are potential areas for stagnation of food debris.

In general, surveying the cast with the occlusal plane horizontal is preferred because:

1. A single path of insertion and removal is obtained where this is possible.

2. Clasps may be designed to provide maximum retention in the plane where displacement is most likely to occur.

The main exceptions to this generalisation where model tilting is required are:

1. To tilt the anterior aspect of the cast downwards where a free-end saddle exists, so that the distal surface of the abutment tooth can be used as a guide plane (Fig. 5.11).

2. To try to bring parallel oblique abutments into a vertical alignment, and so eliminate the need for blocking out undercuts.

SUBSEQUENT PROCEDURES

Following surveying of the cast, the final design of the denture can be considered, including particular types of clasp most suitable to the survey lines produced. These aspects are further considered in Chapters 14 and 15. The position of the retentive tips of clasp arms relative to the survey lines will

require the use of the undercut gauges, as described above. In general, more flexible materials can engage deeper undercuts, e.g. a long wrought gold alloy clasp arm can engage an undercut of up to 0.75 mm without exerting damaging forces on the clasped tooth during withdrawal of the denture. On the other hand, a cast cobalt–chromium clasp must not engage an undercut in excess of 0.25 mm.

Finally, in association with a knowledge of the occlusion between the opposing teeth, a decision regarding the need for, and the position of, any rest seat preparation and other forms of tooth modification should be made and carried out. It is, of course, essential that all preparation of the mouth be completed before attempting to obtain an impression to produce the working cast on which the denture will be constructed.

STUDY CASTS FOR EDENTULOUS MOUTHS

Apart from the function of providing a means for producing special trays in order to obtain a working impression, there are two further principal situations where study casts for edentulous mouths may be required.

1. Where lack of space appears to be a possible problem. In this case, study casts should be mounted on an adjustable articulator using a record of the retruded jaw relationship. This type of problem is most frequently seen in the posterior part of the mouth, and an adjustable articulator will give an opportunity to assess the tissue proximity during mandibular excursions. A knowledge of the health status of the patient, radiographs of the region concerned and, following discussions with the patient, a decision to adopt a surgical approach prior to denture construction might be made. Alternatively, a modified denture base might be considered — possibly by not including the region concerned in the denture outline.

2. Where unyielding undercuts are present, especially when bilateral. A common site for this to occur is in the tuberosity region of the upper denture bearing area. By using the surveyor, the extent of the undercuts will be revealed.

Where undercuts are minimal, it may be decided to eliminate the undercut on one or both sides by means of plaster of Paris applied to the cast, and subsequently using a chisel or trimmer on the surveyor in order to minimise the area of the denture base which will be affected.

For deeper undercuts, surgery may need to be considered and/or modification of the denture base outline. Alternatively, where surgery is contra-indicated and the use of an undercut is required for adequate retention, the flange of the denture may be constructed using a soft lining material.

FURTHER READING

Atkinson HF 1953 Partial denture problems. Designing about a path of withdrawal. Austral J Dent 57: 187
Axelsson, G 1988 Orthopantomographic examination of the edentulous mouth. J Prosthet Dent 59: 592
Boitel RH 1971 Problems of old age in dental prosthetics and restorative procedures. J Prosthet Dent 26: 350
Bremner VA, Grant AA 1971 A radiographic survey of edentulous mouths. Aust Dent J 16: 17
Coy RE, Arnold PD 1974 Survey and design of diagnostic casts for removable partial dentures. J Prosthet Dent 32: 103
Ettinger RL 1981 Xerostomia — a complication of ageing. Aust Dent J 26: 365.
House MM 1958 The relationship of oral examination to dental diagnosis. J Prosthet Dent 8: 208
Jones JH 1973 The oral mucous membrane markers of internal disease. Br Dent J 134: 81
Katulski EA, Appleyard WN 1959 Biological concepts of the use of a mechanical cast surveyor. J Prosthet Dent 9: 629
Keurr JJ, Campbell JP, McCarthy JF, Ralph WJ 1987 Radiological findings in 1135 edentulous patients. J Oral Rehab 14 183
Langer A 1979 Prosthodontic failures in patients with systemic disorders. J Oral Rehab 6: 13
Neill DJ, Walter JD 1977 Partial denture prosthetics. Blackwell, Oxford
Rothwell PS, Wragg KA 1972 Assessment of the medical status of patients in general dental practice. Br Dent J 133: 252
Schole MC 1959 Management of the gagging patient. J Prosthet Dent 9: 578
Szymaitis DW 1977 Considerations in treatment of alcoholics. J Am Dent Assoc 95: 592

6. Diagnosis and treatment planning

INTRODUCTION

In principle, diagnosis and treatment planning for dentate and edentulous patients seeking prosthodontic treatment are similar.

Following the history-taking and examination procedures, the basic reason for the patient seeking treatment will become apparent. Indeed, where natural teeth are missing, the patient will often ask for a specific type of treatment, e.g. for partial or complete dentures, and may be unaware that such treatment may be inappropriate, or that other treatment may be required before their requirements can satisfactorily be met. Thus, having obtained all the relevant information regarding the dental condition of the patient, consideration is next given to the possible alternative forms of treatment which are available. Any preliminary treatment required to bring the mouth to an optimal state of health is then carried out.

Details of the prosthodontic treatment can then be planned, including any necessary modifications of the hard or soft tissues of the mouth.

Diagnosis is the identification of a disease state by its signs and symptoms. For prosthodontic treatment, the term 'diagnosis' must take into account any conditions which might necessitate preliminary treatment, such as the presence of any pathology, and also modifications of any hard or soft tissue which might mitigate against effective treatment. (The consideration of alternative forms of treatment which might be available to a patient can be regarded as a differential diagnosis.)

Treatment planning refers to the order in which the proposed treatment is to be carried out, and includes an outline of the clinical techniques to be used in the various stages of treatment.

While the principles are similar, there are considerable differences in detail between dentate and edentulous mouths in respect of diagnosis and treatment planning, and they will be considered separately.

Plaque control

Wherever natural teeth are present, the damaging effects of plaque must be borne in mind, and also that the capacity for the retention of plaque by removable dentures is well established. The risks of the effects of this on the remaining dentition and supporting tissues may outweigh any possible benefits of the denture. It is, therefore, basic to the success of removable denture therapy that the establishment of plaque control and instruction in appropriate oral hygiene procedures are given at the outset of treatment. Plaque control must be established for all patients as an integral part of removable denture treatment.

Poor plaque control in the dentate patient may result in periodontal breakdown, with the ultimate loss of the natural teeth. The edentulous patient wearing complete dentures must also be aware of the need for plaque control, in order to avoid soft tissue lesions such as those resulting from trauma caused by the build up of plaque on the fitting surface of dentures, and candidal infection.

WHERE NATURAL TEETH ARE PRESENT

The treatment alternatives for the patient who has lost some natural teeth are:

1. No prosthetic treatment.
2. The provision of fixed appliances.

3. Removable partial denture treatment.

4. Extraction of some or all of the remaining teeth and the provision of partial immediate dentures, overdentures or complete dentures. A common means by which the conversion of a dentate patient to a complete denture wearer is achieved is by the provision of immediate dentures. This topic is considered in detail in Part IV of this book — special aspects relating to immediate denture treatment (pp. 245–291).

5. The provision of implant treatment. This topic is considered in Chapter 40.

No prosthetic treatment

Health

In some circumstances, it might be considered to be in the best interests of the health of the patient not to replace missing teeth by means of a removable partial denture. Where a patient is known to be severely epileptic, for example, the presence of a removable denture in the mouth might represent a danger to the patient. Similarly, where a functional but incomplete dentition exists in a patient who, by virtue of physical or mental handicap, is incapable of inserting or removing a denture from the mouth, it might be considered better not to provide prosthodontic treatment by means of a removable appliance.

The number and position of the missing teeth

Both must be considered. In a mouth from which only the third molars are missing, it is unlikely that a denture would be required. Where the second and third molars have been lost from one side only of the upper or lower arch, in the absence of over-eruption of the opposing teeth it might be considered preferable not to replace the missing teeth using a removable denture.

Age

The age of the patient may also be a factor to be considered. An elderly patient, having several teeth missing and an adequate number of opposing teeth to provide for effective mastication, may find adjust-ment to a denture difficult. In addition, the extra care of the mouth and the appliance required might represent too difficult a task to be undertaken on a regular basis. Chronological age is not of itself the criterion on which to base decisions of this nature. It is the biological age of the patient which is important in this context.

Plaque control

This important factor has already been considered above. It is repeated here to remind the reader that where there is a lack of appreciation of the need for good oral hygiene, the provision of a removable partial denture may have a harmful rather than a beneficial effect on the dental status of the patient.

The provision of fixed appliances

Where acceptable conditions exist, a bridge which is permanently cemented into the mouth is in every way a more acceptable form of treatment than that using removable partial dentures. Bridges occupy a similar amount of space in the mouth to the teeth they replace, and this is rarely true of a removable denture. Being entirely tooth-borne, they may withstand greater masticatory force than a mucosa-borne denture. A further advantage is that the patient is never conscious of bridge movement, whereas some patients may detect partial denture movement during function. Where anterior teeth are involved, and excessive loss of residual alveolar bone has not occurred, the aesthetic result achievable with fixed bridgework may be superior to that obtained using removable partial dentures.

Where feasible, bridgework is the method of choice in the treatment of handicapped patients, e.g. the physically handicapped patient who is unable to manipulate a removable partial denture, or in severe epilepsy where a denture may become dislodged.

Fixed bridgework, however, is only recommended for use over relatively short spans, depending on the suitability of the abutment teeth to which the bridge is cemented. It is always necessary to prepare the abutment teeth for crowns to provide retention and, where such teeth are free of any lesion, the loss of tooth substance from a healthy tooth may not be acceptable.

Where fixed bridgework is contemplated, it must be borne in mind that adaptation of the appliance to further tooth loss is often impossible. Thus, where the life expectancy for other teeth is limited, this can be an important consideration.

In addition to being somewhat less versatile, in that partial dentures are usable over a wider variety of clinical conditions, the clinical time required for the preparation of the abutment teeth involved tends to make bridges more expensive than dentures, so that an economic factor may also need to be considered.

Removable partial denture treatment

Where the dentition is incomplete, its restoration by removable partial denture treatment may be contemplated. There are a number of clinical circumstances in which removable partial denture treatment may be indicated:

1. Where fixed bridgework is contraindicated, e.g. if the span of the edentulous ridge is too long for the available abutments, or where periodontally involved teeth remain which would benefit from cross-arch bracing, or where the contemplated abutment teeth are unblemished.

2. Where excessive loss of residual bone has followed tooth loss, e.g. in the anterior region, as the aesthetic requirements in such cases cannot be met by bridgework.

3. Where there is need for replacement of posterior teeth, in patients having an abutment tooth at one end of the edentulous ridge only.

4. In children and adolescents where growth of the jaws or tooth roots might still be taking place.

5. Where it is required to attach an obturator, e.g. for a cleft palate patient, to the denture.

6. Where there is a short life expectancy for other remaining teeth.

7. As a transitional prosthesis, e.g. where total tooth loss is anticipated and it is desired to accustom the patient to denture management before the provision of complete dentures, or where alteration to the vertical dimension is indicated and the decision as to the permanent form of restoration is to be guided by the reaction of the patient to a temporary appliance.

Extraction of some or all of the remaining teeth and the provision of partial immediate dentures, overdentures or complete dentures

Where it is found to be necessary for only some of the remaining teeth to be extracted from one or both jaws of a patient, the most appropriate treatment will often prove to be the provision of a partial immediate denture (or dentures) to replace the teeth requiring extraction, along with other missing teeth. Provision of a more permanent type of removable partial denture (or dentures) may then be indicated, once the major degree of alveolar resorption has occurred in the immediate extraction area.

Where, instead, examination suggests there is a need for all of the remaining teeth to be removed from one or both jaws of a patient, it must be appreciated that this is an irreversible procedure which can have very serious implications. It must never be undertaken lightly and should only be carried out where alternative forms of treatment are inappropriate.

The principle reasons for the loss of several teeth are trauma, advanced caries, and loss of bony support for the teeth. The condition of the mouth of a patient on examination will also have been subject to many other factors. For example, the attitude of the patient to dental treatment and home dental care will have been factors of long-term influence, as will the nature and quality of the dental care provided for the patient.

The age of the patient may also be a factor of some significance, where the long-term prognosis for the retention of the natural teeth is poor. In such circumstances it is important to remember that the older patient requires, in general, a longer period for adaptation to dentures than a younger one.

In some cases, an older patient may be beyond the point where control of dentures can be learned and, consequently, all patients beyond the middle 50s in age should be carefully assessed with this in mind. It may be more desirable from a long-term point of view to convert these patients to complete denture wearing while they can learn new muscular activities. No such problem exists where the prognosis for retention of the remaining natural teeth is good.

Where only a few pairs of opposing natural teeth can be retained, they may provide the basis for better masticatory effectiveness than complete dentures.

Caution should be exercised in considering a complete denture in one jaw opposed to natural teeth in the other. The prognosis for a complete upper denture opposed by natural teeth can be fair, provided that there is a minimum of potential displacing contacts between the teeth and the denture. Modification of the natural tooth surfaces may be required to achieve this. The situation in which natural upper teeth oppose a lower complete denture should be avoided, as the small surface area covered by the denture does not allow for protection of the underlying mucosa from the high masticatory forces developed.

One of the common problems presented by a patient with only a few teeth remaining is the very long clinical crowns of the teeth, resulting from bone resorption in the edentulous regions. Such teeth may be susceptible to tilting forces because of their crown length, and may be mobile. This does not necessarily mean that the teeth must be extracted as, by endodontic treatment where necessary, and reduction of the length of the tooth crown, the tooth may be rendered suitable for use in the support of an overdenture. Similarly, a tooth with advanced damage of the crown by caries can be considered for retention as an abutment for support of an overdenture. This form of treatment is considered in more detail in Chapter 39.

TREATMENT PLANNING WHERE NATURAL TEETH ARE PRESENT AND A REMOVABLE PARTIAL DENTURE IS TO BE PROVIDED

Following the history-taking and examination procedure, and having reached a decision concerning the overall treatment to be undertaken, a detailed treatment plan can be drawn up.

This will consist of:

1. Immediate measures for the relief of pain or any acute condition present.
2. Details of the treatment to be undertaken in respect of the provision of removable partial dentures.
3. The details of the proposed treatment which must be noted include:

a. Treatment of any oral lesions such as denture stomatitis, ulceration, candidal infections, etc.

b. Treatment of the periodontal condition and instruction and motivation to effective oral hygiene.

c. Any surgical and conservative treatment necessary to prepare the mouth for removable partial dentures. This will include any necessary extractions and restorations. The provision of any rest seats, modifications to guiding planes or additional retentive regions will have been decided upon with the examination of the study casts. Any conservative treatment must be carried out with reference to that phase of planning.

d. The impression procedure to be used should be planned on the basis of clinical conditions present (see Ch. 9).

e. Any special aesthetic requirements must be noted.

f. The type of artificial teeth to be used, including the material from which they should be made, must be noted (see Ch. 12).

g. The type of articulator required for mounting the working casts and setting the teeth should be recorded (see Ch. 11).

h. The base material of which the denture is to be made — whether metallic or non-metallic, and any requirements for stress breaking using precision attachments or other elements — must be noted.

i. The proposed final design of the removable denture(s) must be recorded on a prescription form in such a manner as to be clearly communicated to the dental technician without possible misinterpretation (see Ch. 16).

WHERE NO TEETH ARE PRESENT

The treatment alternatives where no natural teeth are present are:

1. No prosthetic treatment
2. The provision of complete dentures
3. The provision of complete dentures in conjunction with dental implants.

No prosthetic treatment

Where all the teeth have been lost from one or both jaws, it is unusual for a patient to be prepared to suffer the deprivation and indignity of edentulousness without seeking denture treatment.

Contraindications to complete denture treatment are rare, and include some advanced neuromuscular disorders and certain mental disorders and other conditions where cooperation of the patient cannot be obtained.

The provision of complete dentures

A detailed treatment plan for the edentulous patient must encompass all treatment necessary to bring the mouth to an optimal condition for the provision of complete dentures.

This will involve:

1. Immediate measures for the relief of pain or any acute conditions present.

2. Treatment for any oral lesions present such as denture stomatitis, candidal infection, ulceration or any other inflammatory condition. This will include the correction of any condition resulting from ill-fitting dentures and may require the modification, or withholding, of the existing dentures as a preliminary measure prior to undertaking further treatment (see Ch. 7).

3. Any surgical treatment required to prepare the mouth for complete dentures (Ch. 7).

4. Where a single complete denture is opposed by the natural dentition, any tooth modification required to eliminate or reduce occlusal contacts which might tend to displace the denture.

5. The selection of an impression procedure based on the clinical conditions present (see Ch. 9).

6. Whether any change in vertical dimension from that provided by an existing denture is required. Where a gross change in vertical dimension is required, it may be necessary to consider incremental changes using the existing dentures, with suitable occlusal adjustment over a period of time.

7. Any special aesthetic requirements of the patient should be noted.

8. The type of articulator required for mounting the working cast and setting the teeth should be recorded (see Ch. 11).

9. The type of artificial teeth to be used, including the material from which they should be made, must be noted (see Ch. 12).

10. The base material from which the dentures will be constructed must be recorded. In some circumstances, a soft lining material may be prescribed.

Soft lining materials

Denture base materials are generally of a rigid nature, being of a rigid polymer or, less frequently, of metal. Occasionally, the forces transmitted to the underlying mucosa via the denture base are such as to produce pain during functions such as mastication.

The use of a soft material under that part of the denture which contacts the mucosa overlying the residual alveolar ridge may afford relief to the patient. This is considered to occur by virtue of energy absorption of the soft material as it distorts when the masticatory force is applied.

Soft lining materials are most effective where the mucosa is thin and overlies a smooth alveolar crest. They are generally used under complete lower dentures, but may occasionally be used with the upper denture where it is considered essential for the denture base to enter an unyielding undercut.

FURTHER READING

Anderson JN, Storer R 1981 Immediate and replacement dentures, 3rd edn. Blackwell, Oxford
Beeson PE 1970 The mouth examination for complete dentures: a review. J Prosthet Dent 23: 482
Carlsson GE, Hedegard B, Koivumaa KK 1970 The current place of removable partial dentures in restorative dentistry. Dent Clin North Am 14: 553
Curtis TA, Langer Y, Curtis DA, Carpenter R 1988 Occlusal consideration for partially or completely edentulous skeletal class II patients, Treatment concepts. J Prosthet Dent 60: 334
Dawson PE 1974 Evaluation, diagnosis and treatment of occlusal problems. CV Mosby, St Louis
Stern N, Brayer L 1975 Collapse of the occlusion — aetiology, symptomatology and treatment. J Oral Rehab 2: 1
Zarb GA, Bolender CL, Hickey JC, Carlsson GE 1990 Boucher's prosthodontic treatment for edentulous patients, 10th edn, CV Mosby, St Louis
Wright PS 1976 Soft lining materials: their status and prospects. J Dent 4: 247

7. Preparation of the mouth for prosthodontic treatment

INTRODUCTION

Only when the mouth is in a healthy state should prosthodontic treatment be undertaken. Even when the oral tissues have been brought to as healthy a condition as possible it is often necessary for further treatment to be undertaken to facilitate and maximise the benefits of prosthodontic treatment for the patient.

There are many conditions of a general nature having oral manifestations. The operator must be able to recognise general disease states having oral signs and symptoms. Reference should be made to the relevant literature on this important topic, which is considered to be outside the scope of this text. Clearly, any such condition must be recognised and treatment instituted before any dental treatment is undertaken.

For descriptive purposes, the common conditions which necessitate treatment prior to denture production have been grouped together. It must be appreciated that there may be overlap between these groups, as the treatment required may embrace both surgical and non-surgical procedures.

NON-SURGICAL PREPARATION

Soft tissue preparation

Nutrition and the oral tissues

The nutritional status of the oral tissues is of some importance when considering the provision of removable dentures, especially for those which will be supported by the soft tissues.

While gross nutritional deficiency is rare in Western society, there are a number of circumstances in which nutritional status may be compromised. These include lack of teeth, painful teeth or dentures, ill-fitting dentures, some degenerative disease states, anorexia nervosa, self-prescribed dietary supplements, and socio-economic factors which may lead to inappropriate dietary practices. Deficiencies of the B complex of vitamins and ascorbic acid may be related to chronic alcohol intake. As pointed out in Chapter 1, nutritional factors play an important role in the maintenance of the bony skeleton.

It is generally conceded that the ability of the oral tissues to withstand the stresses induced by removable dentures is greater if the patient consumes a well-balanced and varied diet and is well nourished. Indeed, dentures which in all other respects are well produced may prove to be unsatisfactory for a patient because of poor tolerance by the oral tissues.

Some relatively common conditions may be related to nutritional inadequacies and should be borne in mind when considering a differential diagnosis. These include angular cheilitis, glossitis, atrophy of the filiform papillae of the tongue, gingival tenderness and bleeding, reduced salivary flow and the 'burning mouth' syndrome.

Where nutritional factors are suspected to influence the condition of a patient or their capacity to tolerate removable dentures, reference to a general medical practitioner for dietary advice and counselling should be undertaken as a preliminary to prosthodontic treatment.

Periodontal treatment

Where natural teeth are present in the mouth of a patient seeking denture treatment, periodontal treatment is likely to be required. Any calculus present will need to be removed at the outset of treatment, so that an accurate assessment of the gingival tissues can be made. Even where the teeth are to be extracted, calculus removal will be required prior to surgery. Treatment of the periodontal condition of denture patients may require scaling and polishing, together with oral hygiene instruction and/or reinforcement, or more advanced forms of periodontal therapy might be indicated. A thorough understanding of this topic is essential to successful restoration of the mouth, and reference to the literature should be made for its full consideration.

The potential denture patient should be required to show evidence of adequate plaque control before treatment is proceeded with.

Tissue distortion

Where continuous use of a soft-tissue-supported denture which has become ill-fitting has occurred, the uneven forces directed to the mucosa via the denture will result in deformation of the tissues from their resting form. Distortion of the form of tissues occurs to the greatest extent where thickened mucoperiosteum is present, and usually some signs of inflammation of the tissues may be seen. Return of the tissues to their resting contour is a time-dependent phenomenon, and the simplest and most effective method for achieving this is by removal of the denture until the tissues have recovered.

Even where there are no obvious signs of tissue deformation in patients having thickened mucoperiosteum, up to 90 minutes may be required to allow the tissues to achieve stable contours following removal of the existing denture (Fig. 7.1). It is, therefore, desirable that this interval be allowed to elapse before impressions are taken.

Denture stomatitis

This is a condition in which chronic irritation of mucoperiosteum contacted by the denture base has produced an inflammatory response. Denture stomatitis is most commonly seen in association with upper dentures, and may appear as a vivid inflammation over an area coincident with that covered by the denture. In less severe cases, small discrete areas of pinpoint inflammation, often associated with the ducts of the palatal mucous glands,

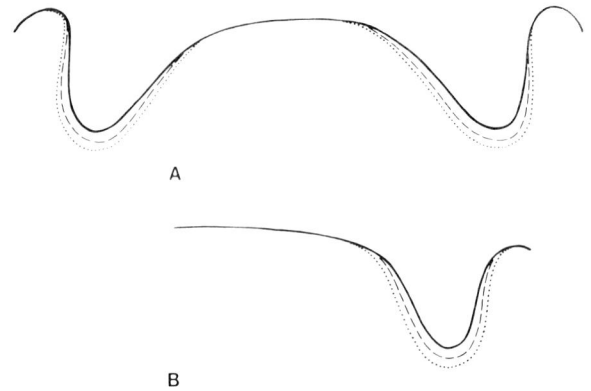

Fig. 7.1 **A** Coronal section through the first molar region and **B** sagittal section through the incisor region for an edentulous patient, showing the surface contours at several times following removal of a complete upper denture. Solid line, immediately following removal; dashed line, 30 minutes following removal; dotted line, 90 minutes and all subsequent times to 150 minutes following removal.

may be present. Between these two extremes, inflammation of varying extent may be present. A further form of denture stomatitis is described as papillary hyperplasia, in which a nodular, hyperaemic surface of the mucosa of the denture-bearing area is seen. Papillary hyperplasia occurs commonly in the central palatal region and, more rarely, may extend over the entire denture-bearing area.

A large number of causative factors have been implicated in the aetiology of denture stomatitis, including:

1. Trauma, usually associated with an existing denture.
2. Endocrine disturbances, e.g. associated with climacteric; diabetes
3. Deficiency states (e.g. certain vitamins)
4. During antibiotic therapy
5. Associated with xerostomia (dry mouth).

The first of these factors is by far the most common. The trauma induced by a denture may result from occlusal or articulation faults such as premature tooth contacts, roughness of the denture base, poor denture hygiene, faulty adaptation of the denture to the underlying tissues, or incorrect vertical dimension of occlusion. These factors can cause undesirable effects from movement between the mucosa and the denture base, and this trauma produces an inflammatory response in the mucosa.

This inflammation is often associated with infection by *Candida albicans*, invasion of which appears to be stimulated by trauma to the tissues, and also by the nature of the denture base, particularly in the presence of poor oral hygiene.

Treatment is directed towards the elimination of trauma and control of the candidal infection. Denture-induced trauma is best eliminated by removal of the denture. Where only relatively minor faults are present in the denture, it may be possible for a patient to continue to use the appliance following correction of the faults which are present. The use of a tissue-conditioning material may also be required. Details relating to these materials should be obtained from the literature. Control of candidal infections will involve the use of suitable antifungicides on both the oral mucosa and the denture.

Angular cheilitis

This is a condition in which a painful inflammation of the corners of the mouth is present. It occurs commonly as a result of constant wetting of the angles of the mouth by saliva, because of: lack of lip support following tooth extraction; a poorly designed denture flange lacking the capacity to provide adequate lip support; or loss of occlusal vertical dimension of a denture or a natural dentition lacking opposing posterior teeth. The skin at the angles of the mouth cracks and becomes infected, producing painful fissures. Other causes of angular cheilitis include vitamin deficiency and iron deficiency states. Angular cheilitis may be associated with an intra-oral candidal infection.

Angular cheilitis may require antibacterial or antifungal therapy, and appropriate medication where a deficiency state exists. It must also be taken into account in planning the design of a new denture.

Denture hyperplasia (denture granuloma)

This condition is characterised by the presence of one or more rolls or flaps of soft tissue, usually associated with the border of a denture flange. It generally results from resorption of the residual alveolar ridge so that the flanges of the denture become overextended with respect to the functional sulcus, and the hyperplasia follows the resultant severe tissue irritation.

The treatment of this condition involves removal of the source of irritation, i.e. removal of part or the whole of the denture flange in the region concerned, or removal of the denture, when resolution may occur over a period of weeks. Should resolution fail to take place, surgery may have to be considered.

Other soft tissue conditions

Other soft tissue conditions which will require investigation and treatment prior to denture treatment include:

Hyperkeratosis
Aphthous ulceration
Pseudomembranous candidosis ('thrush')
Chronic hyperplastic candidosis
Leukoplakia
Lichen planus
Tumours.

A suitable text on oral medicine should be consulted for details of the recognition and management of these conditions.

Tooth preparation

A sound restorative condition of all the teeth is required so that individual restorations throughout the mouth must be of a high standard.

Rest seats, guide planes and undercuts

The exact site for these types of preparation will have been decided during detailed treatment planning, and study casts must be available at the chairside when tooth modification is being undertaken. In some instances, restorations may exist in teeth in sites where modification to accommodate the planned denture elements is required. In other cases, new restorations may be required in positions where rest seats, guiding planes or undercuts are planned and the new restorations must be designed accordingly. It may be necessary to replace existing restorations or, where they are suitable, surface modifications may be adequate to achieve the required feature.

Where a rest seat or guide plane is to be prepared in an unrestored sound tooth, the preparation must remain within the thickness of the enamel. After suitable preparation, the abraded surface must be polished and topical fluoride applied. Suitable forms for rest seats are considered in Chapter 14.

If an undercut region is required to assist direct retention, a cervical inlay incorporating a dimple may be produced. A ball-ended clasp can be constructed to engage the dimple (see Fig. 14.28, p. 114). A further method for producing an undercut region is to modify the tooth contour by means of a composite restorative material, which is attached to the enamel surface following etching of the tooth by a suitable acid. This method has the advantage of leaving the tooth structure intact.

Modification of the occlusion

Because of occlusal relationships which may have developed following the loss of some teeth, it may not be possible to obtain the required occlusal balance between the opposing teeth and removable dentures during treatment. Overeruption of a tooth or teeth, or the presence of a grossly irregular occlusal plane, are examples which might suggest the need for occlusal modification. The treatment required might vary from the reduction of the cusps of a tooth, or an increase or reduction in the crown height of a tooth or teeth requiring full-coverage crowns. Where the occlusal discrepancy is gross, tooth extraction may need to be considered.

Orthodontic treatment might also be considered as a means of reducing anomalies in tooth relationships prior to denture treatment.

SURGICAL PREPARATION

Treatment of pathological entities

Whenever pathological entities are disclosed during the clinical or radiographic examination of the mouth, their treatment may be indicated. Retained roots and unerupted teeth are possibly the most common problems encountered. Where infection or other pathology is present, treatment is mandatory. Where retained roots and unerupted teeth are in contact with the overlying soft tissues, their removal will usually be required. A root or tooth deeply buried in the bone of the jaws and showing no associated pathology will allow a level of election regarding surgery. The basis for a decision concerning treatment will relate to such factors as age, health status and whether removal will be to the benefit of the patient.

Other conditions such as cysts and soft or hard tissue tumours will require surgical treatment prior to denture treatment.

Modification of the oral tissues

There are a number of surgical procedures which may be useful in providing a better basis for successful dentures than that present in the mouth of the patient on examination.

Soft tissue surgery

Surgical procedures involving only the soft tissues of the mouth, and which may facilitate denture treatment, include the following.

Frenectomy. Where prominent labial or buccal frenae will interfere with the production of an effective peripheral seal, or might predispose a denture to fracture by virtue of the deep notch required to accommodate the tissue, removal or repositioning of the frenae may be undertaken.

Hyperplasia. If hyperplastic tissue associated with a denture fails to resolve on removal of the denture, its surgical removal may be required.

Fibrous enlargement of the tuberosities. Excessive amounts of fibrous tissue can produce problems, e.g. in respect of tooth positioning for a denture by occluding the space required for artificial teeth. The enlargement may also preclude full extension of the denture base. Surgical reduction of the soft tissue may be considered in such cases.

Sulcus extension. Deepening the sulcus at the borders of the denture-bearing area on the labial and buccal aspects may be considered as a means of increasing the denture-bearing area in edentulous jaws. The method used involves the use of an epithelial inlay, formed by lining the surgically opened sulcus with an epithelial graft obtained from a suitable skin surface. The technique has most favourable results where some alveolar bone remains, and the danger of obliteration of the newly formed sulcus as extended healing proceeds is ever present.

Flabby ridges. Where a very mobile ridge is present, such as may occur in the upper anterior region of the edentulous maxilla where a denture has been opposed by natural lower anterior teeth, surgery is occasionally recommended. Surgery is, however, to be avoided in these circumstances where little or no residual alveolar bone remains beneath the mobile tissue.

Hard tissue surgery

Alveoplasty. This is the term applied to altering the form of the residual alveolar ridge by shaping the bony tissue. In its simplest form, alveoplasty involves smoothing irregularities of the ridges. The irregularities may take the form of undercut 'knobs' of bone, or a very sharp 'knife edge' ridge form, which may occur especially in the lower anterior region following the extraction of severely periodontally involved teeth. Lack of intermaxillary space may preclude the provision of denture base coverage and the tuberosity and retromolar pad region are common sites for this problem. It is clearly important to distinguish between large tuberosities present as a result of excess bone from irregularities resulting from fibrous enlargement, before attempting treatment for reduction. Occasionally, a general reduction of ridge height is required so that space can be provided for dentures. However, it must be borne in mind that lack of bony support is often productive of difficulties for denture patients later in life, and careful planning with a generally conservative approach is always required.

Exostoses. Torus palatinus or torus mandibularis may require removal when excessively lobulated, or undercut, or so large as to cause a severe reduction in tongue space when covered by a denture base.

Mylohyoid ridge resection. This is really a form of sulcus extension and involves removal of the mylohyoid ridge and the portion of muscle attached to it. A sharp, prominent, mylohyoid ridge can be a source of considerable discomfort to a patient. Similarly, the superior genial tubercles may be so prominent, and covered with very thin mucoperiosteum following resorption of the mandibular residual alveolar ridge, that their removal may be indicated.

FURTHER READING

Arendorf RM, Walker DM 1987 Denture stomatitis: a review. J Oral Rehab 14: 217

Cecconi BT 1974 Effect of rest design on transmission of forces to abutment teeth. J Prosthet Dent 32: 141

Druyon ME 1988 Imbalance in nutrition advice. Gerodontics 4: 176

Gunne HJ, Wall AK 1985 The effect of new complete dentures on mastication and dietary intake. Acta odontol Scand 43: 257

Harrison A 1981 Temporary lining materials. A review of their uses. Br Dent J 151: 419

Hopkins R, Stafford GD, Gregory MC 1980 Preprosthetic surgery of the edentulous mandible. Br Dent J 148: 183

Klein I, Miglino J 1966 Uses and abuses of tissue treatment materials. J Prosthet Dent 16: 1

Lytle RB 1959 Complete denture construction based on a study of the deformation of the underlying soft tissues. J Prosthet Dent 9(4): 539

Miller EL 1977 Clinical management of denture induced inflammations. J Prosthet Dent 38: 362

Österberg T, Steen B 1982 Relationship between dental state and dietary intake in 70-year-old males and females in Göteborg, Sweden. J Oral Rehab 9: 509

Quayle AA 1979 The atrophic mandible: aspects of technique in lower labial sulcoplasty. Br J Oral Surg 16: 169

Rauta K, Tuominen R, Paunto I, Sepponen R 1988 Dental status and intake of food items among an adult Finnish population. Gerodontics 4: 32

Sandström B, Lindquist LW 1987 The effect of different prosthetic restorations on the dietary selection in edentulous patients. A longitudinal study of patients initially treated with optimal complete dentures and finally with tissue-integrated prostheses. Acta Odontol Scand 45(6): 423

Walker DM, Stafford GD, Huggett R, Newcombe RG 1981 The treatment of denture induced stomatitis. Br Dent J 151: 416

Wilkie ND 1975 The role of the prosthodontist in preprosthetic surgery. J Prosthet Dent 33: 386

Winkler S 1987 Essentials of complete denture prosthodontics 2nd edn. PSG Publishing, Massachusetts

8. Cross-contamination control in prosthodontic procedures

INTRODUCTION

The prevention of disease transmission is one of the constant responsibilities of dental practice. Three clearly recognized routes of infection apply to all dental procedures: patient to clinical staff, clinical staff to patient, and patient to patient.

In prosthodontic practice in particular, a further potential route for cross-contamination exists. This is the possible transmission of infection between the dental laboratory and the surgery. Failure to maintain adequate infection controls can lead to infected substances passing between clinical and laboratory personnel.

Thus, a cycle of cross-contamination may develop which could involve clinician, patient, surgery assistants, dental technicians and reception staff. This is illustrated diagrammatically in Figure 8.1.

Awareness of the incidence and mode of transmission of viral and bacterial disease has sharpened a realization of the need for stringent cross-contamination control. For example, it is generally accepted that dental personnel are at some four-fold higher risk of contacting hepatitis B than is the general population. Prosthodontists have been shown to be next to oral surgeons in the prevalence of hepatitis B serological markers amongst dental personnel.

Table 8.1 lists some of the diseases which may be transmitted in prosthodontic practice; this table is incomplete and could include the many common bacterial and viral diseases to which man is subject.

Blood is a common contaminant of impressions, especially where some or all of the teeth are present. It should be borne in mind that as little as 0.000 000 1 ml (0.1µl) of hepatitis B surface antigen

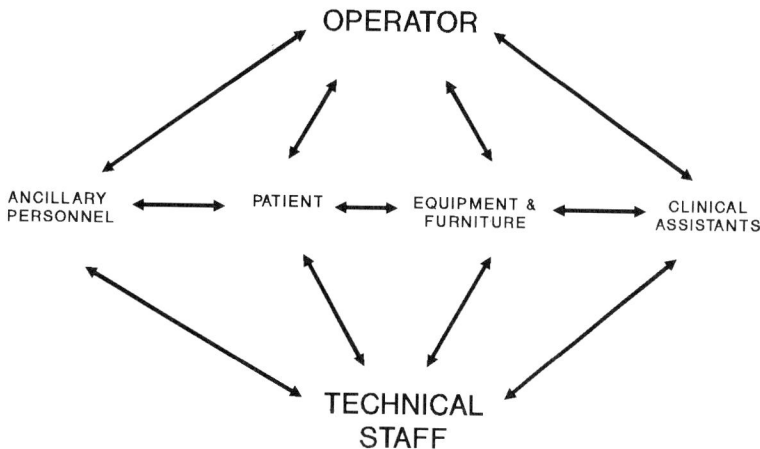

Fig. 8.1 Diagram to illustrate the personnel and objects which contribute to the cycle of cross-contamination.

Table 8.1 Some diseases which may be transmitted in prosthodontic practice

Disease	Causative agent	Route of transmission
Hepatitis A	Virus	Oral or faecal
Hepatitis B	Virus	Saliva, blood, droplets
Hepatitis (non-A, non-B)	Virus	Saliva, blood, droplets
Acquired immunedeficiency syndrome (AIDS)	Virus	Direct sexual contact, blood
Herpes simplex	Virus	Blood, possibly saliva
Herpetic whitlow	Virus	Saliva, blood, droplets
Herpetic conjunctivitis	Virus	Saliva, blood, droplets
Tuberculosis	Bacteria	Saliva, droplets
Infectious mononucleosis	Virus	Saliva, blood, droplets
Legionella	Virus	Respiratory
Pneumonia	Bacteria	Respiratory, blood
Tuberculosis	Bacteria	Saliva, droplets

(HB_sAg)-positive serum can transmit hepatitis B — such a volume would be invisible to the naked eye.

With regard to human immunodeficiency virus (HIV)-infected patients, the principal risk in the dental surgery is the danger of the associated infections which may be carried into the clinic. These include hepatitis B, herpes, candidiasis, oral hairy leukoplakia, venereal disease and tuberculosis.

Because of the difficulty of detecting the presence of these and other disease states, particularly in the early stages, it is considered desirable to treat all patients as if they presented a serious infection risk. Thus, sterilisation and other cross-contamination procedures must be adopted which will ensure the safety of the patient and the whole dental team. In this way, the dangers attendant with the asymptomatic carrier of disease will also be minimised.

GENERAL CONSIDERATIONS

Personal hygiene and protection

A high standard of personal hygiene is an obvious requirement.

The maintenance of clean short fingernails, scrubbed hands and wrists and the covering of any breaches of the skin with waterproof dressings should be routinely practised.

Routine wearing of operating gloves by all clinical staff is required. Gloves must be changed if punctured and also after any treatment which results in blood contamination. Where treatment has not involved blood contamination, the gloved hands may be washed between patients using a similar handwashing method to that used for the ungloved hands, aided by the use of a chemical handwash.

It should be noted that the possibility of glove permeability increases with time of wearing, so that gloves require changing regularly and cannot be worn indefinitely.

Once gloved, the operator should not touch any object which is not directly associated with treatment, such as pens, record cards, switches, etc. A disposable film such as a paper towel may be used to turn tap handles, operate switches or adjust operating lights, etc.

Face masks and eye protection are required, especially when rotating cutting instruments are to be used.

Clinic organization

Clinic design should incorporate clear separation of those areas which will be used in direct treatment procedures from those having secondary or auxiliary functions.

The materials working area, in which items from the laboratory are placed and adjusted for use in the mouth, is a direct treatment area. All instruments placed there must be sterilized prior to their introduction to this area, and all prosthodontic work placed in it must be disinfected prior to and after use.

The work surfaces should be smooth, impermeable and capable of disinfection. After use, they should be cleaned, wiped down with 70% isopropyl alcohol solution and subsequently misted with a solution containing 1000 parts per million (p.p.m.) of available chlorine.

Other items ancillary to direct treatment — such as record cards and containers for transportation of work to and from the laboratory — must be provided for in a site remote from the materials working area.

All switches and handles for equipment must be capable of disinfection or covering with disposable protection.

Sterilisation and disinfection

Sterilisation is the complete destruction of all microbial forms, including viruses and microbial spores. This is best achieved by means of steam under pressure in an autoclave.

Disinfection refers to the destruction of pathogenic microorganisms. As many of the objects and materials used in prosthodontic procedures are heat-labile — impression materials, special trays, wax rims, trial dentures, etc. — a cold chemical type of disinfectant is required.

A frequently recommended disinfectant is a 2% aqueous solution of glutaraldehyde. This has been shown to be very effective but requires prolonged immersion of the articles to be disinfected and has a taste and smell which some find disagreeable. Another disinfectant solution which has been adopted by other authorities contains 1000 p.p.m. of available chlorine. This latter solution has been found to be safe, effective and convenient, following 10 minutes of immersion of the objects to be disinfected. It is suitable for most impression materials (some alginates may be adversely affected and consequently should be avoided), wax, baseplate shellac and acrylic resins. All these items should be subjected to complete immersion in the solution for 10 minutes before their use, and again before their removal from the surgery.

The disinfection of clinical materials is the responsibility of the clinician and must under no circumstances be left to laboratory staff to carry out.

In the laboratory, brushes, mops and wheels should be disinfected and pumice slurry made up with liquid disinfectant and changed between patients. Technical staff should be well informed on the problems of cross-infection, particularly in relation to their own personal hygiene and protection.

All lathes, lathe attachments and polishing equipment should be provided with shields and appropriate extraction and filtration.

Disposal of infected waste material must be undertaken promptly and safely.

Stages of denture treatment and infection control

Impressions. Stock trays should be autoclaved. The impressions should be washed in running water to remove adherent mucous and blood. They should then be immersed for 10 minutes in a solution containing 1000 p.p.m. available chlorine.

Impression compound should be separately prepared for each patient and should never be recycled for use, unless it has been autoclaved.

Special Trays. Following thorough cleaning, they should be immersed in the disinfectant solution for 10 minutes before use.

Occlusal rims. These should be cleaned and then immersed in the disinfectant solution for 10 minutes. Casts should be treated as indicated below.

Casts and Articulators. These should be cleaned and sprayed with the disinfectant solution before leaving the laboratory. A spray made of plastic components of the type commonly used for spraying domestic plants has been found to be useful for this purpose. No wax residue or stains should be apparent on these items — while they may not be infected, such artefacts could convey to the patient an idea that the items are not clean.

Trial and completed dentures. These should be immersed in the disinfectant for 10 minutes prior to their insertion, and, in the case of the trial dentures, also prior to their replacement on the articulator.

While chlorine-containing solutions are highly corrosive to metals, the concentrations and times recommended above have been found to be satisfactory for use with the metallic components of dentures — provided that they are thoroughly washed immediately following their removal from the solution.

FURTHER READING

BDA 1987 Guide to blood borne viruses and the control of cross-infection in dentistry. BritishDental Association,London
Burke FJT, Wilson NHF 1990 The incidence of undiagnosed punctures in non-sterile gloves. Br Dent J 168: 67

Chiayi Shan, Jarid NS, Colaizza FA 1989 The effect of glutaraldehyde base disinfectants on denture base resins. J Prosthet Dent 61: 583

Grant AA, Walsh JF 1975 Reducing cross-contamination in prosthodontics. J Prosthet Dent 34: 324

Leung RL, Schonfeld SE 1983 Gypsum casts as a potential source of microbial cross-contamination. J Prosthet Dent 49: 210

Runnells RR 1988 An overview of infection control in dental practice. J Prosthet Dent 59: 625

Scully C 1985 Hepatitis B: an update in relation to dentistry. Br Dent J 159: 321

Scully C, Cawson RA, Porter SR 1986 Acquired immune deficiency syndrome: a review. Br Dent J 161: 53

Tullner JB, Cornette JA, Moon PC 1988 Linear dimensional changes in dental impressions after immersion in disinfectant solutions. J Prosthet Dent 60: 725

Wilson SJ, Wilson HJ 1987 The effect of chlorinated disinfecting solutions on alginate impressions. Rest Dent 3: 86

9. Principles of impression procedures

INTRODUCTION

In removable denture prosthodontics, an impression is an accurate negative likeness of the denture-supporting tissues associated with the upper or lower jaw.

The impression represents a stage in the prosthodontic treatment of a patient, and its planning is equally as important and demanding as that of the other stages of denture treatment.

The significance of accuracy of adaptation of the denture base to the dental tissues, and also that of the need for the development of a properly designed border seal, has already been considered in Chapter 2. In this chapter, a general consideration will be given to principles directed towards the attainment of these objectives.

Just as there is an infinite variety of clinical oral conditions, so there is a large number of impression techniques, as the procedures used are related to the clinical conditions present. Most impression methods, however, fall into relatively few types and it is not intended to consider all possible variations within these groups.

IMPRESSION TRAYS

In order to carry the material used to obtain the impression into intimate contact with the oral tissues in the desired manner, impression trays are used. To obtain the degree of accuracy required to produce the cast on which the denture will be produced, an individually prepared impression tray called a special tray is used. The special tray is made on a cast of the patient's jaw and to produce this it is necessary to use a ready made impression tray, which is known as a stock tray.

Stock trays

These trays can be purchased in a variety of sizes and shapes and may be made of metal or of a plastic material. The metal trays are strong and rigid and, being sterilisable, they may be reused. Plastic trays are disposable and not intended for reuse. Only those plastic trays designed to provide maximum rigidity are considered suitable for use, as any distortion of a tray at any stage of the impression procedure will result in distortion of the contained impression.

There are three main types of stock trays:

1. Box trays, used to obtain impressions of dentate mouths.
2. Trays for obtaining impressions of the edentulous mouth.
3. Combination trays, which are used where only anterior teeth are present in the jaw to be impressed. The anterior section is of a box form and the posterior section is similar to that used for the edentulous mouth.

Trays for the edentulous mouth have a curved form of the body of the tray, whereas those where teeth are present have a square or box section, to allow for additional impression material around the teeth. Lower trays differ from upper trays in having space provided to allow the tongue to remain uncovered when taking the impression (Fig. 9.1).

Perforations may be present, to provide a measure of mechanical retention which is required to secure some impression materials in the tray. Special adhesives are also required for some impression materials, to aid their retention in the tray. It has been shown that perforations alone are not always reliable for this purpose. Any loss of retention of the

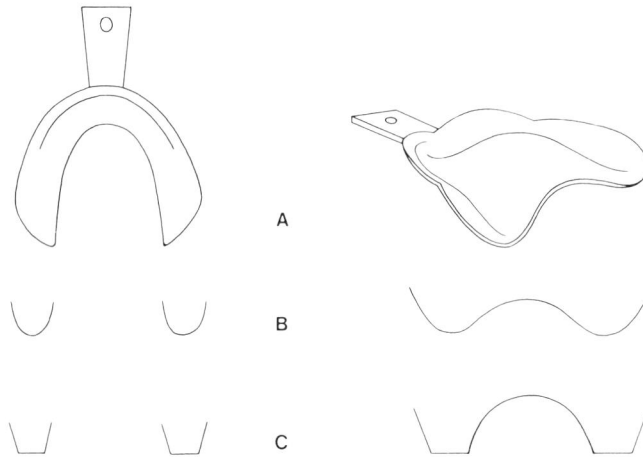

Fig. 9.1 Stock impression trays (lower trays on the left and upper trays on the right); **A** Trays for edentulous mouths. **B** Sections through trays for edentulous patients; **C** Sections through trays for dentate patients.

material in the tray will result in distortion of the impression contained therein.

Despite the variety of sizes of stock trays available, they will only very rarely fit the mouth accurately. For example, the trays may have flanges shorter than those required to support the impression material for the clinical conditions present, or the tray may be too large and distort the cheeks and lips, thus altering the form of the functional sulcus.

Perhaps the most common cause for the resultant inaccuracy of fit associated with stock trays is that they do not provide for an even layer of impression material between the tray and the tissues of the mouth. It has been shown that the capacity of impression materials to reproduce accurately the form of the tissues depends on an even and controlled layer being used.

As the preliminary impressions produced using stock trays are required to be as accurate as possible, various methods for modifying the form of the trays are used. Examples of modifications for box-type trays appear in Chapter 16.

Special trays

These are constructed on casts produced using the preliminary impressions obtained by means of stock trays. As the name implies, they are specially constructed for the patient being treated.

Special trays may be made of metal, heat-cured or cold-cured acrylic resin, baseplate shellac, or impression compound. The materials commonly used for their construction are heat-cured and cold-cured acrylic resin and baseplate shellac. Perforations may be required, depending on the nature of the impression material to be used. Provision of controlled space is provided for the impression material during the construction of the tray. The space will depend on the material to be used for the impression. Where space is provided, stops or small areas of contact with the tissue to be impressed are fitted. The stops are equal in thickness to the space intended for the impression material. They should be placed in regions of firm tissue, which will not be easily displaced during the impression procedure.

The handle provided for the special tray should be centrally placed and must not interfere with lip action. The tray should be rigid, accurately made, and free of undercuts which would interfere with its insertion and withdrawal from the mouth. It should also be finished with smooth surfaces, free from any potentially injurious sharp edges and corners.

A guide to some aspects of special trays is presented in Table 9.1.

DISPLACEMENT OF TISSUES

Impressions for dentures are frequently described according to whether they involve pressure, selec-

Table 9.1 Some examples of aspects of special tray design in relation to clinical requirements

Clinical conditions	Secondary impression material	Suitable tray material	Spacer thickness required	Perforations	Adhesive
Edentulous jaw Minimal undercuts Average salivary flow	Plaster of Paris	Shellac	2 mm	No	No
Edentulous jaw Minimal undercuts Average salivary flow	Zinc oxide–eugenol	Acrylic resin	0.5 mm	No	No
Edentulous jaw Deep unyielding undercut	Alginate	Acrylic resin	3 mm	Yes	Yes
Dentate mouth Average tooth inclination	Alginate	Acrylic resin	3 mm	Yes	Yes
Dentate mouth Severe undercuts	Elastomer	Acrylic resin	1.5 mm	Yes	Yes
Selective pressure impression	Compound/zinc oxide–eugenol	Acrylic resin/compound	As determined by clinical conditions	Provision for escape of material is required	No

tive pressure, or minimal pressure between the impression material and the soft tissues covering the residual alveolar ridge.

Pressure impressions

Proponents of pressure impressions consider that as the soft tissues contacted by the denture are displaced by the forces transmitted to them via the denture during mastication, the mucosa should be similarly displaced during the impression procedure. In this way, the denture made using an impression obtained under pressure will fit the tissues during functional activities. It is, however, considered that non-predictable displacement of the teeth or soft tissues will occur during function, since such forces are applied in dynamic and transient circumstances. On the other hand, the forces applied during impression taking under pressure are static and continuous. They are likely, therefore, to produce distortion of the tissues involved. The distorted tissue will always be stressed when a denture produced on such an impression is in the mouth and, therefore, tending to return to its resting state when no forces are acting. Thus, a denture prepared using this type of impression may tend to be dislodged under resting conditions.

Pressure techniques may be open-mouth techniques or closed-mouth procedures, depending whether the pressure is applied by the operator's fingers or via the patient's masticatory muscles. Generally, it is considered that closed-mouth techniques are fraught with potential difficulties, because of the inability of the operator to control the setting impression directly once the tray has been placed in the mouth of the patient. In particular, closed-mouth techniques do not permit close control of border moulding procedures.

Selective-pressure impressions

In many cases, there will be clinical circumstances involving marked differences between the displaceability of the soft tissues covering the various regions of the denture-bearing area. This situation can be approached by attempting to control the forces used in obtaining the impression, so that the softer areas, and those requiring protection from the high forces developed during mastication, are stressed least during function. When the denture produced using such an impression is subjected to masticatory and other functional contacts, the aim is to distribute the transmitted forces selectively over the basal tissues to those regions considered best able to withstand them.

Minimal-pressure impressions

The objective with impressions obtained using minimal pressure is to obtain an accurate record of the tissues in the resting relationship with each other. In normal circumstances, functions in which high forces are exerted on the denture-supporting tissues operate for only a fraction of the time that a denture is in position in the mouth. Proponents of minimal-pressure impressions, therefore, consider that an appliance constructed using such an impression will fit accurately in relationship to the tissues for the greater part of the day. Where differences in tissue displaceability occur over the denture-bearing areas, relief areas are provided in the denture base to accommodate these differences. The extent of relief required is carefully judged by palpation of the denture bearing tissues, and relief equal to the difference in displaceability between the harder and softer areas is provided over the clinically determined extent of the hard areas.

INSERTION AND REMOVAL OF IMPRESSION TRAYS

Impression trays should be inserted into the mouth by a rotational movement about the angle of the mouth. Where the patient is seated upright, the lower tray is brought to the region of the mouth with the tray oriented at right angles to the sagittal plane, and the junction of the handle and body of the tray by the left angle of the mouth. The operator, standing in front and usually to the right of the patient, uses the left forefinger to retract the right angle of the patient's mouth, and the tray is rotated about the left angle, past the orifice into the mouth.

With the upright patient, the upper tray is inserted into the mouth with the operator placed behind the patient. The junction of the handle and body of the tray is placed to the right angle of the mouth, and the left forefinger retracts the left angle of the patient's mouth while the tray is rotated into position.

A similar approach may be made with the supine patient. However, if the lower tray is inserted from the cranial direction, with the patient supine and the operator positioned cranially, adequate mandibular support is difficult to achieve.

Once the tray has been inserted into the mouth, it should be held in position and a careful check of the tissue covered by the tray made to ensure inclusion of all the required denture bearing area, and at the same time freedom from interference with the reflected tissue.

SUPPORT FOR THE MANDIBLE

It must constantly be borne in mind that any force applied to the mandible must be adequately reciprocated by support from the operator's fingers or thumbs, otherwise possible damage to the temporomandibular joint may result. Similarly, during removal, it is particularly important for all impressions, and especially where high-viscosity materials which enter undercuts are used in the mouth, that the patient should be instructed partially to close the mouth before applying the removal force to the lower impression. This will allow the condyle to retract into the glenoid fossa and minimise the possibility of trauma to the temporomandibular joint.

It is also pertinent to note that it is not good practice for the patient to be encouraged to hold the mandible in a forced open position during the lower impression procedure, as measurable medial approximation of the lateral segments of this bone will occur under these conditions. Wide opening of the mouth also tends to distort the form of the sulcus and makes the provision of an adequate peripheral seal impossible.

FURTHER READING

Atkinson HF 1966 The physical principles of impression techniques. Aust Dent J 11: 145
Douglas WH Wilson HJ Bates JF 1965 Pressures involved in taking impressions. Dent Pract Dent Rec 15: 248
Frank RP 1970 Controlling pressures during complete denture impressions. Dent Clin North Am 14: 453
Lee RE 1980 Mucostatics. Dent Clin North Am 24: 81
Regli CP Kelly EK 1967 The phenomenon of decreased mandibular arch width in opening movements. J Prosthet Dent. 17: 49
Rehberg JH 1977 The impression tray — an important factor in impression precision. Int Dent J 27: 146
Stephens AP 1969 Special trays for full denture impressions. J Irish Dent Assoc 15: 31
Storer R, McCabe JF 1981 An investigation of methods available for sterilizing impressions. Br Dent J 151: 217
Tucker KM 1971 Personalised impression trays. Part I. Dent Dig 77: 70
Tucker KM 1971 Personalised impression trays. Part II. Dent Dig 77: 154

10. Principles of registering jaw relationships

INTRODUCTION

As pointed out in Chapter 1, a jaw relationship may be defined as the positional relationship which the mandible bears to the maxilla, and is considered in terms of a vertical and horizontal component. These two components are interdependent, and one cannot be changed without changing the other. The mandible is capable of adopting an infinite number of positions in both the vertical and horizontal planes, and in removable denture production it is essential that the required relationship is established accurately in accordance with the anatomical and physiological needs of the patient.

Once established, the jaw relationship is registered or recorded so that the casts of the patient's jaws can be related in a similar manner to that which pertains in the mouth. The correctly located casts can then be transferred to an articulator. This is an instrument designed to simulate some actions of the jaws and is considered in Chapter 11.

THE VERTICAL COMPONENT OF THE JAW RELATIONSHIP

It has already been pointed out that when the mandible is in the rest jaw relationship the opposing teeth are not in occlusion, being separated by the distance known as the interocclusal distance. When the natural teeth are present in the jaws and in a state of normal occlusion, contact between the opposing teeth determines the vertical dimension of occlusion. Where there is no tooth contact possible because of the absence of teeth, for example, then the vertical dimension must be estimated.

The basis for estimation of the vertical dimension of occlusion is the rest vertical dimension. It is

known that the rest jaw relationship, which determines the rest vertical dimension, may be subject to variation from a number of causes, both short- and long-term. In general, as the rest jaw relationship is maintained by a balance of the muscle forces acting on the mandible, factors which influence muscle activity will affect the rest jaw relationship.

Short-term factors which influence the rest jaw relationship

1. Head posture. As indicated in Chapter 1, tilting the head backwards will increase the rest vertical dimension, while inclining the head forwards will result in a decreased value.

2. Stress. This tends to decrease the rest vertical dimension, as a result of increased activity of the elevator muscles attached to the mandible.

3. Mouth contents. There is a tendency for the rest vertical dimension to decrease following extraction of the natural teeth, and for a new postural position to develop following the insertion of a lower denture.

4. Pain about or within the mouth, or in the muscles supporting the mandible, may affect the rest vertical dimension as a protective posture may be assumed.

5. Respiration produces minor variations in the rest jaw relationship.

Long-term factors which influence the rest jaw relationship

1. Age and health status. These factors may produce a change in the rest jaw relationship. With advancing age, where natural teeth or dentures have

gradually worn down, or a prolonged period of edentulousness has occurred, a decrease in the rest vertical dimension may result. Chronic neuromuscular disorders may also produce a change in the rest jaw position.

2. Bruxism, and the developments of habits related to abnormal occlusion, are often associated with muscular hypertonicity, with a resultant decrease in the rest vertical dimension.

VERTICAL DIMENSION OF OCCLUSION

In the determination of the vertical dimension of occlusion, in the absence of natural teeth or of acceptable tooth contacts, the procedure first involves the establishment of the rest vertical dimension. The vertical dimension of occlusion is then obtained by subtracting from the rest vertical dimension an allowance of 2–4 mm, to provide for an adequate freeway space or interocclusal distance. Thus: rest vertical dimension – freeway space = vertical dimension of occlusion.

ASSESSMENT OF THE VERTICAL DIMENSION

There are many methods in current use which attempt to determine an absolute value for the rest vertical dimension. The variety of methods available is, of itself, an indication of the difficulties involved in assessing this important value. Some of the methods used include the following.

Swallowing. Niswonger (1934) observed that, in swallowing, the mandible moves from the rest position to centric jaw relation, and returns to the resting position on completion of the act. In adapting this observation to estimation of the vertical dimension, the patient is seated and the head supported with the ala–tragal line parallel to the floor. Two marks are placed on the face in the midline – one on the upper lip and the other on the chin. The patient is instructed to swallow and relax, and the distance between the marks measured. This distance represents the rest vertical dimension. The difficulties associated with this approach relate to movement of the marks consequent on movement of the skin, and obtaining adequate relaxation of the patient.

Facial measurements. A number of methods which utilise measurements between various anatomical landmarks have been suggested. Willis considered that the distance from the pupil of the eye to the rima oris was equal to the distance from the base of the nose to the inferior border of the chin, at the vertical dimension of occlusion. The Willis bite gauge was introduced to assist in measuring the above distances. In other methods, it has been suggested that the face can be considered in terms of 'equal thirds' in respect of the forehead, the nose, and the lips and chin.

These and other methods based on facial measurement have been shown to be of little practical value, because of the vague nature of the measuring 'points', and also because of individual variation in facial features.

Phonetic methods. Some phonetic methods are based on the 'closest speaking distance' (without tooth contact occurring) which is assumed by the mandibular teeth in relation to the maxillary teeth during the production of sounds such as 's' or 'ch'. It is considered by users of this approach that the near contact position is close enough to be used as a measure of the vertical dimension of occlusion. Obviously, the correct relationship between the teeth, lips and tongue would need to be developed for the application of this method, and it is considered to be best used as a check on an established vertical dimension at the trial stage of denture production. In another phonetic method, the production of the letter 'm' is used. When this sound is produced, measurement between a mark placed on the upper lip or nose, and another on the chin, is considered to represent the rest vertical dimension.

Appearance. Some operators simply attempt to judge the rest vertical dimension on the basis of the appearance of the patient. Such an approach is very subjective.

Biting forces. Boos (1952) considered that the maximum biting force was developed at a degree of jaw separation equal to the rest vertical dimension, and he developed an instrument (the 'Bimeter') to enable biting forces to be measured. This method has not been shown to produce reliable results for all operators.

Other methods. These include tactile methods in which a jack-screw can be adjusted vertically between the jaws, until the patient considers the degree of jaw separation correct. This is then checked by the operator for reasonableness. A further approach utilises electromyographic recordings, on the basis that minimal muscular activity occurs when the mandible is in the resting or postural position.

No reference has been made here to pre-extraction records which could be obtained before the loss of the natural vertical dimension 'stop' has occurred, such as would be available for use in the production of immediate dentures (see Part IV).

A method for assessing the vertical dimension

The recommended method consists of a combination of some of the above methods.

Markers should be attached to the midline of the face — one on the nose and the other on the chin. As pointed out above, the action of the muscles of facial expression may produce skin movement, so that the sites chosen for attachment of the markers should be observed carefully, and only positions which do not appear to show movement independent of the skeleton should be used. Suitable markers may be of self-adhesive paper, or marks produced by a chinagraph pencil. The patient should be seated upright with the head erect. Measurement between the markers is made with the patient in a relaxed and comfortable position. This can be very difficult to achieve. Requesting the patient to moisten the lips and bring them into light contact may be helpful. Asking the patient to swallow and relax the jaws may be attempted. Observation of the patient's face for signs of muscle activity should be carried out continuously, while suitable encouragement of the patient to be as relaxed as possible should be undertaken. The patient's appearance in a more general sense should be observed also, to take into account the general proportions of the face. Verification of the measured dimension by asking the patient to say 'm' may be helpful. Measurements can be made conveniently using a Willis gauge, for example. This instrument carries a scale and can be readily sterilised (Fig. 10.1).

For an edentulous patient, a lower denture, if available, should be in the mouth during measurement of the rest vertical dimension, to reduce the error resulting from the effect of the absence of

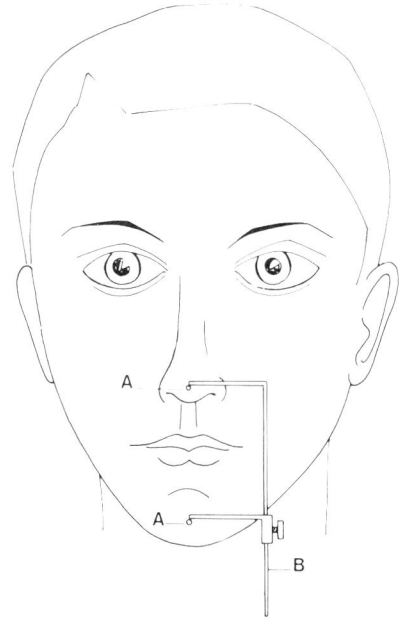

Fig. 10.1 Measurement of vertical dimension of the face using the Willis gauge. A, markers; B, Willis gauge.

teeth from the lower jaw.

The above description provides no indication of the difficulties which may accompany the procedure, particularly in respect of achieving, or recognising, the resting posture of the mandible. Considerable experience may be required for successful determination of the rest vertical dimension.

The next step is to estimate the amount of freeway space to be provided, as the vertical dimension at which the jaw relationship will be registered is the vertical dimension of occlusion. On the average, the freeway space will be some 2–4 mm in the premolar region. In the absence of suitable guidance, e.g. tooth contacts adequate to establish the vertical dimension of occlusion, dentures which may provide a guide in relation to occlusal wear or show the effects of over- or underestimation of vertical dimension, it is common practice to provide the average amount of freeway space. At a later stage of removable denture treatment — the trial denture stage — a re-estimation of the adequacy of the freeway space provided is made and, if necessary, reregistration of the jaw relationship at a newly established vertical dimension of occlusion is made. This aspect is further considered in Chapters 19 and 26.

The importance of accurate estimation of the vertical dimension of occlusion cannot be over emphasised.

Errors in the vertical dimension of occlusion

It is essential that provision for the correct vertical dimension of occlusion be made, as excessive or deficient vertical dimension can produce serious consequences.

Excessive vertical dimension

Excessive vertical dimension will result in deficiency or elimination of the freeway space and the effects may include:

1. Increased risk of trauma to the tissues contacted by the denture. In the absence of freeway space, the teeth will be continually clenched. Muscle forces are increased for the first few millimetres of increased vertical height. These two factors may give rise to considerable discomfort. The oral mucosa overlying the denture seating areas may become painful and inflamed and muscle pain, particularly involving the masseter muscle, may also result.

2. It has been postulated that a decreased or absent freeway space may result in accelerated resorption of the residual alveolar bone.

3. The teeth are liable to contact during speech, resulting in an audible clicking sound.

4. Speech defects may arise because of difficulties in bringing the lips together to produce such sounds as 'p', 'b' and 'm'.

5. Poor aesthetics may be apparent. The lips and cheeks are constantly stretched, and an open mouth posture may be apparent.

6. Symptoms of temporomandibular joint dysfunction syndrome may develop, as a result of increased stress to the tissues related to the joint.

Deficient vertical dimension

A deficient vertical dimension of occlusion is sometimes referred to as 'overclosure' and may result in:

1. Poor aesthetics — lack of proper lip and cheek support, together with protrusion of the chin on closure of the jaws may be apparent. This produces a premature aged appearance.

2. Masticatory efficiency is reduced, because the muscles which are substantially vertical in their fibre direction are required to operate at a reduced length, thus reducing the forces generated on contraction.

3. Lack of support at the angles of the mouth may result in dribbling of saliva, thus favouring the development of angular cheilitis.

4. The risk of cheek biting is increased, because of bunching of that tissue.

5. Symptoms of temporomandibular joint dysfunction syndrome may develop, as a result of increased stress to the tissues related to the joint.

HORIZONTAL JAW RELATIONS

Once the correct vertical dimension is determined, and allowance for the necessary interocclusal distance or freeway space has been made, the jaw relation in the horizontal plane must be established. This will be considered in two sections because, in the production of removable prostheses, a distinction is made between the horizontal relationships of the jaws, depending on the presence or absence of acceptable natural tooth contacts.

Dentate patients where natural tooth contact is accepted

For the patient having natural teeth in sufficient numbers and relative positions to provide a definite intercuspal relationship in the horizontal plane at an acceptable vertical dimension, the maximal intercuspal position is the horizontal relationship to be recorded.

Patients lacking acceptable tooth contact

In all cases where acceptable natural tooth contact is absent, the retruded jaw relationship is that which must be determined and recorded at the vertical dimension of occlusion. These include:

1. All edentulous patients.
2. Dentate patients lacking acceptable tooth contact. Where changes in the normal occlusal relationships have occurred following tooth extraction, e.g. drifting of teeth into edentulous spaces, rotation

or overeruption of teeth, the maximal intercuspal contact presented may be achieved by deflection from the normal path of closure, following premature contact between opposing teeth. In situations such as these, occlusal modification will be required as part of the planned treatment for removable partial dentures.

3. Dentate patients requiring a change in the vertical dimension of occlusion from that provided by natural tooth contact. As a result of tooth loss, there may be no occlusal contact between teeth in opposing jaws, or because of gross attrition or abrasion of opposing teeth, contact may only be achieved at an inadequate vertical dimension of occlusion.

While the absolute value of the difference between the maximal intercuspal position where natural teeth are present, and the retruded jaw relationship is relatively small (approximately 1 mm), it is considered by many authorities to be significant in clinical terms, where normal occlusal contacts are absent or cannot be maintained.

Reasons for acceptance of the retruded jaw relationship

1. The retruded jaw relationship is reproducible. Only when opposing tooth surfaces in substantially normal positions are present in the mouth is the position of maximal intercuspation reproducible.

2. The apparatus used for reproducing some jaw movements and setting the teeth operate basically from the retruded position. Commonly used articulators are incapable of reproducing a retrusive mandibular action.

3. Denture instability will result from abnormal contact between dentures, or dentures and natural teeth, when set up with the casts in other than the retruded jaw relationship. The non-reproducibility of positions other than the retruded position makes the achievement of balanced occlusion and articulation unlikely.

4. The vertical dimension of occlusion may be altered during function, when the teeth are set with casts of the jaws in other than the retruded jaw relationship.

5. Abnormal temporomandibular joint activity, related to attempts by the patient to modify chewing

action to accommodate incorrect occlusal relationships, may result in joint dysfunction.

RECORDING AND TRANSFER OF JAW RELATIONSHIPS

Having established the vertical and horizontal components of the jaw relationship, it is essential that the recording of this relationship (the registration), and the subsequent transfer of the jaw relationship record to the articulator, is carried out without error.

Clearly, any errors introduced at this stage will be retained in the subsequent stages of denture production, and appear as occlusal errors in the completed appliance. It is known that inaccurate occlusal relationships constitute the most common cause of denture failure and tissue damage.

The clinical techniques adopted for recording the above jaw relationships will be considered in Chapters 17 and 24, together with the precautions which should be taken to ensure accuracy.

OTHER JAW RELATIONSHIPS

Protrusive and lateral jaw relationships may also be recorded. These relationships are used primarily to assist in the adjustment of the condylar guidance mechanism of the articulator.

A protrusive jaw relationship pertains when the mandible is postured forward of the accepted retruded jaw relationship. Lateral jaw relationships occur when the mandible is postured towards the right or left side. In each of these movements, one or both condyles is caused to travel downwards and forwards from the retruded position in the glenoid fossa. In addition, lateral movements include a total lateral shift of the condyles.

The form of the bony elements of the temporomandibular joint do not of themselves govern the path taken by the condyles. Most articulators have a straight path which the equivalent of the condyle follows in its movement, and this differs from the path taken by the mandibular condyle in its movements. This situation arises because records obtained for adjusting the mechanism of the articulator utilise two static records, and the assumption is made that the pathway between these positions is straight. Thus, the protrusive movements of the simple adjustable articulator are not identical to those of the mandible. Such records do, however, offer refinements in the development of occlusion between artificial teeth, and artificial and natural teeth, and also provide opportunity for the study of the occlusion of natural teeth.

Protrusive relationships are more commonly used for condylar mechanism adjustment, although some clinicians use both protrusive and lateral records, while others use left and right lateral records only.

The method of adjustment of the condylar mechanisms of an articulator using the protrusive record utilises the phenomenon observed by Christensen at about the turn of the century. Christensen noted the development of a gap in the molar region of patients having natural teeth, during protrusion of the mandible while contact between the anterior teeth was maintained. This wedge-shaped space between the opposing occlusal planes of the upper and lower teeth results from the downward movement of the condyle (Fig. 10.2) and is used as a means of determining the gross downward and forwards movement of the condyle during protrusion.

In practice, an interocclusal record between the upper and lower teeth, or their equivalent, is obtained in wax or other suitable medium. This record (protrusive registration) is then transferred to the articulator in which casts of the jaws have been mounted in the appropriate retruded jaw relationship. The condylar mechanism of the articulator is then adjusted to permit the reproduction of the protrusive record between the casts of the patient's jaws. Following adjustment of the horizontal condylar inclination of the articulator, with some articulators adjustment for Bennett movement may be made in accordance with Hanau's equation (see Chapter 11):

$$L = \frac{H}{8} + 12 \; ,$$

where L is the lateral condylar inclination and H is the horizontal condylar inclination.

Thus, when the horizontal condylar inclination is found to be 24°, the lateral condylar inclination would be 15°. The articulator pillars supporting the condyle mechanism would, therefore, be rotated 15°, and this would influence the extent of the provision for Bennett movement by the articulator (Fig. 10.3). As this adjustment is also of a mechanical type dependent on the geometry of the instrument in use, it will be seen that both condylar guidance and Bennett adjustment represent approximations to the patient's mandibular movements.

To date, no mechanism has been devised which can accurately imitate the complex movements which can occur in the temporomandibular joints.

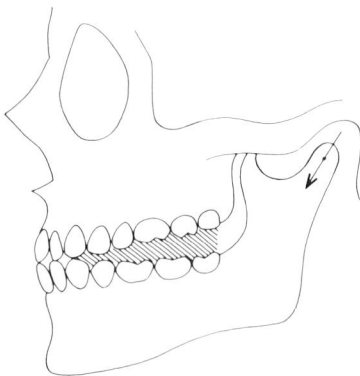

Fig. 10.2 Christensen's phenomenon in protrusive jaw relationship. The arrow indicates the downwards and forwards excursion of the condyle. The wedge-shaped gap between the opposing occlusal planes, which develops on protrusion of the mandible, is shown as a hatched area.

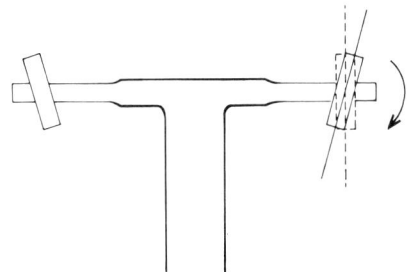

Fig. 10.3 Plan view to illustrate adjustment of the condyle mechanism of an articulator for Bennett movement.

FURTHER READING

Bates JF, Huggett R, Stafford GD 1991 Removable denture construction, 3rd edn. Wright, London.
Dyer EH 1973 Importance of a stable maxillomandibular relation. J Prosthet Dent 30: 241

Gilboe DB 1983 Centric relation as the treatment position. J Prosthet Dent 50: 685

Hickey JC, Williams BH, Woelfel JB 1961 Stability of mandibular rest position. J Prosthet Dent 11: 566

Lammie GA, Laird WRE 1986 Osborne and Lammie's partial dentures, 5th edn. Blackwell Scientific, Oxford

Lawson WA 1959 An analysis of the commonest causes of full denture failure. Dent Pract Dent Rec 10: 61

Swerdlow H 1965 Vertical dimension literature review. J Prosthet Dent 15: 241

11. Dental articulators and their selection

INTRODUCTION

A dental articulator is an instrument in which casts of the upper and lower dentate or edentulous jaws can be attached for reproducing jaw relations and movements of the lower jaw relative to the upper.

The simplest form of articulator consists of two arms or bows united by a hinge. This type of instrument enables an accurate record of a single static relationship between the jaws to be maintained, and the only movement which can be made is an opening and closing one about the hinge. It is known as a simple hinge or plane-line articulator. More complex articulators are able to assume relationships other than a single static one, and instruments capable of assuming such eccentric positions are known as 'adjustable' or 'anatomical' articulators. These articulators vary considerably in their capacity to simulate jaw movements and relationships, and may be considered as falling into several classes of instruments.

CLASSIFICATION OF DENTAL ARTICULATORS

1. Simple hinge or plane-line articulators
2. Average value articulators
3. Adjustable articulators, which may be either:
   a. Simple adjustable or
   b. Fully adjustable.

A SHORT HISTORY OF ARTICULATORS

As an aid to understanding articulators, it will be useful to have an insight into their development. This will be considered on the basis of significant changes rather than a complete history.

The plaster slab

The earliest known device used for relating casts of the upper and lower jaws was by modification of the posterior aspects of the casts to produce a fixed relationship between them. This 'plaster slab' or 'occludator' arrangement is associated with the name of Pfaff (1755) (Fig. 11.1).

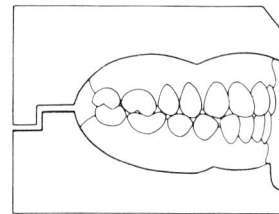

Fig. 11.1 Plaster slab articulator.

Simple hinge articulators

It is believed that the simple hinge-like cast relator was invented by Gariot in 1805. Opening and closing movements about a convenient, but not anatomically related, axis were provided for. The Gariot instrument consisted of two metal frames or bows to which the casts could be attached. These were joined by a simple hinge mechanism, and a stop or screw to hold the bows a fixed distance apart was provided (Fig. 11.2).

Many forms of this instrument have been, and continue to be, employed. Some forms incorporate, for example, remounting devices and adjustable bearings, but the basic features of the instrument remain essentially similar to that designed by Gariot.

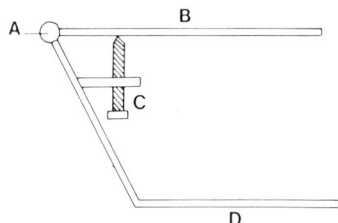

Fig. 11.2   Diagram to show the essential features of the simple hinge articulator. A, hinge; B, upper bow; C, vertical stop mechanism; D, lower bow.

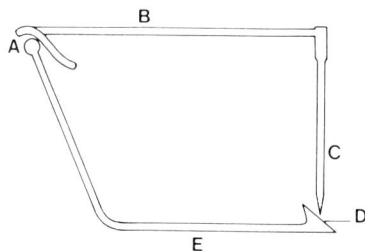

Fig. 11.4   Essential features of the Gysi 'simplex' articulator. A, condylar guidance mechanism; B, upper bow; C, incisal guide pin; D, incisal guide plate; E, lower bow.

Average value articulators

In 1840, Evans patented an articulator having a hinge connection between the upper and lower bows, and a slot arrangement which allowed a sliding motion at the joint, but it is generally considered that the first instrument incorporating a mechanism meant to reproduce the mandibular movements was that of W. G. Bonwill (1858). Bonwill's 'anatomical' articulator was based on his theory that the distance between the condyles and the mid-incisal point of the mandible was an equilateral triangle of 4 inch side. A sliding ring and spring mechanism about the horizontal 'condylar' element allowed for opening, protrusive and lateral components of movement (Fig. 11.3).

In practical terms, this was the first of the average value articulators, and it allowed the possibility of serious points of interference between cusps of teeth to be detected and eliminated, thus permitting a semblance of balanced occlusal relationships to be developed. The 4 inch equilateral triangle concept is now known to be inaccurate and the horizontal condylar mechanism inappropriate, but Bonwill's

work was significant in recognising the need to relate articulator design to condylar activity.

Gritman, in 1899, produced an articulator having the condylar guides inclined at 15° to the horizontal, to allow for the effect of the articular eminence in joint activity.

The Gysi 'simplex' articulator, which was produced in 1914, incorporated curved condylar guidance in recognition of the form of the glenoid fossa, and was provided with an incisal guide pin and an incisal table set at a fixed value of 60° (Fig. 11.4). The incisal guidance mechanism was an important development, which significantly assisted setting up of the artificial teeth by stabilising movements of the upper bow of the articulator.

A further average-value-type articulator of interest was that of Monson (1918), which evolved from the concept that the biting surfaces of the upper and lower teeth move over each other as over the surface of a sphere with a radius of 4 inches. The centre of the sphere was considered to be in the region of the glabella. This development represented a philosophical divergence from the accepted role of the condyles in mandibular movement, in that it placed the whole emphasis on the teeth as being the guiding influence for mandibular movement once tooth contact occurred. The Monson concept survives in the form of various metal templates, some of which are based on the 4 inch radius sphere, to which artificial teeth are set in an attempt to produce occlusal balance.

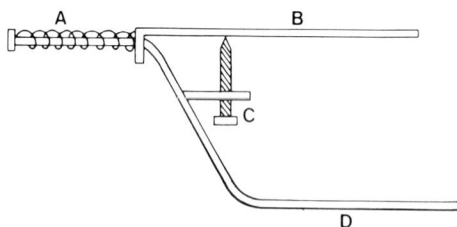

Fig. 11.3   Essential features of the Bonwill articulator. A, horizontal sliding mechanism; B, upper bow; C, vertical stop mechanism; D, lower bow.

Adjustable articulators

While the above instruments simulate movements of the mandible for the 'average' patient, it is clear

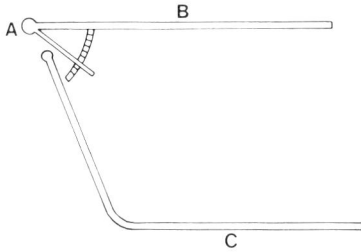

Fig. 11.5 Essential features of the Walker articulator. A, adjustable condylar mechanism incorporating a vertical stop; B, upper bow; C, lower bow.

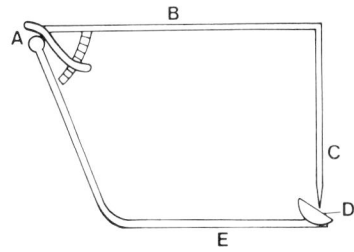

Fig. 11.6 Essential features of the Gysi adaptable articulator. A, adjustable condylar mechanism; B, upper bow; C, incisal guide pin; D, adjustable incisal guide plate; E, lower bow.

that the patient as an individual must be catered for in many instances.

W.E. Walker (1897) noted the balance achieved by dentures produced using Bonwill's articulator did not always balance in the mouth of the patient. As a consequence, he developed an articulator having individually adjustable condylar guidance (Fig. 11.5).

The Christensen articulator (1901) incorporated adjustable condyle paths which could be set by means of intra-oral registrations of eccentric jaw positions. Christensen also introduced the intra-oral records used to assist the articulator adjustments.

Snow, in 1900, produced an articulator similar to the Gritman instrument, and introduced the face-bow at this time to relate the intercondylar axis to the maxillae. All adjustable articulators from this time onwards made provision for use of the face-bow.

The Gysi adaptable articulator (1910) included a curved condylar guidance which was variable both vertically and horizontally. Variable intercondylar width was introduced and an incisal guidance mechanism was incorporated (Fig. 11.6). The Gothic arch method for establishing the most retruded relationship of the jaws from which lateral movements could be made was also introduced about this time.

The Wadsworth articulator (1919) had condylar posts which could be moved laterally to match that dimension of the patient, and also incorporated removable remounting plates so that casts could be removed from the articulator and replaced accurately as required.

The Hanau articulator (model H) introduced in 1922, and the Dentatus (1944), have condylar

adjustments in both the vertical and horizontal (or lateral) planes, and incorporate allowance for the Bennett movement. A variable incisal guidance mechanism is also provided on both instruments. The variable condylar path is arranged in such a manner that alteration of the slope of the path does not alter the distance between the upper and lower bows of the articulator. Remounting of casts is provided for by means of replaceable plates which are screwed into position.

Hanau devised a mathematical relationship following experiments with registrations of protrusive and lateral relations between the maxilla and mandible such that

$$L = \frac{H}{8} + 12 \ ,$$

where L is the lateral inclination of the condyle path and H is the horizontal inclination. Using this formula, the inclination of the condylar guides in the lateral direction can be set, when the horizontal inclination has been established using a registration of protrusive relationship. Variation in the lateral condylar inclination varies the amount of Bennett movement provided for.

Many more adjustable articulators have been, and continue to be, produced, and it is likely that developments in this field will continue. Some types have very complex mechanisms and aim to simulate as faithfully as possible the movements of which the temporomandibular joint is capable. Such instruments often require extremely demanding clinical methods to be followed to produce the records necessary for adjustment of the mechanism.

On the other hand, a form of compromise between the average value and the simple adjustable articulator has been provided for by some manufacturers. This type of articulator has a fixed condylar slope, generally of the order of 30°, and is provided with an adjustable incisal guidance table. The condylar mechanism may include some provision for Bennett movement. Used in conjunction with a face-bow, these articulators are superior to the average value instruments, while lacking the capacity for the individual adjustment provided for in other simple adjustable instruments. For removable denture prostheses, and particularly those which are borne by soft tissues, little advantage will accrue from the use of a highly sophisticated articulator, since the resilience of the tissue underlying such an appliance will usually permit gross movement of the denture, in excess of the finer adjustment settings of the instrument.

An instrument of the Dentatus type, permitting individual condylar angle variation, Bennett adjustment and incisal guidance adjustment may be regarded as a satisfactory general-purpose articulator for removable prostheses. The detailed adjustment capacity of the more complex articulator is more suited for specific clinical methods related to diagnosis and restoration of the occlusion of the natural dentition.

Only an outline of important developments in this large field has been included in the foregoing. The reader is recommended to consult the literature for a fuller treatment of this topic.

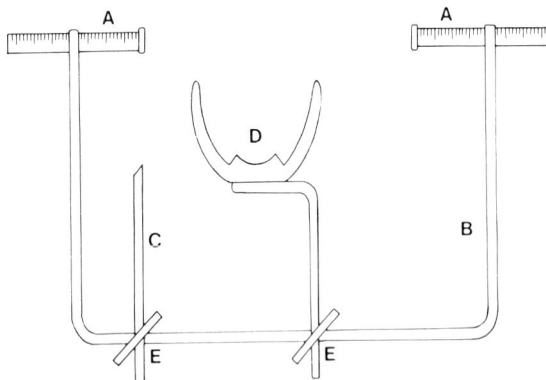

Fig. 11.7 The simple face-bow. A, calibrated condyle indicators; B, body; C, orbital pointer; D, fork; E, universal joints.

FACE-BOW REGISTRATION

The face-bow is a caliper-like device which is used to record the relationship between the intercondylar axis and either the maxillary or mandibular arch. Once established, this relationship can be transferred to an articulator, so that casts of the patient's jaws will assume the same relationship to the hinge axis of the articulator as that of the upper or lower jaw of the patient to the intercondylar axis.

Two types of face-bow exist:

1. The simple face-bow
2. The hinge axis face-bow.

The simple face-bow

This instrument was introduced by Snow in approximately 1900. Modern simple face-bows are similar to that of Snow, but with the addition to many of them of an orbital pointer. The pointer serves to identify an anterior point of reference which, in conjunction with the condyles, forms a horizontal plane of reference.

The face-bow consists of a U-shaped body having calibrated adjustable condyle indicators at each side (Fig. 11.7). The body of the face-bow carries a joint for securing a fork having an offset rod attached, and another for the orbital pointer.

Use of the simple face-bow

This will be considered in some detail, as this is the most commonly used face-bow.

The lateral poles of the condyles are located by a combination of estimation of their positions and palpation. The average anatomical position of the condyle is some 12 mm from the posterior point of the tragus of the ear, along a line joining the upper border of the external auditory meatus and the outer canthus of the eye. After determining this point, the ball of the finger should be placed over it and the patient asked to make small mouth opening and closing movements, when movement of the tissues overlying the lateral pole of the condyle will be appreciated. Some corrections of the position of the finger may be required where variation from the estimated position is present. The site as determined should be marked on the skin of the face, using

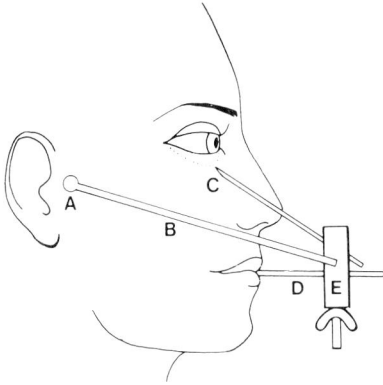

Fig. 11.8 The face-bow in position on the face as seen from the lateral aspect. A, condyle indicator; B, body of face-bow; C, orbital pointer; D, rod of fork; E, universal joint.

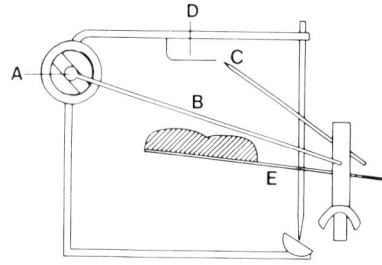

Fig. 11.9 The face-bow in position on the articulator as seen from the lateral aspect. A, condyle indicator; B, body of face-bow; C, orbital pointer; D, orbital locator; E, rod of fork.

a small self-adhesive paper marker or chinagraph pencil. Both condyles should be located.

The fork of the face-bow is attached to the upper occlusal rim or, where natural teeth are present in the upper jaw, to a wax record of the occlusal and incisal surfaces of the teeth. The occlusal rim or wax record is placed in position in the mouth, leaving the rod of the fork protruding from the mouth. All joints on the body of the face-bow are loosened and the joint for the face-bow fork is slipped into position. The condylar indicators are placed in contact with the previously recorded marks. An assistant will be required for this procedure. Centring of the face-bow is carried out by ensuring that the condyle indicators show equal graduations while maintaining contact with the skin markers. The fork joint is then tightened.

Where an orbital pointer is used, the patient is instructed to close the eyes while the tip of the pointer is carried towards the lowest part of the orbit (orbitale). The joint on the body for the orbital pointer is tightened. After slackening off the condyle indicators, the face-bow, together with the upper occlusal rim or wax template, is removed from the patient (Fig. 11.8).

Mounting the models on the articulator

The condyle markers of the face-bow are placed in position on the joint mechanism of the articulator. Provision for face-bow attachment is made on average value and adjustable articulators. The

condyle indicators are then centred, so that equal graduations appear on both indicators.

Where an orbital indicator has been used, the pointer is made to contact the appropriate site near the top of the articulator, in order to fix the horizontal plane of the record (Fig. 11.9).

Where an orbital pointer is not used, other methods may place the plane of occlusion parallel to the ala–tragus line; or to a line joining the tragus of the ear and the anterior nasal spine; or approximately parallel to the base of the articulator.

Once the horizontal disposition is established, the face-bow is supported steadily in position. The cast of the maxillary ridge or teeth is firmly seated into position in the upper baseplate carrying the occlusal rim assembly, or the wax record as appropriate. This cast is then luted to the upper bow of the articulator using plaster of Paris. The upper cast has now been attached to the upper bow of the articulator in the same relationship to the hinge of the articulator as the maxilla of the patient bears to the intercondylar axis.

The mandibular cast can then be attached to the lower bow of the articulator by means of a record of retruded jaw relationship, obtained as considered in Chapter 10.

The hinge axis face-bow

This instrument was introduced by McCollum in 1930 and is used to determine the centre of rotation or hinge axis of the condyles.

The fork of the hinge axis face-bow is attached to the lower jaw (Fig. 11.10) and, during opening movements, styli, which are located in the region of

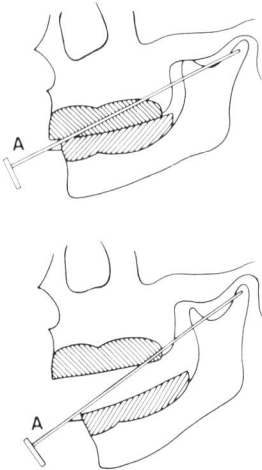

Fig. 11.10 Diagram to illustrate the action of the hinge axis face-bow (A). Jaws closed (upper) and open (lower).

the condyles, are adjusted until rotation of the styli is observed without any translation. The points so determined are marked on the skin as the 'hinge axis'.

Many complex variations of this instrument exist. It is not as commonly used for removable denture prosthetics as the simple face-bow. The validity of the hinge axis concept is considered to be controversial.

THE BASIS FOR SELECTION OF AN ARTICULATOR

This will be considered in terms of the classes of articulator considered above.

Simple hinge articulators

These instruments can only open and close in a hinge-like action. Teeth set up on such an articulator for complete dentures will not always balance in contact positions in the mouth, other than the single position in which the casts were related together. This arrangement would be suitable only for a patient whose masticatory and other functional activities are of a simple hinge-like nature.

In complete denture construction, the use of a template based on average occlusal contours to which the teeth are set improves the possibility for

limited occlusal balance. A range of templates is available, some of which are based on the 4 inch radius used by Monson in conjunction with his articulator. Such methods require posterior teeth of the flat cusp or inverted cusp type to be used, so that good conformation of their occlusal surfaces to the template can be developed.

A further technique in which the surface of special occlusal rims are modified by the patient grinding the rims together in the mouth ('chew-in' technique) may be used. This provides a more individual template to which flat cusped teeth may be set, to assist in providing balanced contact with the opposing teeth. This method, while occasionally useful, is not commonly used because patients often have difficulties in producing suitable 'templates' during the 'chew-in' phase.

Average value articulators

These articulators provide for 'average' mandibular excursions. Used in conjunction with a face-bow record, better results are achievable than with the hinge articular, but detectable error in eccentric movements of the mandible in relation to occlusal balance will occur in many cases because of variation between the geometry of the instrument and the anatomical form of the patient.

Adjustable articulators

When adjusted to the individual requirements of the patient, this class of articulator will provide the best occlusal balance attainable. From the clinical point of view, the records required to adjust the articulator, in addition to the retruded jaw relationship, will include a protrusive registration and a face-bow registration.

Where it is desired to match exactly the occlusal relations of natural teeth which are present, the more complex articulators may need to be considered as the variation in occlusal form of the natural teeth is much wider than that of artificial teeth. In many instances, average value instruments may be used where the numbers and positions of the remaining teeth are such that a clear guide to the position and form of the missing teeth exists. However, in the majority of these cases, an adjustable incisal table is required, because the overbite and overjet relations of the natural teeth are frequently outside the range of the fixed incisal guidance instruments.

FURTHER READING

Bergstrom G 1950 On the reproduction of dental articulation by means of articulators. Acta Odont Scand 9: suppl 4

Celenza FV 1979 An analysis of articulators. Dent Clin North Am 36: 305

Thorpe R, Smith DE, Nicholls J I 1978 Evaluation of the use of a face-bow in complete denture occlusion. J Prosthet Dent 39: 5

Weinberg LA 1961 An evaluation of the face-bow mounting. J Prosthet Dent 11: 32

Weinberg LA 1963 An evaluation of basic articulators and their concepts. Part I. Basic concepts. J Prosthet Dent 13: 622

Weinberg LA 1963 An evaluation of basic articulators and their concepts. Part II. Arbitrary, positional, semiadjustable articulators, J. Prosthet Dent 13: 645

Weinberg LA 1963 An evaluation of basic articulators and their concepts. Part III Fully adjustable articulators, J Prosthet Dent 13: 873

Weinberg LA 1963 An evaluation of basic articulators and their concepts. Part IV. Fully adjustable articulators, J Prosthet Dent 13: 1038

12. Principles of tooth selection

INTRODUCTION

The selection of artificial teeth to replace lost natural teeth can be a difficult phase of removable denture production. Where partial dentures are involved, a clear guide may be provided by the remaining natural teeth. For complete dentures and removable partial dentures where many teeth require replacement, in the absence of accurate pre-extraction records no such guide is available. No infallible method of selection exists, and the teeth which are to be used must be chosen to harmonise with the aesthetic and functional characteristics of the patient.

The requirements for a patient may have special facets in respect of the anterior and/or posterior artificial teeth, and these will be considered separately.

THE SELECTION OF ANTERIOR TEETH FOR REMOVABLE DENTURES

The factors to be taken into account in the selection of anterior teeth include:

1. Size
2. Form
3. Texture
4. Colour
5. Material.

Size

Where a removable partial denture is to be produced, and a tooth requiring replacement has the corresponding tooth from the opposite side of the arch still in situ, determination of the exact size of the tooth required is a simple matter of measurement. Bodily movement or tilting of the remaining teeth may complicate the use of artificial teeth of the same size as their natural predecessors, and it might be necessary to overlap teeth on the one hand, or provide spacing on the other hand, in order to achieve the degree of balance in size required between the right and left sides of the arch. It is occasionally necessary to use a tooth of a different size to those remaining, but generally the aim is to replace a missing tooth with one of the same size, since it is very uncommon to find corresponding teeth on the left and right sides of the natural dentition which differ in size.

Where no natural anterior teeth remain, the selection of artificial teeth presents the same difficulties as are met in the edentulous patient.

When pre-extraction records are available, they may provide very useful guides to tooth selection. Study models including the patient's natural teeth will give a clear guide to the size and form of the teeth. Clinical photographs can be an equally accurate guide and, while photographs obtained from the family album will rarely provide clear detail of the anterior teeth, they may be very useful as a guide to the relative proportion of the size of the teeth and face of the patient. Other pre-extraction records which can be a helpful guide to tooth size include radiographs of the patient's teeth, and also extracted teeth which have been retained by the patient.

In the absence of any pre-extraction guides, a great deal will depend on the judgement of the dentist. The difficulties experienced during this phase of denture production have resulted in many average value measurements and formulae based on anatomical features being suggested.

General guidelines subject to wide, individual variation suggest that the larger the person, the larger the teeth will be, and that the teeth of women tend to be somewhat smaller than those of men. More specific aspects of anterior tooth selection will be considered in terms of the length and the width of the teeth.

Length

Generally, the incisal edges of the natural central incisors extend below the lowest part of the relaxed lip. For a young person, some 2–3 mm of the upper central incisors may be visible, while for an elderly patient only a fraction of a millimetre of tooth may be seen beneath the relaxed lip. There is, of course, wide variation between individuals in this respect.

Some of the factors responsible for differences in the amount of tooth visible include:

1. Age. With increasing age, tooth wear tends to shorten the clinical crowns.

2. Length of the upper lip. Where a patient has a short upper lip, up to half the length of the crown of the central incisors may be exposed beneath the relaxed upper lip. On the other hand, a long lip may completely cover the incisors, even in a young patient.

3. Overbite. Where a deep overbite exists, more of the upper anterior teeth tend to be exposed.

At the gingival aspect, the high lip line may be taken as a guide. The high lip line is the maximum vertical excursion of the upper lip during functions such as smiling. Thus, a combined estimation of the position of the incisal edge and the high lip line will provide a guide to the length of the central incisors.

Alternatively, determination of tooth length may be approached by estimating the width of the anterior teeth, and then utilising the proportion between the length and width of the teeth provided by the manufacturer for a given tooth form in relation to the length and width of the patient's face (see p. 89).

Width

There have been many methods suggested for determining the width of the upper anterior teeth. Most methods provide a value for the six anterior teeth together, rather than for individual teeth. Some of these methods are listed below:

1. Canine eminence. If this anatomical feature is well defined, the distance between lines drawn on the cast of the upper jaw at the distal aspect of the eminences, may be taken as the mesiodistal breadth of the upper anterior teeth.

2. Bizygomatic width. It has been suggested that the combined breadth of the six upper anterior teeth may be estimated by dividing the maximum bizygomatic width of the skull by 3.3; and that the width of the upper central incisor is one-16th of the bizygomatic width. A face-bow may be used as a caliper, in conjunction with a ruler, to determine the bizygomatic width. The results of these calculations represent the proportions frequently found in pleasant looking natural dentitions.

3. Cranial circumference. The cranial circumference has been found to have a direct relationship to the width of the six upper anterior teeth, in a high proportion of cases. The horizontal circumference of the cranium, about a plane passing through the glabella and the maximum occipital point, is said to be ten times the width of the six upper anterior teeth.

4. Corner of the mouth. The distal surface of many natural upper canines is positioned at the corner of the relaxed mouth. The method used to record this position, in a patient lacking natural teeth, requires a properly contoured upper occlusal rim to be in position in the mouth, in order to provide correct lip support. The patient is requested to relax with lips in light contact, and a pointed instrument is passed to the occlusal rim at each corner of the mouth, and a mark recorded on the rim (Fig. 12.1). The distances between these marks, following the contour of the rim, is taken to represent the width of the six upper anterior teeth.

5. Width of the nose. Parallel lines extended from the lateral surfaces of the ala of the nose onto the properly contoured upper occlusal rim will give an indication of the position of the cusp tip of the upper canine teeth (Fig. 12.2). In practice, the distance between the lateral extremities of the ala can be measured with dividers and then transferred to the rim. The mesiodistal width of the teeth, between the tip of the cusps of the canine teeth, is then measured around the contour of the occlusal rim.

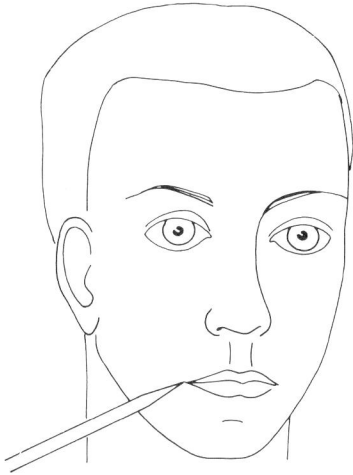

Fig. 12.1 Marking the position of the corner of the mouth on the occlusal rim.

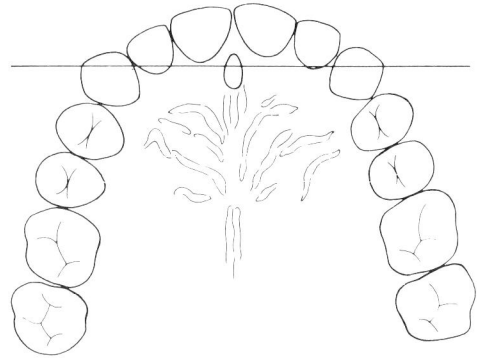

Fig. 12.3 Occlusal view of the upper arch showing the relationship between the incisive papilla and the tip of the cusp of the canines in the coronal plane.

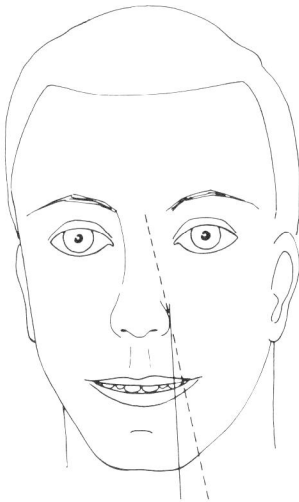

Fig. 12.2 Establishing the position of the canine teeth. The broken line gives an indication of the position of the distal aspect of the canine. The solid line indicates the position of the tip of the cusp.

6. Lateral surface of the nose. A further, and perhaps more commonly used guide utilising the ala of the nose, requires the projection onto the properly contoured upper occlusal rim of an imaginary line along the lateral surface of the nose, through the centre of the brow-line, and contacting the lateral aspect of the ala. The line on the occlusal rim gives an indication of the position of the distal aspect of the canine tooth, at the point where the projected line passes the occlusal plane (Fig. 12.2).

7. The incisive papilla. It has been demonstrated that a line parallel to the coronal plane, and passing through the incisive papilla, contacts the natural canine teeth near the tips of the cusps (Fig. 12.3). This may be used as a guide to determining the width of the anterior teeth and positioning the canine teeth, when used in conjunction with a properly contoured occlusal rim.

Form

The overall shape of the teeth is important to the development of harmony of form with the face. A method of long standing usage in the selection of aesthetically acceptable tooth form is that developed by J. Leon Williams. The theory introduced by Williams was that the shape of the crown of the upper central incisor corresponded to the outline form of the face. If the outline form of the central incisor is enlarged and inverted, so that the incisal edge is placed in the region of the hair line, with the neck of the tooth corresponding to the outline of the chin, Williams claimed that the form of the tooth and that of the face will coincide (Fig. 12.4). He classified the form of the face as square, tapering or ovoid — a basic classification which was later added to by combining the basic types to increase the variety of forms (Fig. 12.5).

It has now been demonstrated that the relationship described above occurs only rarely. However, it

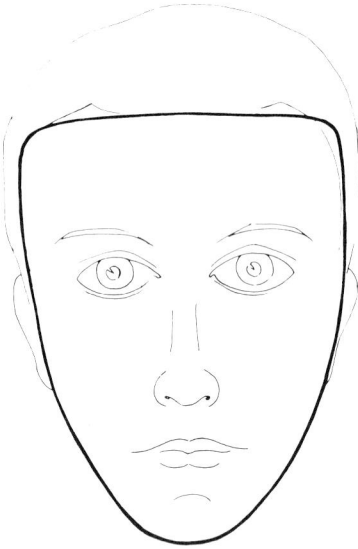

Fig. 12.4 Superimposition over the face of an inverted and enlarged form of the crown of the central incisor.

is clear that the application of Williams' method can produce aesthetically satisfactory results.

Age, sex and personality factors have been cited as relevant to selection of tooth form. For example, the wearing down of natural teeth which accompanies advancing age, and the softer, more rounded, contours of the teeth of women, are factors to be considered.

The contours of the labial face of the teeth is also important in considering tooth form, and this often relates to the form of the profile of the patient. A patient having a strongly convex profile may require the teeth to have a strongly convex labial surface, for example.

Texture

When viewed in detail, most natural anterior teeth possess very complex labial surface features, and these are important to the appearance of the teeth. Smooth-surfaced artificial incisors reflect light evenly and have a lifeless appearance because of the lack of a suitable surface texture. In the production of an aesthetically pleasing restoration, artificial teeth which incorporate reproductions of such features as imbrication lines, surface facets, hypoplastic areas, etc., are superior to those having smooth, featureless surfaces.

Artificial teeth should be unobtrusive, and the texture of the tooth surface contributes to the harmonious blending of the teeth with the patient's tissues. In this respect, surface texture contributes

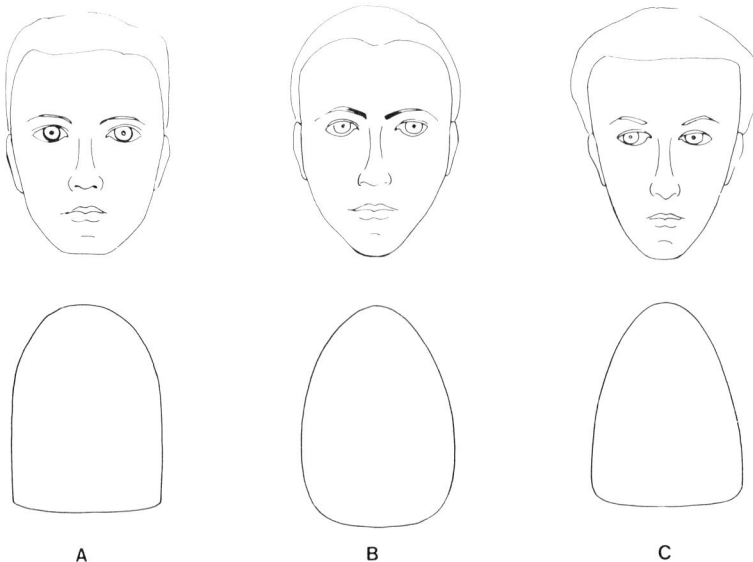

Fig. 12.5 Classification of facial forms as a guide to the selection of tooth form: **A** square; **B**, ovoid; **C**, tapering.

as much as colour selection and tooth arrangement to the overall 'natural' appearance of a denture.

Texture is a quality of particular importance in removable partial denture service, where anterior teeth are missing unilaterally. The replacement teeth will need to be careful copies of the remaining natural teeth in respect of surface texture, as well as colour, so that they will not be obviously artificial in appearance.

Colour

The colour variation in natural teeth covers a wide spectrum. There is gradation in the colour over a single tooth, which varies from darker near the gingival margin to lighter and more translucent near the incisal tip. In addition, there is also variation between teeth — the central incisors generally being lightest in overall colour, the lateral incisors slightly darker, and the canine teeth slightly darker again. The colour, or hue, of the teeth must harmonise with the patient's complexion and, in particular, with the skin of the face — and, to a lesser extent, the hair and the iris of the eyes. Skin colour tends to fall into one of three groups, having red, yellow or grey tints.

The basic hue of the teeth is a yellow colour, being derived from the dentine. Colour saturation, i.e. the amount of colour per unit area, is a factor of some importance. If the yellow colour is diluted to white, the tooth will appear light in relation to one having a similar basic yellow, but where black is added the result is a darker, more grey tooth. Variation in lightness and darkness is sometimes referred to as brilliance.

Where the complexion is fair or blonde, the tooth colour tends to be light and, for patients having a darker complexion, darker-coloured teeth predominate. In the mouth of a patient having a very dark complexion, teeth in which grey tones predominate may appear to be light in colour and, in this respect, it is important to appreciate the need for a harmonious balance of basic tooth colour relative to that of the patient's face.

In the natural teeth, the enamel is translucent and provides a thin covering to the dentine near the gingival margin of the crown, and a relatively thick covering at the incisal edge. This results in an apparent gradation of colour over the length of the tooth crown. At the incisal edge, where there may be no dentine underlying the enamel, the translucence of the enamel results in a greyish appearance which varies in apparent hue depending on the tongue, lip and mouth posture. In the better artificial teeth, this translucence is achieved by the manufacturer, and has the effect of blending the various pigments used in colouring the teeth, and also provides for subtle colour variation to occur during functional activity in the mouth, particularly near the incisal edges of the teeth.

It is generally advised that in the selection of the shade for artificial teeth where no natural anterior teeth are present, reference should be made to the skin and also to the hair and the eyes. Of these, skin colour is by far the best guide. The hue and saturation of colour in the teeth must harmonise with that of the skin. Hair colour is useful in the younger patient as a guide, but it should be borne in mind that hair colour may be subject to quite rapid change from both natural and artificial causes. The colour of the iris of the eyes is sometimes useful in a general sense, but this feature is relatively small in proportion to other colours about the face.

Age has a marked effect on tooth shade. With advancing years, tooth wear may result in exposure of dentine which readily takes up extrinsic stains. The reduction in size of the pulp chamber with advancing age produces a yellowing effect, because of the increase in the quantity of dentine. Injury to the tooth and repair of the tooth structure also have an effect on the colour of a tooth.

Manufacturers of artificial teeth produce a wide range of shades for their products. While the available range is generally satisfactory for complete dentures, the enormous variation which exists with the natural teeth is not always satisfied by those available for removable partial denture work. In such circumstances, it might be necessary to resort to the use of the pigments, stains, etc., which are produced for the purpose of modifying the stock teeth produced commercially. The alternative is to accept the nearest available shade, which may not produce an aesthetically harmonious result.

In using the shade guide for artificial teeth as supplied by the manufacturer, the tooth colours are usually observed holding the chosen shade:

1. Outside the mouth against the skin of the face,

and also near to the eyes and the hair of the patient. This is to establish the basic hue, brilliance and saturation of colour.

2. Under the lip, to observe the colour of the tooth in the mouth. Shade selection should be carried out preferably in diffuse daylight, as the light incident on the teeth will influence the apparent colour of the reflected light. The shade guide tooth placed under the lip should be observed with its surface wet.

The selection of tooth shade for an edentulous patient presents a difficult problem, and is dependent to a large extent on the artistic interpretation of the dentist. For the partially dentate patient, only colour matching is required, and this presents difficulty only when suitably shaded artificial teeth are not available.

Material

Artificial teeth are manufactured in porcelain and in plastic materials. Both types are available in a wide range of sizes, shapes, surface textures and colours. It is not the intention of this section to deal with the materials science aspects of the two materials, but it is necessary to touch on these as they affect use of the teeth. Porcelain teeth require mechanical retention to the denture base material, and anterior teeth are usually provided with pins for this purpose. The pins protrude from the tooth and prevent close adaptation of the tooth to the residual ridge, and this is a potential source of difficulty where the space available for placement of the tooth is limited. Where it is necessary to alter the shape of a porcelain tooth, it is extremely difficult to polish the material to reproduce the glazed surface which existed prior to alteration.

Plastic teeth are simple to adjust and repolish, and do not rely on mechanical retention for attachment to denture base resins. Plastic teeth are also much simpler than porcelain teeth in respect of alteration of surface texture and incorporation of stains, etc. They are, therefore, much more versatile, particularly where lack of space for tooth placement is an aspect of the denture being produced.

From the aesthetic and functional points of view, both porcelain and plastic teeth may be regarded as equally satisfactory for replacement of anterior

teeth. A table (Table 12.1) citing the relative merits of porcelain and plastic teeth will be found on page 96.

SELECTION OF POSTERIOR TEETH

The selection of posterior teeth will be considered in relation to:

1. Size
2. Form
3. Colour
4. Material.

Size

The selection of the appropriate posterior tooth size is based on the space available for the replacement teeth, and, where upper premolar teeth are involved, the aesthetic requirements must also be considered.

The space available for posterior teeth may be defined in three dimensions:

1. The mesiodistal dimension
2. The occlusogingival dimension
3. The buccolingual dimension.

Mesiodistal dimension

For bounded saddles, where natural teeth are present in the mouth, the mesiodistal dimension is readily defined as the distance between the distal surface of the mesial abutment and the mesial surface of the distal abutment. It is important that this mesiodistal space is occupied to provide for the development of effective contact points between the denture and the remaining natural teeth, in order to minimise the possibility of food packing and the occurrence of stagnation areas about the abutments. Generally, the same number of artificial teeth as that of the natural teeth lost from the dental arch will be provided, but this may not be possible as a result of drifting, tilting or rotation of the remaining teeth, and a compromise will be required.

Where complete dentures are concerned, the mesiodistal dimension available for artificial teeth extends between the distal surface of the lower canine and the mesial end of the retromolar pad. Because of the potential displaceability of the thick layer of soft tissue comprising the retromolar pad, artificial teeth must not be placed over that structure as instability of the lower denture will result during chewing when the denture is loaded in this region, and the denture consequently is displaced tissuewards. Where the alveolar crest of the lower residual alveolar ridge slopes steeply upwards anterior to the retromolar pad, the mesiodistal dimension for the teeth will need to be reduced. Placing an artificial tooth over such a steeply inclined plane will result in the development of resolved forces during chewing, which will tend to displace the denture anteriorly. These principles also apply to the selection of teeth for free-end saddle partial dentures.

Having obtained by measurement the dimension available, reference to a manufacturer's selection guide will give an indication of the teeth available to satisfy this size requirement.

Occlusogingival dimension

Artificial teeth of similar mesiodistal dimension are available in various lengths. In general, the longest tooth which can be used in the vertical space available should be selected. This is particularly important in respect of the upper premolar teeth, which are often visible during speech, laughing, etc. Where a premolar tooth is used which is significantly shorter than the canine tooth next to it, when viewed from the buccal aspect, the result is aesthetically unacceptable. In removable partial denture treatment, where an upper premolar is to be replaced, it may be necessary to substitute a canine tooth for the premolar in order to provide a tooth of adequate length for the aesthetic requirements of the patient.

Buccolingual dimension

The buccolingual space available for artificial teeth is limited by the cheek and tongue tissues, and also by the load-bearing capacity of the supporting tissues. In respect of the space between cheek and tongue tissues, earlier artificial tooth forms tended to be of similar dimension to the natural teeth they were intended to replace. This, however, ignores biomechanical aspects of posterior tooth replacement. The supporting mechanism for natural teeth

is well adapted to resist the forces applied to them during functional activity. Artificial teeth which are to be used with soft-tissue-borne bases utilise the mucosa covering the residual alveolar ridges and palate for support, and this tissue is unable to tolerate without damage the forces capable of acceptance by the natural teeth. Where a removable partial denture is of a tooth-supported design, the capacity of the periodontal ligament of the abutment teeth to support additional denture teeth is such as to require the extra loading to be kept to a minimum. As it is essential to provide adequate contact points between the denture and the abutment teeth, the buccolingual width of the denture teeth should be kept to a minimum consistent with the other requirements for a particular patient. By this means, the surface area of the artificial teeth is reduced, so that higher pressures can be developed for a given force generated by the muscles of mastication over the narrow artificial teeth, than would be the case for broader teeth. Thus, it is possible that the masticatory ability of the patient wearing dentures having narrow occlusal surfaces might be maintained without overloading the periodontal ligament of the abutment teeth or the mucous membrane underlying the denture base. Further aspects of this facet of posterior tooth selection are considered in the following section.

Form

Early artificial posterior teeth were hand carved from wood, bone or ivory, and even the crowns of natural teeth were used. When porcelain was introduced in France towards the end of the 18th century, very durable artificial teeth simulating natural teeth were produced. The development of porcelain teeth continued through the 19th century, using natural teeth as the basis for the form of the teeth. By the end of the 19th century, it was realised that natural tooth forms were often quite unsuitable for artificial dentures, and there followed efforts by many workers to produce tooth forms aimed at minimising the difficulties experienced. This development has continued up to the present time and various designs have been introduced to aid in stabilising the denture, increasing masticatory efficiency or minimising trauma to the underlying tissue, or combinations of these objectives.

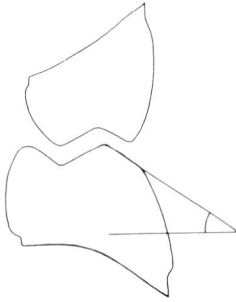

Fig. 12.6 Buccolingual section through 33° molar teeth (Gysi, 1914).

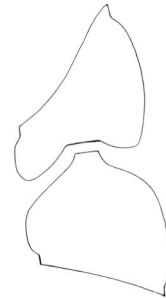

Fig. 12.7 Gysi's 'cross-bite' teeth in buccolingual section.

Some of the developments which have taken place will be described. It is not intended that this represents a review of tooth forms which are or have been available, but the types to be considered are representative of important groups of artificial tooth designs.

Prior to the 20th century, tooth forms were based on 'design', rather than having a basis implicating the factors known to have a relationship to balanced occlusion and articulation.

In 1914, Gysi carved teeth specially for use with his 'simplex' articulator, on the basis that condylar and incisal guidance angles for most patients required a tooth having a cusp angle of 33°. This represented the first 'anatomical' form of tooth to be produced on the basis of research relating the variable factors involved in articulation (Fig. 12.6).

Dr Gysi introduced 'cross-bite' teeth in the 1920s. These teeth were developed because of the realisation that the 33° teeth were not always adequate for a ridge relationship requiring a cross-bite arrangement of the posterior teeth. These teeth (Fig. 12.7) had narrow lower teeth having low cusps, for use with a 10° incisal guidance angle. The upper teeth were without a buccal cusp, so that a 'mortar and pestle' action was produced.

Sear's channel teeth were introduced in 1927. These teeth were produced having a central fossa in the upper teeth which ran mesiodistally through the four posterior teeth. The lowers had a corresponding narrow ridge of approximately 1.5 mm width. Freedom from cusp rise on protrusion of the lower teeth was allowed for, and the buccal and lingual inclined planes limited lateral gliding (Fig. 12.8).

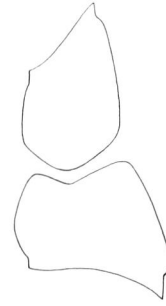

Fig. 12.8 Buccolingual aspect of Sear's channel teeth.

In 1929, Hall introduced his inverted cusp teeth. These teeth were produced having depressions in the surface and were designed to be set to the surface of a sphere, giving freedom of movement in all sliding contacts between the upper and lower teeth. The porcelain surrounding the inverted cusps was intended to act as an effective cutting edge (Fig. 12.9).

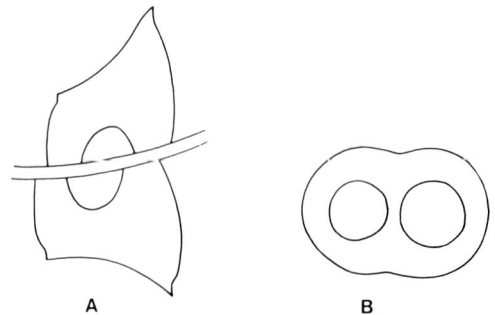

Fig. 12.9 Hall's inverted cusp teeth: **A**, Buccolingual section; **B**, plan view of a molar tooth.

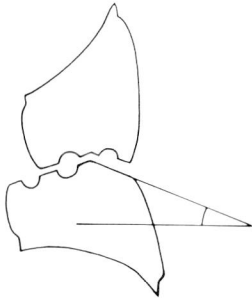

Fig. 12.10   Buccolingual section through 20°-type teeth.

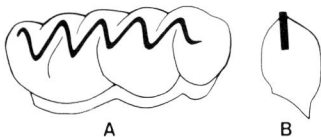

Fig. 12.12   Cook's posterior teeth: **A** viewed from an occlusobuccal aspect; **B** buccolingual section.

In 1935, French introduced his 'modified posteriors' which were of an inverted cusp style, but having the buccal aspect of the lower teeth removed so that contact occurred only with the lingual aspect of the uppers. French considered this design gave better stability to the lower denture than other occlusal arrangements.

Gysi introduced a further tooth form in 1935, having a low (20°) cusp angle and deep grooves and sulci for a modified inverted cusp effect. This represents a type of design which has been quite widely adopted (Fig. 12.10).

Metal inserts in stylised plastic posterior teeth were introduced in 1946 by Hardy. A zig-zag ribbon of Vitallium was present and raised slightly above the embedding plastic, to provide an effective cutting device when opposed by a similar metal ribbon (Fig. 12.11).

The development of vacuum firing techniques for porcelain in 1951 enabled much finer detail of cusp geometry, supplementary grooves, etc., to be retained during manufacture of posterior teeth and so improve shearing efficiency.

Cook, in 1952, suggested the use of cobalt–chromium lower teeth of inverted cusp form, but incorporating sluiceways on the buccal aspect.

These teeth were set against flat porcelain opposing surfaces in the upper teeth (Fig. 12.12).

While being efficient at cutting and dividing food, these teeth suffer from the disadvantage of constantly passing food into the buccal sulcus, from where it may be difficult for the patient to remove it. Also, there was a tendency for some foods to clog the sluiceways.

Bader, in 1957, introduced a 'cutter-bar', which was a metal bar replacing the lower second premolar and the first and second molars. The bar was opposed by flat porcelain upper teeth (Fig. 12.13).

With the exception of the higher-cusped 'anatomical' type of teeth, which simulate the natural teeth in a general way, many of the above tooth types have been developed for complete denture production. In removable partial denture work, the cuspal inclines and arrangement of the remaining natural teeth will determine contact movement paths between the opposing teeth, where some anterior and posterior teeth remain. Where only anterior teeth are present, the incisal guidance angle will, to a large extent, determine the form of posterior tooth to be used. The closer the incisal guidance approaches zero, the wider the choice of

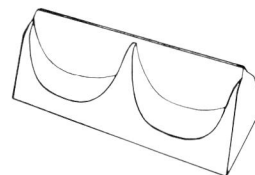

Fig. 12.11   Hardy's V.O. posterior teeth: **A** occlusal view; **B** buccolingual section. The heavy black line represents the metallic insert.

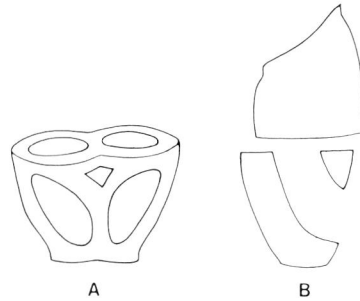

Fig. 12.13   Bader's cutter-bar.

Table 12.1   Advantages and disadvantages of porcelain and acrylic resin teeth

Property	Acrylic resin	Porcelain
Rate of wear	May be rapid	Very slow
Brittleness	Tough and will not chip	Brittle and may chip
Ease of adjustment	Easily ground and repolished	More difficult to grind and repolish
Density	1.18 g/cm^3	2.35 g/cm^3
Aesthetics	Can be excellent	Can be excellent
Ease of modification	Simple to characterise using stains, etc.	Difficult to characterise
Noise during use	Little impact sound on contact	Sharp impact sound
Retention to base	Potential for chemical bond	Mechanical bond only
Transmission of occlusal forces	Considered to transmit reduced forces	Considered to transmit all forces

posterior tooth form becomes and non-anatomical tooth forms may be considered.

If a deeper overbite exists, higher-cusped teeth will be required where posterior occlusal balance is sought. However, it must be appreciated that high-cusped teeth transmit relatively high lateral stresses to the denture base and the underlying supporting tissues, and this is to be avoided wherever possible — particularly where the residual alveolar ridge shows substantial atrophy. In general terms, the lower the crest of the residual alveolar ridge is in relation to the surrounding sulcus, the lower the cuspal angle of the teeth selected should be. Also, as pointed out previously, stresses on the underlying supporting tissue will be minimised by narrowing the occlusal table provided.

Colour

In selecting the colour of posterior teeth for removable partial denture work, the shade of the remaining natural teeth should be matched. Where an exact shade is not available, it is considered preferable to err on the side of selecting the nearest shade on the dark side of that required. Where a lighter option is used, the aesthetic effect may undesirably draw attention to the artificial replacement, even when only posterior teeth are involved.

For complete denture prostheses, the same shade of posterior tooth should be selected as that chosen for the anterior teeth.

Material

With the exception of the tooth forms described above as being made of metal, most types of posterior teeth are available in both porcelain or plastic (acrylic resin). No general rules are available in respect of the choice between porcelain and acrylic resin, except that relating to the available inter-ridge distance. Where this is minimal, acrylic teeth will be required as excessive grinding of porcelain posterior teeth will remove the diatoric holes provided for retention of the tooth to the baseplate. Because of the relatively rapid rate of wear of acrylic resin posterior teeth, some operators would contend that the resultant changes in occlusion would mitigate against their use. Patients seeking replacement dentures, and who have acrylic resin teeth on their existing dentures, may not readily tolerate a replacement denture having porcelain teeth. The simplicity of adjustment of acrylic teeth is often the major factor in their choice by many operators.

The advantages and disadvantages of porcelain and acrylic resin teeth are listed in Table 12.1.

FURTHER READING

Brewer AA, Reibel PR, Nassif NJ 1967 Comparison of zero degree teeth and anatomic teeth on complete dentures. J Prosthet Dent 17: 28
Brewer A A 1970 Selection of denture teeth for esthetics and function. J Prosthet Dent 23: 368

Frush JP, Fisher RD 1955 Introduction to dentogenic restorations. J Prosthet Dent 5: 586

Frush JP, Fisher RD 1956a How dentogenic restorations interpret the sex factor. J Prosthet Dent 6: 160

Frush JP, Fisher RD 1956b How dentogenics interprets the personality factor. J Prosthet Dent 6: 441

Frush JP, Fisher RD 1957 The age factor in dentogenics. J Prosthet Dent 7: 5

Frush JP, Fisher RD 1958 The dynesthetic interpretation of the dentogenic concept. J Prosthet Dent 8: 558

Ray GE 1963 Artificial posterior teeth. Dent Pract Dent Rec 14: 31

Saleski CG 1972 Colour, light and shade matching. J Prosthet Dent 27: 263

Sears VH 1957 The selection and management of posterior teeth. J Prosthet Dent 7: 723

Wehner PJ, Hickey JC, Boucher CO 1967 Selection of artificial teeth. J Prosthet Dent 18: 222

PART II

Special aspects relating to partial denture treatment

13. Introductory considerations

DEFINITION

Of the many definitions which have been proposed for removable partial dentures, the following is felt to be the most apt:

A removable partial denture is an appliance which restores a partial loss of natural teeth and associated tissues, and which receives its retention and support from the natural teeth and/or from the mucous membrane.

This definition is based on one given by Craddock, modifications having been introduced to meet the requirements of UK terminology.

TREATMENT OBJECTIVES

As noted in Chapter 6 — Diagnosis and treatment planning — the provision of a removable partial denture is one of the ways of providing treatment for the partially dentate condition. If, instead, a decision is made to provide no replacement of the missing teeth, it should be borne in mind that a number of problems may develop. These are described below.

1. Increased alveolar resorption

It has been claimed that the lack of any appreciable degree of loading stimulus will cause the alveolar processes in the edentulous regions to resorb at a faster rate than that which occurs when a denture has been fitted.

Gross alveolar resorption, which particularly tends to occur in the mandible, will reduce the prognosis for successful provision of a denture at a later date.

2. Reduction in masticatory efficiency

Manly and Braley have shown that the loss of the third molars reduces the masticatory function of a full complement of natural teeth by 10%. Additional removal of the first molars brings the value down by a further 20%.

Although the majority of individuals can manage to chew most foods satisfactorily when only one or two posterior teeth have been lost, additional loss may produce a noticeable fall in masticatory efficiency.

When multiple loss has occurred, the patient may complain of dietary limitation, and there is also a possibility that digestive disturbances will arise.

3. Effect on aesthetics

Tooth loss can affect aesthetics in two ways. Firstly, there will be an obvious loss of aesthetics where normally visible teeth are absent from the dentition. This will be most noticeable where anterior teeth are missing, but the effect may extend into the premolar regions. Secondly, the support for the lips and cheeks which the teeth provide will be lost. Loss of either anterior or posterior teeth may be evident because an inward collapse of lips or cheeks has occurred.

4. Effect on speech

The various consonants and vowels of the alphabet are produced by placing the lips or tongue in certain positions relative to the teeth, so developing definitive air channels. For example, 'f' and 'v' are made by bringing the lower lip into apposition with the upper anterior teeth (Fig. 13.1). As a conse-

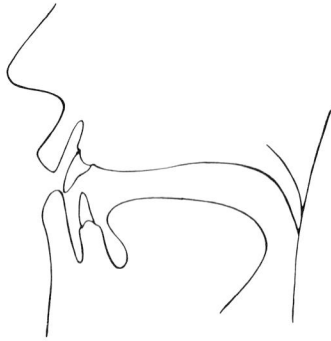

Fig. 13.1 Sagittal section of the oral cavity, showing the position of the lower lip relative to the upper anterior teeth in the formation of the 'f' and 'v' sounds.

quence, loss of the upper anterior teeth will inevitably interfere with the formation of the 'f' and 'v' sounds. Similarly, loss of other teeth from the arches can affect the quality of production of other speech sounds.

It is common to find, though, that in a relatively short time after tooth loss has occurred, a degree of adaptation will develop by, for instance, modification in tongue position, so lessening the effect on phonetics.

It is, in fact, unusual for a patient to attend with a complaint of poor phonetics arising from a partial loss of the natural dentition. Even so, there may well be a residual effect on the quality of speech where multiple tooth loss has occurred, and the provision of a denture in such cases can produce a noticeable improvement.

5. Effect on the integrity of the dentition

There is little doubt that the loss of a single tooth from the intact natural dentition can lead in some instances to general malocclusion, and the loss of the integrity of both dental arches.

There is a natural tendency for the teeth adjacent to the space created by tooth loss to tilt and drift into that space. This results in the opening up of contact areas between teeth in more remote positions in the arch, inviting food packing and plaque accumulation, with consequential increase in the risk of caries and periodontal damage arising. Where tilting occurs, the affected teeth become subject to non-axial loading from the opposing

dentition. This can hasten periodontal breakdown with thickening of the lamina dura, loss of bone from the alveolar crest and deepening of the periodontal pockets. The teeth in the opposing jaw, which are situated opposite to the space, will now lack occlusal stimulation. As a consequence, they tend to overerupt into the space, and the effects thus extend to the opposing jaw.

Eventually, where multiple tooth loss has occurred, disruption of tooth contact between the opposing jaws may reach the point where mandibular overclosure develops. When this happens, the temporomandibular joints may be affected. A detrimental effect on aesthetics may also arise, as the mandible moves upwards and forwards into its new stop position.

Overeruption of unopposed teeth may leave little or no room for the positioning of artificial teeth, where the provision of a removable partial denture is attempted in such a case. In addition, the tilting of isolated teeth may make the positioning of retentive clasp units on such teeth very difficult.

At times, conditions will become so severe that further extractions must be carried out before the provision of a removable partial denture becomes a feasible proposition.

6. Attrition of the remaining dentition

As the volume of the natural dentition is reduced by tooth loss, the remaining teeth will bear an increased masticatory load. Especially in those instances where tooth contact only occurs on the anterior teeth, there is a risk that gross attrition will occur in these teeth. Where this eventuality arises, treatment may necessitate the application of relatively complex procedures.

7. Effect on the neutral zone

Where any sizeable edentulous area is left unrestored for a period of time, it will be found that the tongue tends to occupy a part of the space vacated by tooth loss. Likewise, the cheeks and lips will tend to move inwards into the space.

The size of the neutral zone (or zone of minimum conflict) will thereby be decreased, and this may make the placement of teeth in the zone more difficult in any subsequent denture construction.

An increased risk of denture instability so arises.

8. Effect on masticatory movements

As tooth loss occurs, the necessity to chew on a reduced complement of the dentition may lead to the development of atypical masticatory movements. Facial pain may arise, as a consequence of the onset of temporomandibular joint disturbance. Increased difficulty may also be experienced in registering the correct fully retruded jaw relationship, where denture construction is subsequently carried out.

The formidable size of the above list of the possible consequences of a failure to restore a partial loss of the natural dentition clearly indicates the need for some form of replacement therapy to be applied in most instances. Where it is decided that this shall be achieved by the provision of a removable partial denture, the objectives may be summarised as follows:

1. Restoration of appearance
2. Restoration of masticatory efficiency
3. Restoration of speech to a normal quality
4. Maintenance of the health and integrity of the soft and hard tissues of the oral cavity.

It is likely that a patient would place these four treatment objectives in the order given above in terms of priority. The dental surgeon, though, should place treatment objective 4 at the top of the list of priorities. In that way, he will be best able to satisfy the prime aim of partial denture prostheses as advocated by De Van: 'our objective should be the perpetual preservation of what remains rather than the meticulous restoration of what is missing'.

A well-designed partial denture may meet this objective excellently by, for instance, splinting together the remaining natural teeth and by providing functional stimulus to the edentulous tissue areas. The need for such a biological concept of partial denture provision should be the uppermost consideration in all stages of design and construction.

CLASSIFICATION

Classification of partial dentures may serve one or both of two possible functions:

1. Provide a simple or 'shorthand' description of the features of a case, in terms of the disposition of the natural teeth and edentulous tissue areas in the arch.
2. Provide a guide to denture design, or at least be linked to design.

Many proposals have been made for schemes of classification. Of these, two have been selected for consideration on the basis of their frequency of application.

The Kennedy system

First introduced in 1928, this system fulfils only the first of the above functions, but is very widely used. It may be said to provide only a description of the unrestored natural dentition, rather than relate to the partial denture which is to be provided. Four classes are described:

Class I — the edentulous areas are bilateral, and lie posterior to the standing teeth (Fig. 13.2).

Class II — the edentulous area is unilateral, and lies posterior to the standing teeth on that side (Fig. 13.3).

Class III — the edentulous area is unilateral, and has standing teeth both anterior and posterior to it (Fig. 13.4).

Class IV — a single edentulous area lies anterior to the standing teeth (Fig. 13.5).

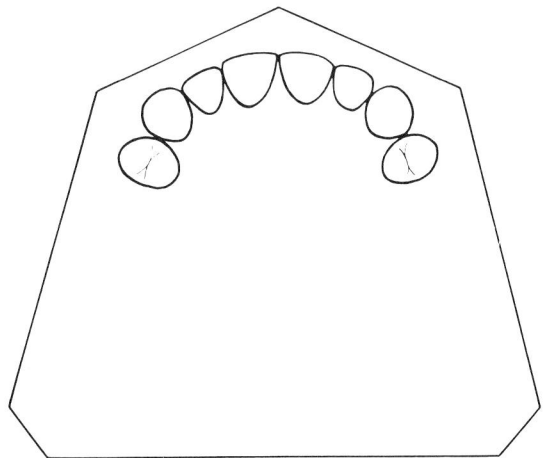

Fig. 13.2 A Kennedy class I dentition.

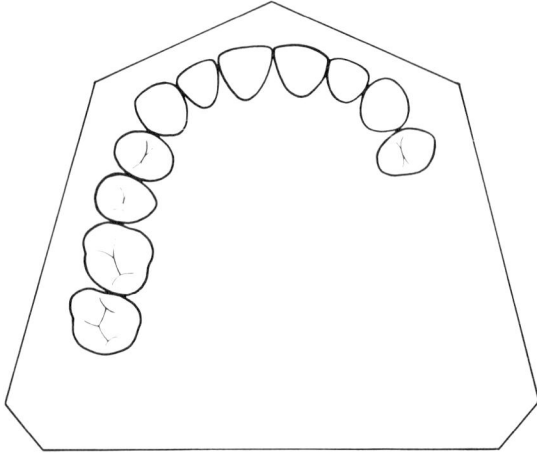

Fig. 13.3   A Kennedy class II dentition.

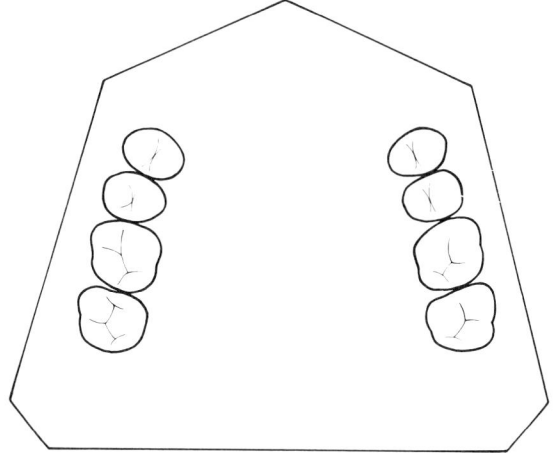

Fig. 13.5   Kennedy class IV dentition.

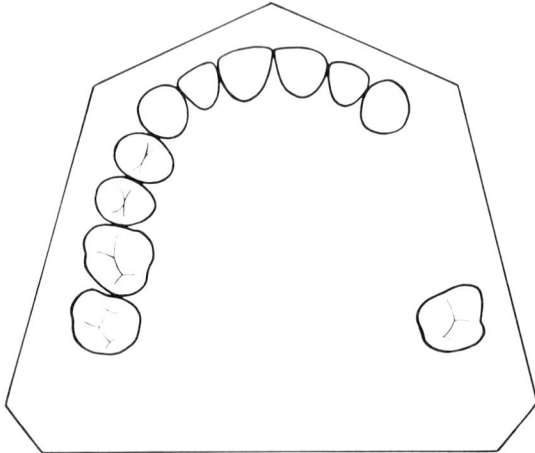

Fig. 13.4   A Kennedy class III dentition.

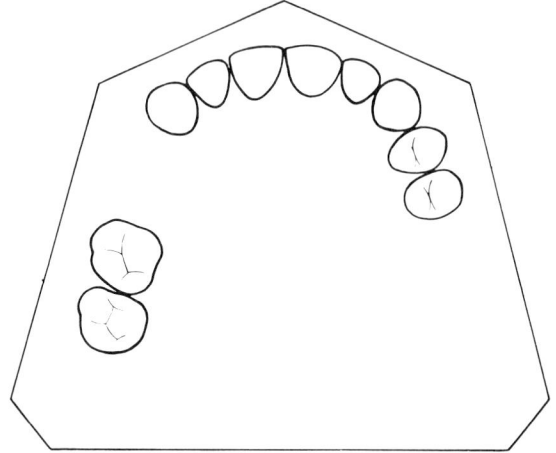

Fig. 13.6   An example of a Kennedy class II, modification 1 dentition.

In addition to the basic class descriptions, modifications are also described for each of the first three classes. These are numbered according to the number of additional edentulous areas which are present, one additional edentulous area being termed 'Modification 1', two additional edentulous areas 'Modification 2', and so on. Examples of cases showing modifications are shown in Figures 13.6 and 13.7.

No modifications are possible in the case of class IV dentitions, as the presence of any additional edentulous areas would bring such a case within the definition of one of the first three classes.

The Craddock system

This system meets, in particular, the second of the possible functions of systems of classification. It is based on earlier proposals of Bailyn, and is linked to the means which are to be adopted for supporting the partial denture on the oral tissues. Three classes are described:

Class I — denture entirely supported on the abutment teeth.

Class II — denture entirely supported on the mucous membrane.

Class III — denture support provided by both the

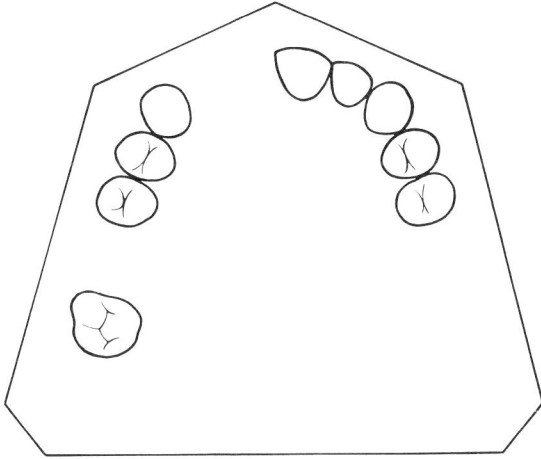

Fig. 13.7   An example of a Kennedy class II, modification 2 dentition.

abutment teeth and the mucous membrane, neither tissue being judged able to bear the applied load alone without sustaining damage.

The existence of various systems of classification necessitates that in all cases where reference is made to a class, a prefix must be applied to indicate the system which is being referred to. For example, one should refer to a 'Kennedy class I' case and not just a 'class I' case.

FURTHER READING

Craddock FW 1951 Prosthetic dentistry: a clinical outline. Henry Kimpton, London
De Van MM 1952 The nature of the partial denture foundation. Suggestions for its preservation. J Prosthet Dent 2: 210
Ettinger RL, Beck JD, Jakobsen J 1984 Removable prosthodontic treatment needs: a survey. J Prosthet Dent 51: 419
Kennedy E 1942 Partial denture construction. Dental Items of Interest New York
Lawson WA, Bond EK 1969 Speech and its relation to dentistry. Dent Pract Dent Rec 19: 150
Manley R S, Braley LC 1950 Masticatory performance and efficiency. Dent Res 29: 448
Silverman SI 1987 Differential diagnosis: fixed or removable prostheses. Dent Clin North Am 31: 347

14. Component elements

INTRODUCTION

The component elements which may be present in a removable partial denture are as follows:

1 Saddles
2 Rests
3 Direct retainers
4 Indirect retainers
5 Connectors
6 Stress-breakers.

All partial dentures contain at least two of these elements — saddles and connectors. The presence of additional elements will confer increasing complexity on the appliance, up to the point where all six elements may be present.

SADDLES

A saddle is that element of a partial denture which carries the artificial teeth. It also performs major functional and aesthetic roles in providing replacement for lost alveolar tissues.

Saddles can be classified as being either bounded or free-end. A bounded saddle has abutment teeth present at both extremities of the saddle. A free-end saddle has only a single abutment tooth at its mesial end.

Support for a saddle may be obtained from the abutment teeth, or from the mucosa underlying the saddle, or from a combination of both. The saddle may be made totally in a polymeric material such as acrylic resin, or in a combination of a metal such as cobalt–chromium alloy and a polymer.

The extension adopted for a saddle is dependent on its mode of support. Where the saddle is to be wholly or partly supported on the mucosa, then the maximum possible area of mucosa should be covered. This is necessary in order to keep the load borne by each unit area of mucosa to a minimum, so reducing the risk of evoking a pathological response in the loaded tissues. Where, instead, the saddle is to be supported on the abutment teeth, the extension developed can often be less, the outline here being dictated by the need to provide replacement for lost alveolar tissues.

RESTS

A rest is an extension from a partial denture which is positioned on the surface of a standing tooth capable of providing resistance to displacement of the rest in a tissuewards direction. Where tooth morphology is favourable, a rest may be placed on an unprepared tooth surface. In many instances, though, preparation of the tooth will be necessary if optimal resting action is to be obtained.

Rests are made in metal, as non-metallic materials such as acrylic resin lack the strength and abrasion resistance in thin section needed for this application. They may be wrought or cast in construction, the preference being for cast rests, as this allows the development of a better fit where an irregularly shaped rest seat is present.

There are three types of rests:

1. Occlusal rests — used on posterior teeth.
2. Cingulum rests — used on anterior teeth.
3. Incisal rests — used on anterior teeth.

Occlusal rests

Occlusal rests are normally positioned on the mesio-occlusal or disto-occlusal fossa of a posterior tooth. They find wide application in the construction of tooth-supported and tooth-and-mucosa-supported partial dentures.

Their outline form is triangular in shape, the base of the triangle lying along the marginal ridge of the tooth, with the apex positioned near the centre of the tooth. Buccolingually, the rest should fill all the available space between the buccal and lingual cusps. The rest is joined to the denture by means of an attachment tag, which may either enter the polymeric portion of an adjacent saddle, or may be an integral part of a cast metal framework for the denture.

The occlusal morphology of a rest should resemble that of the tooth on which it is placed, and should take due account of the occlusion with the opposing dentition. Its thickness must be adequate to provide resistance to distortion and fracture.

Cingulum rests

Cingulum rests can be placed on anterior teeth where a well-developed cingulum is present. This condition is most commonly met in upper central incisors and upper and lower canines. Upper lateral incisors may also present a suitable surface for their placement in some cases. Where the morphology of the tooth is such that a comparatively horizontal surface is present at the superior aspect of the cingulum, then the rest may be placed directly on the tooth surface without preparation (Fig. 14.1).

Problems may be encountered, though, where such direct placement of cingulum rests is used. Firstly, the rest presents a positive build-up on the tooth surface in an area of high tongue activity, and so may give rise to tongue irritation. Secondly, unless the surface on which the rest is placed is at right angles to the long axis of the tooth (and this finding is rare), a horizontal force component will

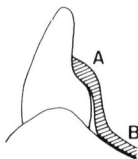

Fig. 14.2 Cingulum rest utilising a prepared rest seat in a lower canine.

arise by inclined plane action when the rest applies load to the tooth. This may cause horizontal tooth movement, which is clearly undesirable. Thirdly, inadequate space may be present for a rest where the anterior tooth relationship is close.

In most cases where a cingulum rest is to be used, preparation of the tooth is thus needed so that a horizontal facet is available for load application (Fig. 14.2).

The use of a rest seat preparation also reduces the build-up effect of the rest on the tooth surface, and thus aids tongue comfort.

Cingulum rests, especially those fitted into prepared rest seats, are nearly always cast.

Incisal rests

Incisal rests can be placed on any anterior tooth. They may, though, give rise to aesthetic problems and, for this reason, their application tends to be limited to those teeth for which the use of cingulum rests is normally not feasible (e.g. lower incisors). They may take various forms:

Form 1. An extension of metalwork on the lingual or palatal surface of an anterior tooth, to provide a thin cover over the whole incisal surface of the tooth (Fig. 14.3). This provides a very

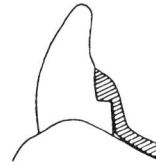

Fig. 14.1 Cingulum rest placed on the unprepared surface of a lower canine. A, cingulum rest; B, attachment tag.

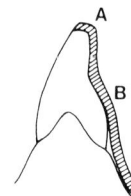

Fig. 14.3 Sagittal view of an incisal rest of form 1 used on a lower incisor. A, incisal rest; B, lingual plate.

positive resting action, but presents an unaesthetic show of metal.

Form 2. A rest seat may be prepared at the mesial or distal incisal corner of a tooth to present a horizontal facet for resting, the metal rest restoring the cut-out portion of the tooth (Fig. 14.4). Attachment of the rest would normally be via lingual or palatal metalwork. Again, aesthetic problems arise.

Form 3. Where the anteroposterior dimension of the tooth is adequate, a corner rest seat can be prepared as in form 2, but with maintenance of the labial enamel surface (Fig. 14.5).

Form 4. Incisal edge metal coverage as in form 1 may be extended into the interproximal embrasures, and onto a small area of the labial surface of adjacent teeth. Such a development is termed an embrasure hook (Fig. 14.6). When properly designed, embrasure hooks serve to splint teeth together and prevent their labial displacement. As with cingulum rests, all forms of incisal rests are normally prepared by casting.

Fig. 14.4 Anterior view of an incisal rest of form 2 used on a lower incisor.

Fig. 14.5 Plan view of an incisal rest of form 3 used on a lower incisor. A, labial surface; B, lingual surface.

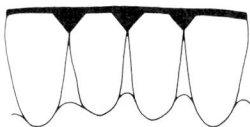

Fig. 14.6 Anterior view of incisal rests of form 4 on 42, 41, 31 and 32. Metal covering the incisal edges of the teeth has been extended interproximally onto small areas of the labial surfaces to form embrasure hooks.

The functions of rests

Function 1. Where a clasp arm is to be placed on a tooth, the presence of an associated rest serves to locate correctly the clasp arm on the tooth in its intended position.

Function 2. A rest can serve as a means of transferring vertical load borne by a denture saddle onto a standing tooth. It can thereby develop a tooth-supported or tooth-and-mucosa-supported characteristic in a saddle.

If it can be arranged that the vertical load applied by the rest to the tooth is transmitted along the long axis of the tooth, a favourable response by the periodontal attachment of the tooth is likely. If, instead, an off-centre load is transmitted to a tooth by a rest, a rotatory torque will arise and this may be less well tolerated by the periodontal attachment. This point should be borne in mind during the planning of the form and positioning of rests, so that the risk of causing periodontal damage will be minimised.

The problem of off-centre loading is particularly encountered where occlusal rests are used. Where design features permit, consideration should be given to the placement of two occlusal rests on a tooth, situated on opposing fossae. A condition approaching axial loading will thereby be achieved. Where only a single rest is to be used, the off-centre loading it gives rise to will be reduced by extending the rest as near to the centre of the tooth as is possible. It will also help if rests are sited in relation to the saddle in such a manner that resistance to tilting of an abutment tooth is present. With bounded saddles, rests should be placed on the fossae of the abutment teeth adjacent to the saddle. The saddle will then be able to act as a brace, resisting tilting of the teeth (Fig. 14.7).

With a free-end saddle, the rest should be placed on the fossa of the abutment tooth remote from the saddle. The tendency for tilting of the abutment tooth which the rest gives rise to will then be

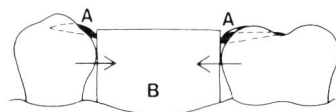

Fig. 14.7 Positioning the rests for a bounded saddle. The saddle resists tilting of the abutment teeth in the directions indicated by the arrows. A, rest; B, saddle.

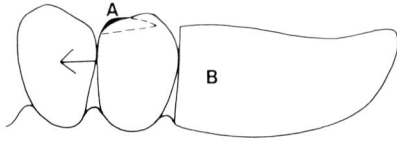

Fig. 14.8   Positioning the rest for a free-end saddle. The contiguous tooth resists tilting of the abutment tooth in the direction indicated by the arrow. A, rest; B, saddle.

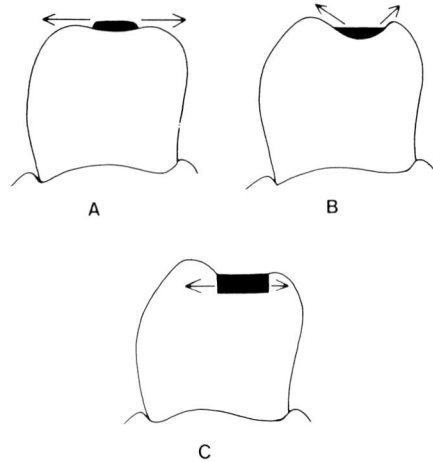

Fig. 14.9   Rest seat forms. **A**, flat form; **B**, saucer-shaped form; **C**, box form.

resisted by the contiguous tooth, or by another saddle where one is present (Fig. 14.8).

In certain circumstances, it may be possible to extend a rest to cover the whole occlusal surface of a posterior tooth. Such a development is referred to as an onlay. Optimal load transfer along the long axis of the tooth will so be obtained. Use of onlays is, however, only feasible where there is a need for the appliance to provide an increase in vertical dimension, either on isolated teeth or over the whole dentition. If used in other circumstances, onlays would produce an unacceptable decrease or even obliteration of the freeway space. In addition, onlays should only be used where the patient is prepared to follow a very strict regime of oral hygiene, as full coverage on an occlusal surface produces a considerable increase in caries risk.

Function 3. A rest can serve as a means of transferring horizontal (mainly lateral) loads from a denture saddle to a standing tooth.

The extent to which such a transfer of load arises will depend upon the form of the rest seat in which the rest is fitted. Where the rest is placed on a flat surface, only minor resistance to horizontal movement will arise from friction. Use, instead, of a saucer-shaped form of rest seat will produce moderate load transfer, whilst maximum load transfer will arise if a box form of a rest seat is used (Fig. 14.9).

Varying the form of the rest seat thus provides a means of controlling the degree to which horizontal (mainly lateral) loads can be transferred from a denture saddle to a rested tooth.

Function 4. Where a rest is placed on a surface of an abutment tooth adjacent to a saddle, and rest and saddle are in continuity, the space between the saddle and the abutment tooth will be covered. This lessens the risk of food packing into the space, with corresponding reduction in the risk of plaque retention and gingival irritation.

A similar benefit can arise where adjacent rests are joined to create a bridge spanning an interdental space (Fig. 14.10).

Interdental spaces of 2–3 mm are not uncommon. They are too small to allow placement of a saddle carrying an artificial tooth and yet, if left unrestored, can be a source of irritation to the patient as a consequence of food packing.

Function 5. By appropriate shaping, a rest may serve to improve the occlusion with the opposing dentition (Fig. 14.11).

This need particularly arises where tilting of teeth has occurred, and is seen most commonly in the relationship of isolated third molars.

Function 6. A rest may act as an indirect retainer (see p. 119).

Function 7. A rest may provide reciprocation for a retentive clasp arm (see p. 115). This is seen most

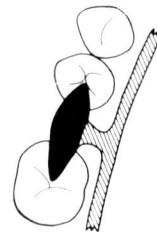

Fig. 14.10   Adjacent rests on 37 and 35 joined to bridge the interdental space.

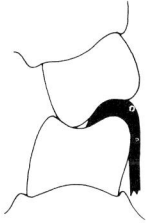

Fig. 14.11 Occlusal rest on a lower molar shaped to improve the occlusion with the opposing upper molar.

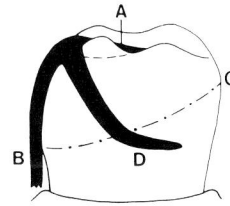

Fig. 14.12 Lateral view of a clasp unit on a lower molar. A, rest; B, attachment tag; C, survey line; D, retentive portion of clasp arm positioned in undercut.

commonly where a cingulum rest on a canine acts as reciprocation for a gingivally approaching retentive clasp arm placed on the labial surface of the tooth.

Function 8. A rest may serve to prevent supraeruption of the tooth on which it is placed, where no opposing tooth is present to perform this function.

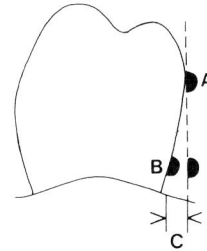

Fig. 14.13 Anterior view of a retentive clasp arm on a lower premolar. A, position of the arm at the survey line; B, position of the arm with the denture in the fully fitted position; C, Extent of flexure of the arm necessary for it to pass over the survey line.

DIRECT RETAINERS

Direct retainers are those elements of a removable partial denture which serve to provide resistance to bodily translation of the denture away from the supportive tissues, when it is subject to the action of gravity or functional forces.

They may be classified as follows:

1. Elements utilised in single-unit dentures;
   a. Clasp units
   b. Precision attachments
2. Elements utilised in sectional dentures:
   a. Hinged flanges
   b. Two-part structures.

Clasp units

Introduction

In a clasp unit, retention is obtained by positioning a flexible metal arm, arising from a suitable portion of a partial denture (e.g. a rest), so that at least part of the arm lies in an undercut zone on a natural tooth (Fig. 14.12).

When a force arises which causes displacement of the denture, the portion of the arm below the survey line has to flex outwards. This results in the

arm applying inward pressure to the tooth, leading to the development of frictional resistance between the arm and the tooth which hinders further displacement. The retaining force will progressively increase as displacement occurs, up to the point where the arm leaves the undercut zone (Fig. 14.13).

Classification of clasp arms

Clasp arms can be divided into two main classes:

1. Those which approach the undercut from the occlusal (or incisal) surface of a tooth. These are termed occlusally approaching or suprabulge clasps (Fig. 14.12).
2. Those which approach the undercut from the gingival aspect of a tooth. These are termed gingivally approaching or infrabulge clasps (Fig. 14.14).

Subclassification of clasps is usually based on the development of a link between the form of the survey line on a tooth and the correspondingly appropriate form of clasp. There are two such systems which are commonly used, the Ney system and the Blatterfein system.

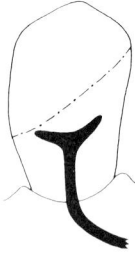

Fig. 14.14 A gingivally approaching or infrabulge clasp arm.

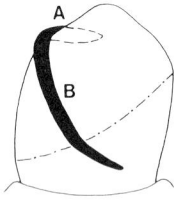

Fig. 14.15 Ney class I survey line and clasp. A, rest; B, clasp arm.

The Ney system. Three basic survey lines are described, along with an appropriate clasp form for each one.

The class I survey line runs diagonally across the tooth surface, its situation relative to the intended rest position being shown in Fig. 14.15.

For this survey line the use of a cast occlusally approaching arm is suggested, the terminal third of the arm entering the undercut.

The class II survey line also runs diagonally across the tooth surface, but as a mirror image of the class I line. Here, the use of a gingivally approaching clasp arm is suggested (Fig. 14.16).

The class III survey line is parallel to the occlusal surface and lies just below it. For this survey line,

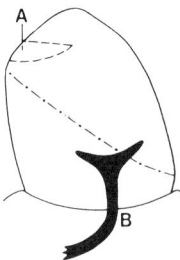

Fig. 14.16 Ney class II survey line and clasp. A, rest; B, clasp arm.

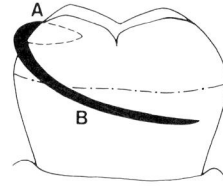

Fig. 14.17 A Ney class III survey line and clasp. A, rest; B, clasp arm.

the use of a wrought, occlusally approaching arm is suggested, with the terminal two-thirds of the arm entering the undercut (Fig. 14.17).

Variants of the Ney class I type of clasp are also described, these being termed back-action, reverse back-action and ring clasps. Back-action and reverse back-action clasps are described for use on premolar and anterior abutment teeth, especially in association with a free-end saddle. They are indicated where the tooth concerned is tilted such that a high survey line is present on one side of the tooth, and a low survey line on the other side (Fig. 14.18). The survey line on side A is too low to allow placement of a retentive clasp arm on that surface without encroaching on the gingival margin. The survey line on side B is too high to allow engagement of the undercut by a short arm placed only on that surface.

Such a condition can best be met by using an arm that extends around three surfaces of the tooth (e.g. lingual, distal and buccal), the attachment to the denture arising from the end of the arm. Where the attachment is placed lingually, the unit is referred to as a back-action clasp (Fig. 14.19). Where, alternatively, the attachment is placed buccally, the unit is referred to as a reverse back-action clasp (Fig. 14.20).

The third variant of the Ney class I clasp, the ring clasp, is described for use on upper or lower

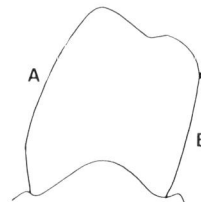

Fig. 14.18 Survey lines on a tilted premolar. The survey line is low on side A and high on side B.

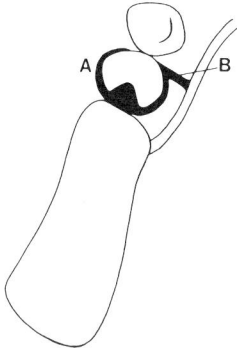

Fig. 14.19 Ney back-action clasp. A, retentive portion of the clasp arm; B, lingual attachment of the clasp arm.

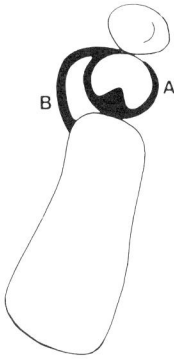

Fig. 14.20 Ney reverse back-action clasp. A, retentive portion of the clasp arm; B, buccal attachment of the clasp arm.

molars which are standing alone, no saddle being required posterior to the tooth. Like the back-action and reverse back-action clasps, it is used where the survey line is high on one side of the tooth (normally, buccally for an upper molar and lingually for a lower molar), and is low on the other side.

It has two occlusal rests, embraces three surfaces of the tooth, and is attached to the denture at the

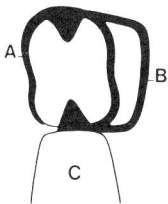

Fig. 14.21 Ney ring clasp. A, retentive portion of the clasp arm; B, optional strengthening element; C, saddle.

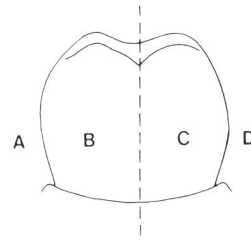

Fig. 14.22 Reference zones used in the Blatterfein system. A, saddle; B, near zone; C, far zone; D, contiguous tooth.

mesial rest. An optional strengthening element may be added, joining the mesial and distal rests on the side of the tooth having the low survey line (Fig. 14.21).

The Blatterfein system. In the Blatterfein system, four types of survey lines are described, along with an indication of suitable clasps for use with each type.

The position of each type of survey line is described in relation to two zones, developed by bisecting the tooth along its long axis. The half of the tooth adjacent to the saddle is termed the near zone, and that adjacent to the contiguous tooth is termed the far zone (Fig. 14.22). The four types of survey lines which are described are as follows:

1. The typical or medium survey line. This extends from the midpoint between the occlusal surface and the gingival margin in the near zone, to a point two-thirds of the distance from the occlusal surface to the gingival margin in the far zone (Fig. 14.23).

Clasps suggested for use where such a survey line is present include occlusally approaching and gingivally approaching arms of the Ney class I and class II types.

2. The atypical A or diagonal survey line. This runs diagonally across the tooth surface from a high

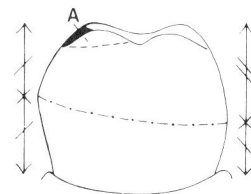

Fig. 14.23 Blatterfein typical or medium survey line. A, rest.

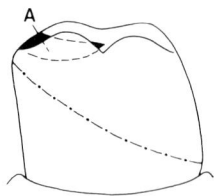

Fig. 14.24 Blatterfein atypical A or diagonal survey line. A, rest.

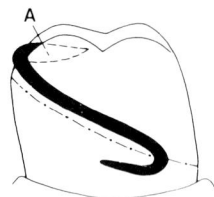

Fig. 14.25 Recurved form of cast occlusally approaching clasp arm used in association with a Blatterfein diagonal survey line. A, rest.

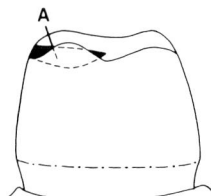

Fig. 14.27 Blatterfein atypical C or low survey line. A, rest.

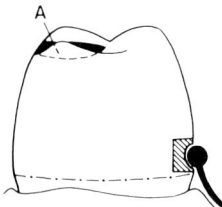

Fig. 14.28 Developing direct retention by the use of a gingivally approaching clasp arm and a class V gold inlay. A, rest.

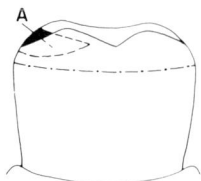

Fig. 14.26 Blatterfein atypical B or high survey line. A, rest.

position in the near zone to a low position in the far zone (Fig. 14.24).

If it is desired to use a cast occlusally approaching arm where such a survey line is present, the arm needs to be of a recurved form to enable the undercut to be engaged at a suitable level (Fig. 14.25).

Gingivally approaching arms may also be used.

3. Atypical B or high survey line. This line is parallel to the occlusal surface and lies close to it (Fig. 14.26). Wrought, occlusally approaching arms of the Ney class III type may be used where this survey line is present. Alternatively, if accompanied by a low survey line on the opposite side of the tooth, clasps of the Ney back-action, reverse back-action or ring type can be used as appropriate.

4. Atypical C or low survey line. Here, the survey line is parallel with the occlusal surface, but lies just above the level of the gingival margin (Fig. 14.27).

This type of survey line contraindicates the placement of a retentive clasp arm on the tooth surface concerned, as the arm would need to be placed too close to the gingival margin for safe application. Where all the usable surfaces of a tooth present survey lines of this type, it is necessary to seek alternative means of obtaining retention.

These methods include:

a. Placement of a crown on the tooth, to artificially develop undercuts.

b. Placement of a class V gold inlay. A dimple is cut in the inlay, and a ball head on a gingivally approaching arm positioned to engage the dimple (Fig. 14.28).

c. An extended arm clasp may be used, where the contiguous tooth offers favourable conditions for retention (Fig. 14.29).

d. Undercut may be developed by adjusting the contour of the tooth by grinding. Caution is essential in applying this procedure as, if the enamel cap of the tooth is penetrated, a considerable increase in caries risk will arise. A simpler, alternative method of developing undercut is to change the contour of the tooth by positive addition to its surface. This can be achieved using acid etch composites, a

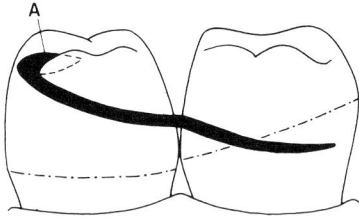

Fig. 14.29 Developing direct retention by the use of an extended arm clasp engaging undercut on the contiguous tooth. A, rest.

procedure which is currently under evaluation. Initial results have been promising, although the life expectancy of the additions is still in doubt.

The functions and design features of clasp units

To achieve optimal efficiency, a clasp unit must be designed to take account of its intended function or functions, which are described below.

Support. In all cases where a clasp arm is to be placed on a tooth, some form of rest should be placed on the tooth to locate correctly the clasp arm in its designated position.

Retention. As previously noted, retention is obtained by the placement of a flexible element of a clasp arm into undercut. This must be done in such a manner that three criteria will be satisfied:

1. Sufficient undercut must be engaged to ensure that the required degree of retention is obtained.

2. The force which arises when the clasp arm flexes during insertion and withdrawal of the denture must be within the level of tolerance of the periodontal attachment of the clasped tooth, otherwise damage to the attachment will occur.

3. The force which arises when the clasp arm flexes during insertion and withdrawal of the denture must also be less than that which would cause permanent deformation of the arm to occur.

Satisfying these criteria requires the engagement of an undercut appropriate to the length, cross-section, form and material of construction of the arm. Measurement of undercuts should always be made by use of appropriate undercut gauges in the cast surveyor. As an approximate guide only, cast occlusally approaching clasps in cobalt–chromium alloy should engage only 0.25 mm undercut. Cast

occlusally approaching clasps in gold alloy may engage 0.50 mm undercut as may wrought occlusally approaching clasps in stainless steel or cast gingivally approaching clasps in cobalt–chromium alloy. Wrought occlusally approaching clasps in gold alloy may engage 0.75 mm undercut if of adequate length (on a molar, for example), and this undercut may also be engaged by gingivally approaching clasps in gold alloy.

Bracing. Bracing is the provision of resistance to lateral displacement of the denture, and is a function performed jointly by the rest and by the clasp arms in a clasp unit. All clasp arms will provide some degree of bracing. For an occlusally approaching arm, bracing will be at a maximum at the rigid portion close to the origin, and will decrease along the length of the arm to the free end. The bracing provided by a gingivally approaching clasp arm will normally be much less than that of an occlusally approaching clasp arm, since only the flexible, terminal portion of the former lies on the tooth. The required level of bracing in a clasp unit may be achieved by the action of the rest, plus that arising from one or more arms placed for retention, where these are of the occlusally approaching type. Where a gingivally approaching clasp arm is being used for retention, it is usually necessary to place an occlusally approaching arm on another surface of the tooth to achieve an adequate level of bracing in the unit. Such an arm will lie above the survey line.

Both bracing and retention should be opposed across the arch to obtain optimal value — where retention or bracing is obtained on the buccal surface of the teeth on one side of the arch, it must also be obtained on the buccal surface of the teeth on the other side of the arch. Alternatively, lingual or palatal retention or bracing on one side should be accompanied by lingual or palatal retention or bracing on the other side.

Reciprocation. In all cases where a retentive clasp arm is positioned on one surface of a tooth, then some suitable element must be provided on the opposite surface to act as a reciprocating balance. This is necessary since if the flexible retentive arm was accidentally bent by the patient (e.g. when cleaning the denture), the arm could apply a constant force to the tooth when the denture was in position. Such a force could give rise to tooth movement or damage the periodontal attachment of the tooth, and these are not intended functions of a partial denture. The provision of a reciprocating element provides opposition to the potential displacing force, and avoids the risk of tooth movement or other damage occurring.

Reciprocation may be provided by another retentive clasp arm, or by a bracing arm. In the case of anterior teeth, a rest may be used, and for both anterior and posterior teeth, where a connector lies on a tooth surface, it may also function as a reciprocator.

Biological acceptability. It is important that the clasp unit be designed on biologically sound principles, if it is to function satisfactorily. As previously noted, it must avoid excessive force application to the tooth by ensuring that form and undercut engagement are correctly linked. It must cover the minimum tooth substance compatible with other requirements, so as to reduce the risk of food stagnation to a minimum. The arm should be kept free of the gingival margin of the tooth, by at least 2 mm, to minimise the risk of it causing gingival trauma. In all cases where an arm needs to cross the gingival margin (in the gingivally approaching type), the arm should be relieved from direct contact with the gingival tissues.

Attachment to denture. Adequate attachment must be provided between the clasp unit and the rest of the denture. This is normally achieved by means of a tag, which is either firmly embedded in the polymeric area of a saddle, or is attached by soldering, welding, or unit cast construction to a metal framework, where one is being used.

Mechanical acceptability. The dimensions of the elements making up a clasp unit must be adequate to achieve a structure which will be resistant to permanent deformation and fracture. Only materials possessing adequate mechanical properties should be used, and their handling should be such that optimal properties will be achieved. This will include the application of appropriate heat-treatment procedures where gold alloys are used. Where fabrication is by casting, porosity must be avoided. Where fabrication is by wrought work, care should be taken not to leave plier marks or other imperfections on the metalwork, as these can act as stress-concentrators and increase the risk of fracture occurring.

Precision attachments

Introduction

Precision attachments consist of two units, one being attached to an abutment tooth, the other being attached to the denture saddle. When the two units are fitted together, they provide direct retention by means of a combination of friction and spring action.

Relative to the use of clasp units as tooth-bearing direct retainers, precision attachments may be said to offer certain advantages:

1. They can provide excellent transfer of vertical and horizontal loads from the denture saddles to the abutment teeth on which they are placed
2. Good aesthetics are obtainable, with no clasp arms visible, for instance.
3. They may be more hygienic, with minimal external components present to trap food and accumulate plaque.
4. They are generally well tolerated by patients, as their form normally avoids irritation of the tongue, lip or cheeks.
5. Unlike the position with clasp units, use is not dictated by the presence or absence of undercuts on a tooth.

Disadvantages which may arise from the use of precision attachments include the following:

1. Their application is usually much more time-consuming in both the clinical and laboratory areas. In addition, the intrinsic cost of many of the attachments is high. Thus, their use may need to be limited by economic considerations.
2. Placement of an attachment on an abutment tooth may necessitate the removal of a considerable amount of sound tooth substance.
3. Special problems can arise where a precision attachment is to be used to provide retention of a free-end saddle. If an attachment is used which provides a rigid link between the saddle and the abutment tooth, then destructive overload of the periodontal attachment of the abutment tooth can occur. Instead, it is usually recommended that an attachment of a more complex (and hence expensive) type should be used, which provides some form of flexible link between the saddle and the abutment tooth, as well as providing direct reten-

tion. Attachments of this type are referred to as stress-broken attachments. Doubt has been expressed about their ability to maintain their initial flexibility over a long period of wear.

Classification and form

A primary classification of precision attachments may be made on the basis of the site of attachment to the abutment tooth:

Class 1 — coronal attachments
Class 2 — root face attachments.

For class 1, subclassification may be made on the basis of the site at which retention is achieved:

Class 1A — extracoronal attachments
Class 1B — intracoronal attachments.

For class 2, subclassification may be made on the form of the attachment:

Class 2A –· stud type
Class 2B — bar type.

It is usual for precision attachments to be purchased in a prefabricated form. A wide range of attachments is available within each of the above classes. In this text, it is only possible to provide examples of the attachments in each class. A more detailed consideration will be found in specialist texts.

Class 1A — extracoronal attachments. Here, the retentive element lies external to the crown of the abutment tooth. An example is provided by the Roach ball attachment (Fig. 14.30).

A rod, arising from an inlay set in the abutment tooth, carries a ball at its free end. A sleeve is set into the associated end of the saddle. As the denture is inserted, the sleeve slides over the ball and develops frictional grip retention.

Class 1B — intracoronal attachments. These are generally much more complicated in form than the extra-coronal attachments. The female unit of the attachment is set within an abutment inlay, or crown, and presents a dovetailed slot. The male unit presents a correspondingly shaped projection, and is attached to the denture saddle. When the two units slide into each other they provide frictional grip retention, which may be augmented in some

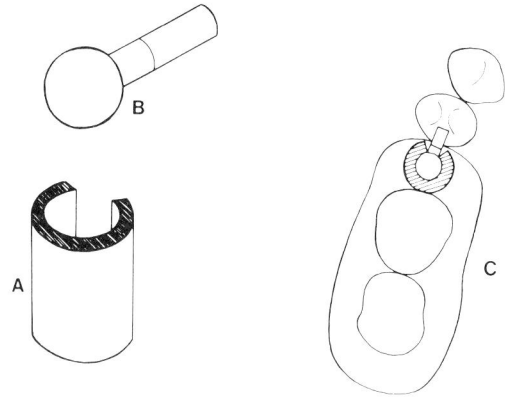

Fig. 14.30 The Roach ball extracoronal attachment. **A**, sleeve set in the saddle; **B**, Rod set in an inlay; **C**, Plan view of the attachment.

types by a spring action. An attachment of this type is illustrated in Figure 2.8C.

A large restoration, such as a three-quarter crown, is required to provide adequate retention of the restoration carrying the female unit. When, as is usual, a number of such units are to be used for denture retention, they need to be accurately paralleled by use of a surveyor technique at the stage of placement within the wax patterns of the abutment retainers.

Class 2A — stud-type attachments. As a preliminary to the use of such attachments, root treatment of the abutment tooth is carried out and the crown is cut off near to the level of the gingival margin. They are particularly indicated for use where the periodontal status of the root is adequate, but the condition of the crown is judged to be unsuitable to allow placement of a coronal attachment. A cast metal post and diaphragm are prepared for the root, the diaphragm offering retention for the base unit of the stud, either via use of soldering or by screw attachment.

As an example of the form of a stud attachment, the Dalbo is illustrated in Figure 2.8A. The male unit is attached to the root face diaphragm and carries a ball-shaped head. The female unit is placed within the denture saddle, and has a hemispherical cavity to provide frictional fit on the ball head of the male unit. Vertical slits in the female unit allow a degree of flexibility, and provide grip action as the two units are fitted together.

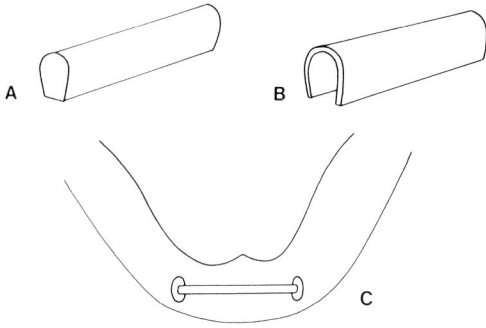

Fig. 14.31 Dolder bar attachment. **A**, Bar unit A; **B**, Bar unit B; **C**, Plan view of bar unit A attached to diaphragms on 43 and 33.

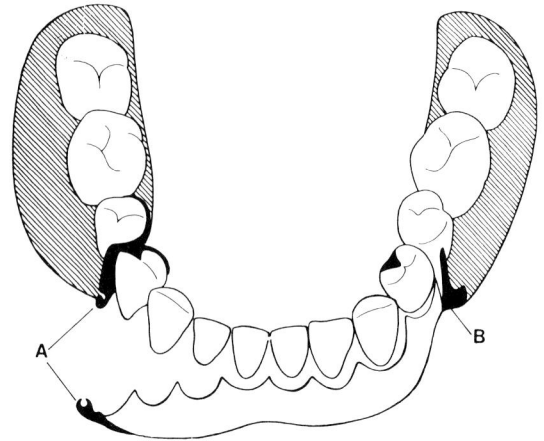

Fig. 14.32 Denture of the 'swinglock' type, showing the labial connector in the open position. A, clasp fastener; B, hinge.

Class 2B — bar-type attachments. As in the use of attachments of the class 2A type, abutment teeth are root filled and the crowns removed near to gingival level. Posts and diaphragms are again prepared.

The attachment takes the form of a bar which extends between and is attached to each of two diaphragms. An example of an attachment of this type is provided by a Dolder bar. This is most commonly used to link the root faces of two lower canines, as illustrated in Figure 14.31.

Unit A bar is pear shaped in section, 3 mm deep and 2.2 mm wide. It is fitted so that its base lies just in contact with the oral mucosa between the diaphragms to which it is attached. Unit B is carried within the denture saddle. It clips into position over unit A, the side pieces extending below the points of maximum convexity of unit A, so gaining retention.

Sectional dentures utilising hinged flanges

Retention is here obtained by using a combination of lingual (or palatal) and labial connectors, the latter being positioned to engage tissue undercuts. If such a combination of connectors was employed in single-unit denture construction, undercuts would prevent seating of the denture. By joining the labial connector to the denture by means of a hinge at one end, and by using a clasp fastener at the other end, the labial connector can be hinged outwards to allow seating of the rest of the denture, and can then be closed. Such a system is utilised in

'swinglock' dentures, an example being illustrated in Figure 14.32.

The labial connector may be made in the form of a metal bar, or may be made in acrylic resin (at least in part) and be brought as a veneer around the gingival margins of standing teeth. Such a veneer is sometimes said to serve as a periodontal splint. It also provides replacement for gingival tissues, where these have been lost by gingival recession or periodontal surgery.

It is important that the denture be properly supported by use of rests, otherwise damage to the tissues covered by the labial connector is liable to occur when the denture receives functional loading. The maintenance of scrupulous oral hygiene by the patient is also essential if tissue damage is to be avoided.

Sectional dentures utilising two-part construction

Here, retention is obtained by designing the denture in two parts, each part having a different path of insertion. When fitted together in the oral cavity and united by means of a locking device, the two parts confer mutual retention on each other.

The principle can be applied to produce small dentures whose extent is limited to a single bounded saddle and the associated abutment teeth. As an example of its use, a case involving replacement of 35 and 36 will be considered.

If a single-unit denture is to be designed to provide replacement of these teeth, it will necessitate interproximal undercuts being blocked out to develop a path of insertion.

Safety factors will also indicate a need for the denture to be extended to the other side of the arch, possibly involving teeth in the design remote from the replacement area.

As an alternative, a two-part denture can be constructed. Each part has a separate path of insertion, enabling it to engage fully the undercut on the proximal surface of the adjacent abutment tooth. A bracing spur extends from the main body of each part to contact the remote surface of the distant abutment tooth (Fig. 14.33B and C).

Fixation of the two parts is usually achieved by the use of a bolt. The sleeve of the bolt runs through the plastic-work attached to one part, and the shank engages a hole prepared in the other part. The relationship of the parts to the bolt is shown in plan view in Figure 14.33A.

The bolt shank can be turned through 90° and may then be withdrawn from the retaining hole.

The two parts of the denture can then be removed

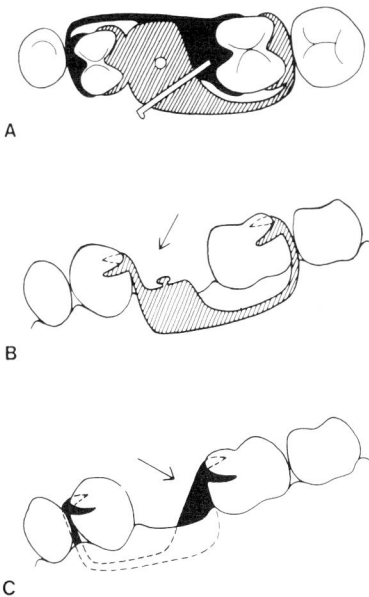

Fig. 14.33 Two-part denture providing replacement of 35 and 36. **A**, Plan view of the assembled denture showing the bolt action; **B, C**, Component parts of the denture. The arrows indicate the path of insertion of each part.

for cleaning. In the fitted position, the handle of the shank is positioned to be flat along the surface of the acrylic flange.

INDIRECT RETAINERS

Indirect retainers are those elements of a partial denture which provide resistance to the rotation of the denture about fulcrum axes. Such axes will be present in all instances where rests have been included in the design to produce a tooth-supported or tooth-and-mucosa-supported type of denture. Theoretical aspects of indirect retention in relation to partial denture design are considered in Chapter 15, (p. 135). Here, consideration will be limited to the form and position of the various types of indirect retainers that are used. They can be divided into two groups according to positioning:

Group A — those indirect retainers that are positioned on the standing teeth, and which may be used in either the upper or lower jaw. They include:

1. Rests
2. Tooth-bearing direct retainers
3. Continuous clasps
4. Cummer arms
5. Tooth-bearing connectors.

Group B — those indirect retainers that are positioned on mucous membrane. These should only be used in the upper jaw. They include:

1. Palatal arms
2. Palatal-bearing connectors.

Rests

The various types of rest (occlusal, cingulum and incisal) may all function as indirect retainers when placed on the opposite side of the fulcrum axis to that on which the displacing saddle is situated. Their form is considered in detail on pages 107–111.

An example of their application is seen in the design of a partial denture for a Kennedy class IV upper dentition, as shown in Figure 14.34.

During the mastication of sticky foods, there will be a tendency for the saddle to move away from the underlying tissues, the denture rotating about an axis joining the rests placed for saddle support. This tendency for rotation can be resisted by placing

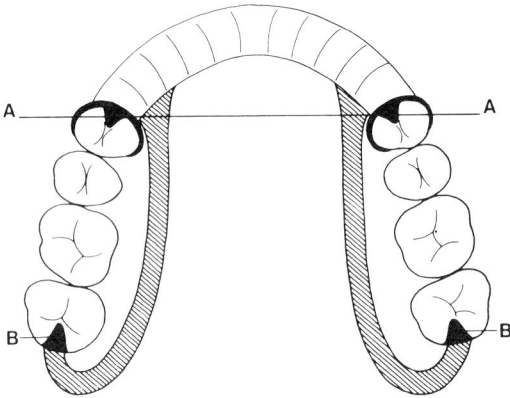

Fig. 14.34 Indirect retention for a Kennedy class IV dentition achieved by posterior placement of occlusal rests. AA, axis of rotation developed by the rests supporting the anterior saddle; B, posteriorly placed occlusal rest.

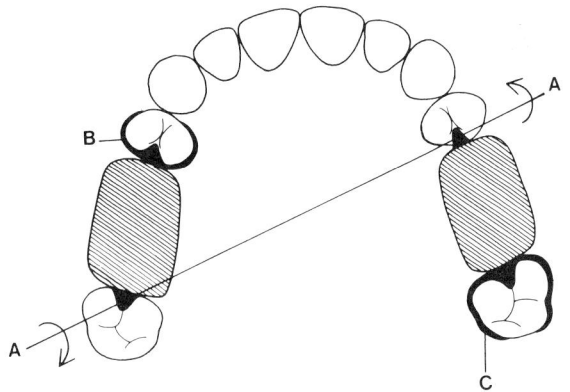

Fig. 14.35 Indirect retention for a Kennedy class III dentition achieved by tooth-bearing direct retainers. AA, axis of rotation; B, clasp unit on 14; C, clasp unit on 27.

occlusal rests bilaterally on the posterior aspects of the last standing teeth. The posterior rests are joined to the saddle by means of anteroposteriorly directed bars lying on the palate.

Tooth-bearing direct retainers

Clasp units (see p. 111) and precision attachments (see p. 116) may also function as indirect retainers. To perform this function, they are placed on the same side of the fulcrum axis as that on which the displacing saddle is situated.

This can be seen in the design of a partial denture for a Kennedy class III, modification 1 dentition replacing 16, 15, 25 and 26 (Fig. 14.35). Consider the potential axis of rotation passing through 17 and 24. During the chewing of sticky foods, the posterior end of the saddle carrying 25 and 26 may tend to rise away from the supporting tissues, the denture rotating in an anticlockwise direction about the axis. This can be resisted by the placement of a direct retainer (e.g. a clasp unit) on 27. Similarly, a clasp unit placed on 14 will resist a clockwise rotation about the same axis, which tends to occur where the anterior end of the saddle carrying 26 and 25 is subject to a displacing force, pulling it away from the underlying tissues. The indirect retainer action obtained in this way, by the placement of tooth-bearing direct retainers, should be regarded as an auxiliary feature to their main function of providing direct retention. Where a need arises in partial denture design for elements to be placed specifically to act as indirect retainers — mainly encountered in the design of partial dentures for Kennedy class I and class IV dentitions — it is rare for tooth-bearing direct retainers to be used.

The continuous clasp

Often referred to as the Beech or Kennedy continuous clasp, this consists of a continuous band of metal positioned on or above the survey lines of the lingual or palatal aspects of the anterior dentition (Fig. 14.36).

The ends of the clasp may join a major connector (e.g. a lingual bar, as illustrated in Fig. 14.36), or may extend posteriorly to terminate in the denture saddles. It is often chosen to provide indirect retention in the Kennedy class I situation. Here, the need often arises for an element to be placed forward of the axis of rotation, to provide resistance

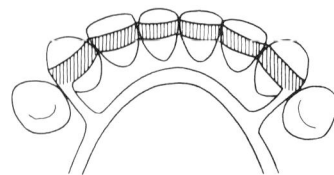

Fig. 14.36 A continuous clasp positioned on 43, 42, 41, 31, 32 and 33.

to rotatory displacement of the free-end saddles. A continuous clasp can perform this function with maximum mechanical advantage, since it extends anteriorly to the limit permitted by the arch form. Also, since it acts on the whole anterior dentition rather than on a single tooth, the risk of it producing tooth movement is minimised.

In addition to acting as an indirect retainer, a continuous clasp can provide other functions:

1. It transfers part of the vertical and horizontal loads borne by the saddle on to the covered anterior dentition. It thus lessens the load applied to the abutment teeth, with corresponding reduction in the risk of the abutment teeth sustaining periodontal damage.

2. It can act as an auxiliary connector of saddles, assisting the major connector, e.g. a lingual bar, in performing this function. This may allow the cross-sectional area of the major connector to be reduced, so aiding its tolerance by the environmental tissues.

3. Where splinting of anterior teeth is required, a continuous clasp can serve as a useful point for the origin of embrasure hooks.

Despite its functional advantages, the continuous clasp also presents a number of possible disadvantages, which must be taken into consideration before a decision is made to include it in the design of a partial denture. These are as follows:

1. It may give rise to problems of tolerance. Usually, this is associated with tongue irritation, but speech problems may also occur. Acceptance by the tongue will be aided by the use of a deep and relatively thin form, in preference to the use of a shallower and thicker form (Fig. 14.37). Upper and lower margins of the clasp should blend in to the tooth form, and not present a ledge to the tongue.

2. The occlusal relationship of the anterior teeth (deep overbite combined with shallow over-jet) may

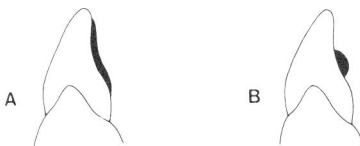

Fig. 14.38 Division of a continuous clasp to avoid the display of metal through a diastema.

be such as to provide inadequate space for placement.

3. Where the anterior teeth are lingually or palatally inclined, there may be insufficient room above the survey lines to allow placement of a continuous clasp.

4. Placement may be difficult where the teeth only present short clinical crowns.

5. Aesthetic problems arise if the teeth are spaced. However, where a single diastema is present, this problem can be overcome by division of the continuous clasp (Fig. 14.38).

6. When long, there is a risk that a continuous clasp will be distorted by the patient during the cleaning of the denture.

Cummer arms

The Cummer arm consists of a metal bar extending anteriorly from a suitable component of the denture (usually a saddle or connector), to terminate on the unprepared palatal or lingual surface of an anterior tooth. They are used bilaterally. The only teeth really suitable for their placement are periodontally sound upper canines, although they are occasionally used on lower canines. If used on other anterior teeth, they are very liable to cause tooth movement.

Like the continuous clasp, they may be chosen for use as specific indirect retainers in the design of partial dentures for Kennedy class I dentitions. An example of their application is shown in Figure 14.39.

They are less effective than the continuous clasp as an indirect retainer, since they are positioned closer to the axis of rotation. They share with the continuous clasp the disadvantage of liability to distortion during cleaning of the denture. Their use is only indicated where long free-end saddles are present, and a continuous clasp cannot be used because of the existence of a close incisor relationship.

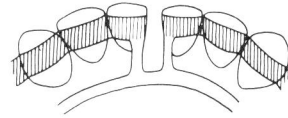

Fig. 14.37 Shaping a continuous clasp to aid acceptance by the tongue. **A**, preferred form; **B**, deprecated form.

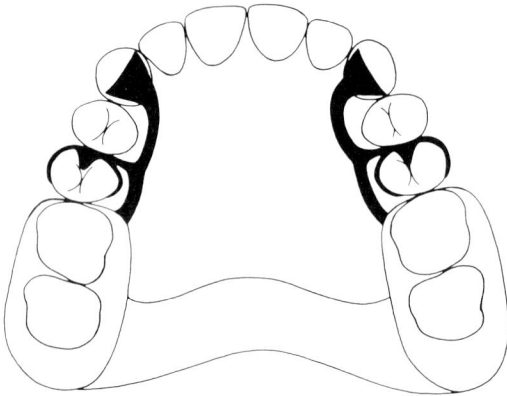

Fig. 14.39   Indirect retention for a Kennedy class I dentition achieved by the use of Cummer arms on 13 and 23.

Tooth-bearing connectors

Two of the tooth-bearing connectors which are used in the design of lower partial dentures offer the advantage of providing auxiliary indirect retention, where this is required. They are:

1. The lingual plate
2. The modified continuous clasp.

The form and positioning of these connectors is considered on pages 127 and 128.

Their auxiliary indirect retainer action can be utilised with benefit when designing lower partial dentures for the Kennedy class I dentition. They will share the effectiveness of indirect retainer action of the continuous clasp, since like that clasp they extend as far anterior of the axis of rotation as the arch form permits.

Palatal arms

The palatal arm consists of an extension from a saddle or palatal connector, usually made in metal, which extends anteriorly forward of the fulcrum axis to lie on the anterior part of the hard palate. They may be used unilaterally or bilaterally to provide indirect retention for free-end saddles. An example of their use is shown in Figure 14.40. As the arms extend on to the rugae they often give rise to irritation of the tongue, and may also interfere with phonetics.

Palatal-bearing connectors

Certain of the palatal-bearing connectors used in the design of upper partial dentures can provide the auxiliary function of indirect retention. These are:

1. The anterior palatal bar. This can be used to provide indirect retention where free-end saddles are present.
2. The posterior palatal bar. This can be used to provide indirect retention where a single anterior saddle is present (Kennedy class IV dentition).

The form and positioning of palatal bars is considered on pages 123 and 124.

The palatal plate connector (see p. 125) can also be used to provide indirect retention by extending it to lie either anterior to the axis of rotation (for free-end saddles), or posterior to the axis of rotation (for a single anterior saddle) — see Figure 14.41.

CONNECTORS

Connectors are those elements of a partial denture which are used to unite other components to form a unit appliance.

They are classified as minor or major connectors according to their length or area of tissue covered. Minor connectors are considered in Chapter 15 (p. 139). In this section, consideration will be limited to major connectors, whose main role is that of joining saddles. They are always designed to be rigid in nature.

They can be divided into two main groups on the basis of the jaw in which they are to be used, and

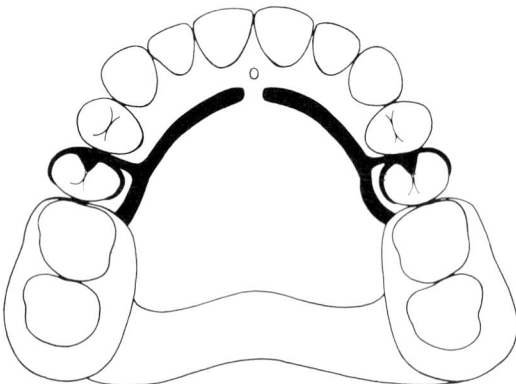

Fig. 14.40   Indirect retention for a Kennedy class I dentition achieved by the use of palatal arms.

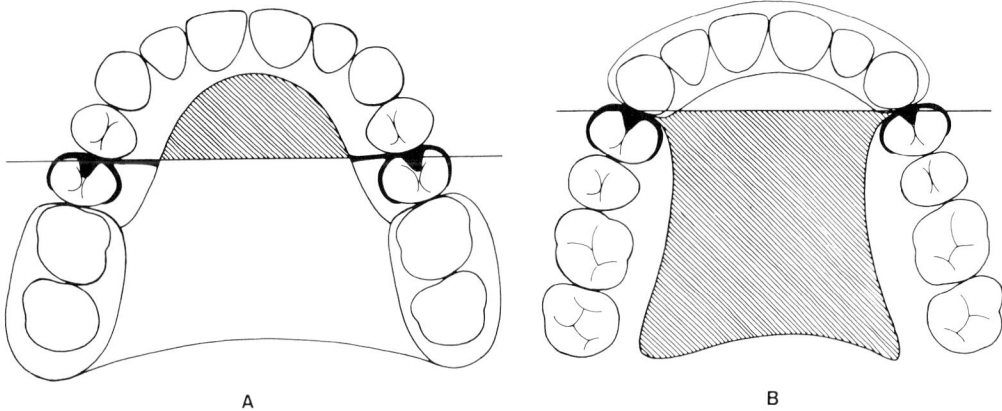

Fig. 14.41 Indirect retention achieved by the use of palatal plate extensions. **A** Extension of the palatal plate anterior to the axis of rotation for a Kennedy class I dentition. **B** Extension of the palatal plate posterior to the axis of rotation for a Kennedy class IV dentition.

then subdivided on the basis of their form and positioning:

Group A — major connectors used in a maxillary denture:

1. Posterior palatal bar
2. Middle palatal bar
3. Anterior palatal bar
4. Palatal plate.

Group B — major connectors used in a mandibular denture:

1. Lingual bar
2. Lingual plate
3. Labial or buccal bar
4. Modified continuous clasp.

The posterior palatal bar

This bar lies on the posterior part of the hard palate. It arises from saddles or direct retainer units on each side of the arch, and extends posteriorly in a smooth curve to terminate at the vibrating line. An example is shown in Figure 14.42.

The anteroposterior dimension of the bar will depend upon the number of teeth being replaced by the denture, and on the physical properties of the alloy used for constructing the bar, the aim being always to achieve rigid connection. It will rarely exceed 1 cm.

Anterior and posterior margins of the bar should

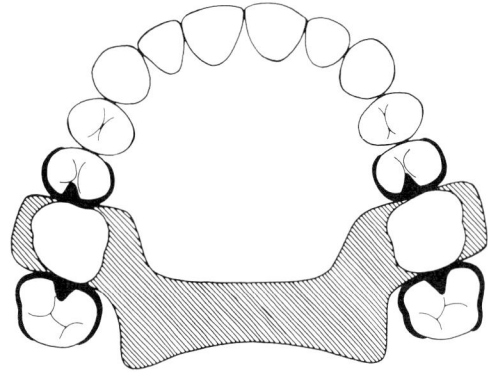

Fig. 14.42 A posterior palatal bar used to connect saddles replacing 16 and 26.

be thinned down to taper into the palate, without developing cutting edges. This will help to avoid irritation of the tongue. The posterior margin, which lies at the vibrating line, should be developed to provide a post-dam as utilised in complete dentures. Other margins of the bar should be provided with a minor dam line, approximately 0.5 mm deep, to aid peripheral seal and reduce the risk of food passing to the fitting surface aspect of the bar.

The posterior palatal bar has the merit of being positioned in an area of the palate where tongue activity is at a minimum. For that reason, it is usually well tolerated by patients. Tolerance will also be aided by use of a thickness not exceeding 1 mm. Increased rigidity, where necessary, should be gained by increasing the anteroposterior dimension rather than by increasing the thickness.

Despite the merit of tolerance provided by the position of a posterior palatal bar, the latter feature can also lead to a problem. This arises from the fact that the bar is positioned on a relatively compressible tissue base. When load is applied to the saddles of the partial denture, it may be found that anteroposterior rocking of the appliance occurs as a consequence of depression of the posterior palatal bar into the underlying tissues. This movement of the bar will be increased if the bar is not a perfect fit on the tissues in its original fitted position. Such lack of fit may occur as a consequence of casting shrinkage, and will be accentuated if the bar is long.

Since the posterior palatal bar terminates at the vibrating line, its position enables it to function as an indirect retainer, resisting rotation of the denture originating from anterior saddles. Its effectiveness in performing this function must, however, be questioned in view of the displaceable nature of the palatal tissues on which it is placed.

The posterior palatal bar may also serve as a means of transferring part of the vertical and horizontal load borne by the denture to the palatal tissues. It may thus be said to have auxiliary supporting and bracing functions. Again, these will be limited in value by the displaceable nature of the covered tissues.

The middle palatal bar

This bar lies on the central portion of the hard palate. The anterior border lies just posterior to the commencement of the rugae on the hard palate. Its path across the palate between saddles or direct retainer units on each side of the arch is more direct than that of a posterior palatal bar. The anteroposterior dimension of the middle palatal bar is usually a little greater than that of a posterior palatal bar. Its form is illustrated in Figure 14.43.

As with the posterior palatal bar, anterior and posterior borders of the middle palatal bar should be thinned to blend in with the palatal tissues. Its situation does not allow the development of a full post-dam, and a minor dam line, approximately 0.5 mm deep, is provided along both the anterior and posterior margins to aid the development of peripheral seal.

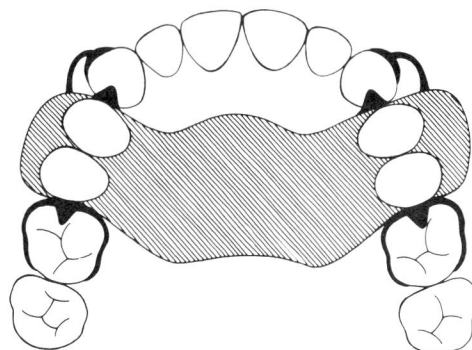

Fig. 14.43 A middle palatal bar used to connect saddles replacing 15, 14, 24 and 25.

Its more direct course across the palate relative to that of a posterior palatal bar results in less liability for casting shrinkage, and hence a better fit is seen in most instances. Also, the palatal tissues underlying the middle palatal bar are usually of a less displaceable character than those under a posterior palatal bar. The problem of anteroposterior rock in function that arises in a posterior palatal bar is thus rarely encountered with a middle palatal bar. The nature of the foundation tissues also enables the middle palatal bar to perform effectively auxiliary supporting and bracing functions. Its more anterior placement in the palate does, though, result in it being a less effective indirect retainer for anterior saddles than the posterior palatal bar, and it is also more likely to give rise to tongue irritation. Despite this, the middle palatal bar is generally well tolerated.

The anterior palatal bar

This bar lies in the anterior, rugal area of the hard palate. In crossing the palate to link saddles or direct retainer units, it should be positioned in the valleys between rugal elevations as far as possible. This is necessary since it lies in an area of high tongue activity and, if placed upon rugal elevations, it may give rise to tongue irritation and phonetic disruption. The need to position it between rugal elevations often necessitates it following a more tortuous path across the palate than that seen with middle or posterior palatal bars. The bar should be as shallow as mechanical considerations will permit.

It is rarely used as a sole connector, normally being used in association with the posterior palatal bar. In view of the problems which may arise from its placement in an area of high tongue activity, it should only be used where special indications apply, which include the following:

1. Where it is needed to develop a connector system of adequate rigidity. Where only one or two short saddles are present and cobalt–chromium alloy is to be used in fabrication of the connector, a posterior palatal bar used alone will often provide adequate rigidity. Where long saddles, or a greater number of saddles than two is present, the use of an extra connector may be required to achieve adequate rigidity. The 'ring' form of connection developed by using a combination of anterior and posterior palatal bars results in a considerable increase in the rigidity of the structure, relative to that obtainable from a single connector. Such a double-connector system will nearly always prove to be necessary where gold alloy is used in construction of the connectors.

2. Where it is needed to act as an indirect retainer for posterior saddles. This need may arise where the occlusal relationship of the anterior teeth prevents use of a continuous clasp or Cummer arms.

3. Where it is needed to provide a convenient point of attachment for an anterior saddle, as illustrated in Figure 14.44.

The palatal plate

Although no strict dividing line exists between the terms 'bar' and 'plate' as applied to palatal connectors, the term 'plate' is usually reserved for those cases where the connector covers an appreciable area of hard palate. Often, the area of coverage would be similar to that which would occur in a hypothetical design involving simultaneous use of all three palatal bar connectors.

The use of a palatal plate is illustrated in Figure 14.45.

Relative to the use of bar connectors, the plate connector has the biological disadvantage of covering a greater area of the hard palate. Where the palatal tissues are covered, they lack the natural stimulus provided by the tongue and salivary flow, with risk of the development of an adverse tissue reaction. Against this must be weighed the advantages arising from increased palatal coverage:

1. An increased proportion of the vertical and horizontal loads which are applied to the denture can be borne by the palate. Where tooth-supported or tooth-and-mucosa-supported designs are being used, such load transfer to the palate can reduce the risk of overloading of the abutment teeth occurring. It also introduces the possibility of using totally mucosa-supported designs in the maxillary denture.

2. It may be possible to achieve adequate rigidity in the connector system using a polymeric denture base material. In distinction, palatal bars are always made in metal. Use of a polymeric denture base

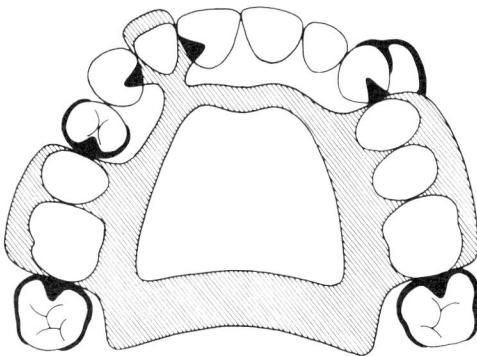

Fig. 14.44 Anterior and posterior palatal bars used to form a 'ring' connector system for a denture replacing 16, 15, 12, 24, 25 and 26.

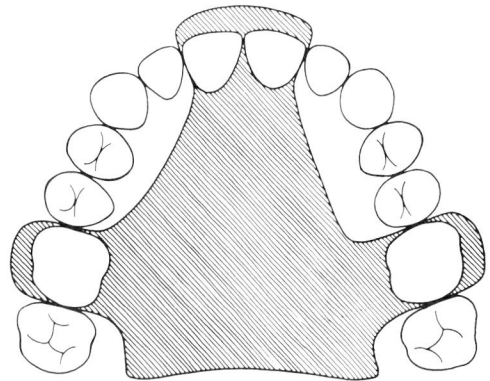

Fig. 14.45 A palatal plate connector used in a mucosa-supported denture replacing 16, 11, 21 and 26.

material for construction of the connector offers advantages in terms of weight, colour and cost.

Wherever possible, a palatal plate should extend posteriorly to the vibrating line and a post-dam should be developed. Along other palatal margins, a shallow dam should be developed, approximately 0.5 mm deep, to aid the development of peripheral seal. The health of the palatal gingival tissues will benefit from the use of designs which avoid coverage of the gingival tissues, as seen in the 'Every' or 'spoon' designs. Comfort will be aided by making the plate as thin as is compatible with achieving the required rigidity. This favours the use of a metal in the construction of a palatal plate connector.

The lingual bar

The lingual bar connects saddles or retainer units on each side of the lower arch, being positioned in close proximity to the lingual alveolar tissues. The bar is usually oval in cross-section, approximately 3 mm deep and 1.5 mm thick, although occasionally a bar of a half pear-shaped section is used.

The bar should be positioned so that its upper border is at least 2 mm below the gingival margins of the standing teeth, and its lower border is not less than 2 mm above the floor of the mouth, as illustrated in Figure 14.46.

Where a lingual bar is to be used, a space of at least 7 mm must thus be present between the gingival margins of the standing teeth and the floor of the mouth. Where the available space is less than 7 mm, the use of a lingual bar is contraindicated and an alternative type of connector must be selected. Where the available space exceeds 7 mm, it is advisable for the bar to be placed as low as

possible, as this lessens the risk of the bar causing irritation to the tongue.

A lingual bar may be wrought using stainless steel or gold alloy, or may be cast in cobalt–chromium alloy or gold alloy. The bar should be relieved from contact with the underlying tissues by a small gap. This allows for minor movements of the bar to occur during the functioning of the denture without causing trauma to the underlying tissues. Except for the provision of this relief, the bar should be positioned to follow closely the contours of the lingual alveolus. There should be no unplanned space between the upper portion of the bar and the alveolar tissues, as a space here would permit food packing. Similarly, there must be no unplanned space between the lower portion of the bar and the alveolar tissues, or the tip of the tongue may enter this space and be irritated. Tongue thrusting into a lower space could also cause displacement of the denture.

One contraindication to the use of a lingual bar has already been noted, that of lack of the necessary space between the gingival margins of the standing teeth and the floor of the mouth. Another arises where retroclination of the lower dentition is present. Like all rigid connectors, a lingual bar must not enter an undercut. Retroclination of the anterior dentition would necessitate the bar being placed away from the alveolar tissues to achieve a free path of insertion (Fig. 14.47), and a lingual bar in this position would almost certainly cause tongue irritation.

Likewise, a grossly undercut lingual alveolus contraindicates use of a lingual bar.

On biological grounds, the lingual bar can be considered to be the most satisfactory of the available types of lower connectors. It avoids contact

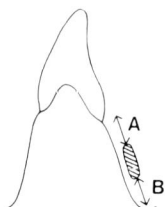

Fig. 14.46 Sagittal section in the lower incisor region illustrating the form and position of a lingual bar. A and B should be equal to or exceed 2 mm.

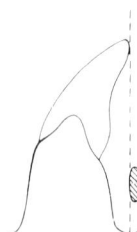

Fig. 14.47 Sagittal section in the lower incisor region illustrating the necessary position of a lingual bar when the incisors are retroclined.

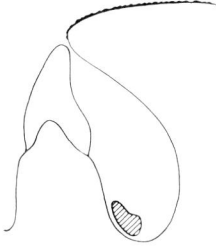

Fig. 14.48 Sagittal section in the lower incisor region illustrating the form and position of a sublingual bar.

with the standing teeth and their gingival tissues and, when correctly positioned, should not give rise to tissue trauma. It does, however, have one major disadvantage, and this is a liability of causing irritation to the tongue. Patients have likened their experience when wearing a denture bearing a lingual bar to that of a horse with a bit in its mouth!

In an attempt to lessen tongue irritation, proposals have been made that a sublingual positioning should be adopted for the bar. In this case, it is usual to use a bar of the half pear-shaped form, the larger element of the bar being positioned at the base and under the tongue, as illustrated in Figure 14.48. Care must be taken to ensure that the base of the bar is kept above the functional level of the floor of the mouth, otherwise severe irritation of the tissues could arise.

The lingual plate

The lingual plate joins saddles or direct retainer units on each side of the lower arch, being positioned in contact with both the lingual surfaces of the anterior teeth and the lingual aspect of the alveolar processes (Fig. 14.49). In the region where it crosses the gingival margins of the standing teeth,

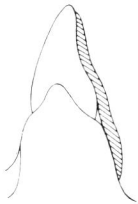

Fig. 14.49 Sagittal section in the lower incisor region illustrating the form and position of a lingual plate.

it should be relieved from direct contact with the tissues by, for example, the placement of foil on the master cast.

The upper border of the plate must be above the survey lines and should extend to a level approximately 2 mm below the incisal edges of the standing teeth, except where full coverage is required for the development of incisal rests or embrasure hooks. The lower margin of the plate should leave a gap of at least 2 mm above the functional level of the floor of the mouth.

Although biologically less satisfactory than a lingual bar since it covers the gingivae, the lingual palate is usually well tolerated by patients. It is particularly indicated for use in those cases where inadequate space exists to permit placement of a lingual bar. The lingual plate also offers another advantage relative to a lingual bar in that the increased dimension of the plate in a vertical direction enables polymeric materials such as acrylic resin to be used in its construction. In distinction, the lingual bar is always made in metal. An economic advantage can so arise, although it should be noted that a metal plate will be more rigid and usually evokes less adverse reaction in the covered soft tissues. With the exception of the relieved gingival margin area, it is essential that a lingual plate should be a close fit on the covered tissues. Otherwise, problems related to food packing may arise.

As with the lingual bar, use of a lingual plate is contraindicated where the anterior teeth are retroclined, or a grossly undercut lingual alveolar process is present.

The labial or buccal bar

This connector is normally only chosen for use where a lingual connector is contraindicated due to retroclination of the dentition.

In form, fitting and construction, it is similar to a lingual bar, except for being placed external to the arch. It is spaced from the gingival margins of the standing teeth, and from the base of the labial sulcus, in a similar manner to a lingual bar (Fig. 14.50).

As the labial bar lies external to the arch, it lies on an arc of greater radius than its lingual counterpart. To achieve the required rigidity, increase in

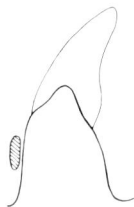

Fig. 14.50 Sagittal section in the lower incisor region illustrating the form and position of a labial bar.

cross-section is necessary relative to that of a lingual bar. This is usually achieved by increase in bar depth rather than in bar thickness. Care must be taken in its placement to avoid contact with the labial and buccal frenae. It should also be provided with slightly more relief from contact with the underlying tissues than is necessary for a lingual bar. Increased relief is especially necessary over the canine eminences.

The labial bar often gives rise to aesthetic problems. It may also cause irritation to the lips and cheeks. On that basis, its use is usually reserved for those cases where no alternative is possible.

The modified continuous clasp

This connector is similar in form to the continuous clasp (see p. 120) but its dimensions, especially its thickness, are increased to develop a level of rigidity enabling it to act as sole connector between saddles or direct retainer units on each side of the arch (Fig. 14.51). Relative to the lingual plate, it has the merit of avoiding coverage of the gingival margins. It can, though, only be used where the teeth have long clinical crowns, as this allows the necessary rigidity to be achieved without undue increase in thickness. Achieving the necessary rigidity will also

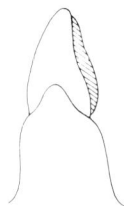

Fig. 14.51 Sagittal section in the lower incisor region illustrating the form and position of a modified continuous clasp.

be aided by the use of an alloy of high modulus of elasticity, such as cobalt–chromium alloy, in its construction.

Of the three lingually positioned lower connectors, the modified continuous clasp is used much less frequently than the lingual bar or the lingual plate, because of the rarity of cases presenting with the necessary length of clinical crowns. One special indication for its use arises where gingival surgery has been carried out, creating the required length of clinical crowns. Often, in such cases, inadequate room remains to permit placement of a lingual bar, and coverage of the gingival tissues with a lingual plate may be considered to be undesirable.

STRESS-BREAKERS

Stress-breakers are those elements of partial dentures which are interposed in a connector system in order to introduce a controlled and intentional degree of flexibility into the structure. Their most common application arises in the design of dentures carrying free-end saddles, where they are used to vary the rigidity of the connection between the saddle and the retainer unit. The principles concerning their application for this purpose are considered in Chapter 22.

Stress-breakers can be classified according to their mode of action:

Type 1 — those utilising a hinge or moveable joint
Type 2 — those utilising flexible connection.

Type 1 stress-breakers

These can be used in association with either precision attachments or clasp units as tooth-bearing direct retainers.

An example of their use with precision attachments is seen in the Crismani combined unit (Fig. 14.52). The alternative use of a type 1 stress-breaker, in conjunction with the use of a clasp unit for the provision of direct retention, can be exemplified by the Wipla unit, shown in exploded view in Figure 14.53.

Type 2 stress-breakers

These are normally used in association with clasp

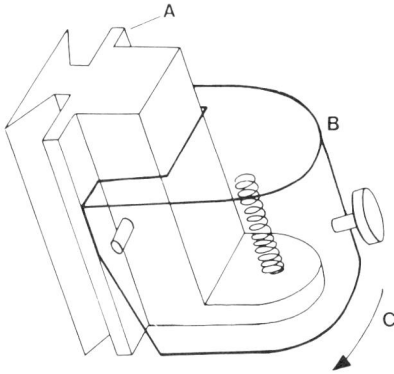

Fig. 14.52 The Crismani combined unit. A, dovetailed element providing intracoronal attachment to an abutment tooth; B, spring-controlled hinged element attached to a free-end saddle; C, movement about the hinge.

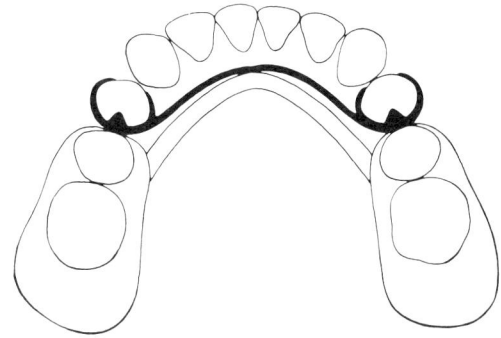

Fig. 14.53 The Wipla hinge unit. A, back plate attached to the tag of the clasp unit; B, axis of rotation of the unit in the direction indicated by the arrow; C, free ends of arms attached to the metalwork of the free-end saddle.

units as direct retainers. Various forms are possible, of which the following are commonly applied.

1. Torsion bars

These may be used in the design of a lower partial denture carrying bilateral free-end saddles. Bars extend anteriorly from the clasp units on each side to join a lingual bar near the midline (Fig. 14.54).

Flexibility can be controlled by varying the cross-section of the torsion bars, the method of construction (cast or wrought) and the material of construction (normally gold or cobalt–chromium alloys).

Disadvantages are associated with the use of the torsion bar structure, in that the double-bar system

Fig. 14.54 Torsion bar stress-breaker used in a lower partial denture replacing 46, 45, 35 and 36.

is liable to trap food and cause irritation to the tongue.

2. Partial division of connectors

The principle can be applied in both upper and lower dentures. For example, in a lower denture, a lingual plate may be partly divided by an antero-posterior slot. The upper portion of the plate is attached to the retainer unit on the abutment tooth, and the lower portion is attached to the saddle (Fig. 14.55). A degree of flexibility between the retainer unit and the saddle is so developed.

3. Mesial placement of occlusal rests

This offers the simplest available approach to stress-breaking. The degree of stress-breaking achieved is,

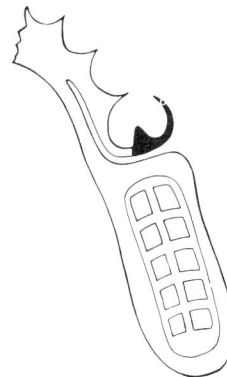

Fig. 14.55 A lower partial denture framework with partial division of a lingual plate to achieve stress-breaking.

though, much less than that available where more complex devices are employed. It may be used in the design of either upper or lower dentures.

By positioning the rest of the clasp unit on the mesial instead of on the distal fossa of the abutment tooth, and by using a minor connector to link the rest to a major connector (e.g. a lingual bar), some flexibility may be introduced into the clasp unit/saddle link (Fig. 14.56).

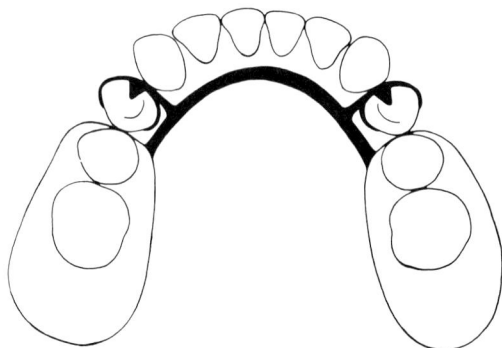

Fig. 14.56 A lower partial denture with mesial placement of occlusal rests to aid stress-breaking.

FURTHER READING

Anonymous 1951 Planned partials. JM Ney, Hartford, CT

Basker RM, Tryde G 1977 Connectors for mandibular partial dentures: use of the sublingual bar. J Oral Rehab 4: 389

Bates JF 1963 Cast clasps for partial dentures. Int Dent J 13: 610

Blatterfein L 1951 A study of partial denture clasping. J Am Dent Assoc 43: 169

Craddock FW 1946 Labial bar partial dentures. NZ Dent J 42: 67

Dolder EJ 1961 The bar joint mandibular denture. J Prosthet Dent 11: 689

Every RG 1949 The elimination of destructive forces in replacing teeth with partial dentures. NZ Dent J 45: 207

Henderson D 1973 Major connectors for mandibular removable partial dentures. J Prosthet Dent 30: 532

Lammie GA, Laird WRE 1986 Osborne and Lammie's partial dentures, 5th edn. Blackwell Scientific, Oxford

Lee JH 1963 Sectional partial dentures incorporating an internal locking bolt. J Prosthet Dent 13: 1067

Preiskel HW 1984 Precision attachments in prosthodontics. The application of intracoronal and extracoronal attachments. Quintessence, Chicago, vol 1

Quinn DM 1981 Artificial undercuts for partial denture clasps. Brit Dent J 151: 192

Reitz PV, Caputo AA 1985 A photoelastic study of stress distribution by a mandibular split major connector. J Prosthet Dent 54: 220

Schuyler CH 1953 Analysis of the use and relative value of the precision attachment and the clasp in partial denture planning. J Prosthet Dent 3: 711

Stileman RDW 1951 Spoon dentures. Br Dent J 91: 294

Wagner GA, Traweek FC 1982 Comparison of major connectors for removable partial dentures. J Prosthet Dent 47: 242

Walter JD 1986 Alternative major connectors for mandibular partial dentures. Rest Dent 2: 82

Wiebelt FJ, Stratton RJ 1985 Bracing and reciprocation in removable partial denture design. Quintess Dent Tech 9: 15

15. Designing partial dentures

INTRODUCTION

Before the designing of a partial denture is commenced, it is essential that all the necessary information should be available. Details of the required information are to be found in Chapter 5. Included is a full knowledge of the clinical condition of the patient. On that basis, it is essential that partial denture designing should be undertaken by the dental surgeon responsible for the patient's care. It is both unwise and unfair for partial denture designing to be delegated to a dental technician who will not be in possession of the necessary clinical findings.

Caution must also be sounded concerning the design procedure which is adopted. All too often, this has involved scanning through the pages of a textbook until an example of design is found where the missing teeth coincide with those in the case under consideration. A request is then made to the technician to produce a denture of similar design. Such a procedure is dangerous since it cannot take into consideration the ruling clinical conditions of the case, and may result in irreparable tissue damage.

The only approach which is acceptable is that of designing from first principles. This involves going through a series of stages in a step-by-step manner. If the order and nature of these stages is understood, even the beginner should experience no difficulty in producing successful partial denture designs.

DESIGN STAGES

There are five stages involved in partial denture design:

1. Classify and outline the saddles.
2. Provide support.
3. Provide direct retention.
4. Provide, where necessary, indirect retention.
5. Unite the various components of the denture with connectors.

Classify and outline the saddles

Note should be made of the number of saddles which are present, their length and their disposition in the arch. Each saddle should first be classified as being either bounded or free-end. A second stage in the classification of each saddle is then to decide on the way that the load borne by the saddle is to be transferred to the available supporting tissues. This secondary classification of the saddles is very important, since it will influence procedures in a number of the subsequent stages of design, and will also play a major part in deciding the success of the denture.

With bounded saddles, the choice lies between:

1. Tooth support
2. Mucosa support
3. Combined tooth-and-mucosa support.

With free-end saddles, the choice is limited to:

1. Mucosa support
2. Combined tooth-and-mucosa support.

The factors taken into consideration when deciding the secondary classification of saddles are:

1. An estimate of the response to loading of the available supporting tissues
2. The jaw for which the denture is to be provided (i.e. maxilla or mandible)

3. The length of the saddles
4. The number of saddles to be carried by the denture.

Factor 1

Information on the likely response to loading of the abutment teeth, and of the mucosa and underlying bone in the saddle areas, will be available from visual, tactile and radiographic examination of the oral tissues. Where the abutment teeth are periodontally sound, a bounded saddle may be tooth-supported. This is preferred where possible, since it develops optimal masticatory efficiency.

The second alternative, that of making a bounded saddle mucosa-supported, should be considered where the periodontal condition of the abutment teeth is suspect, and where it is judged that the tissues underlying the saddle would respond favourably to load-bearing. The latter requirement would be met by:

1. The presence under the saddle of a healthy mucosa of normal and even thickness.
2. The alveolar bone in the saddle area possessing a dense cortical plate, overlying well-developed trabeculae in the cancellous bone.
3. The absence of a history of rapid alveolar bone resorption in the saddle area.

The third alternative of choosing a combination of tooth-and-mucosa support for a bounded saddle is to be deprecated. It introduces the problem of providing equitable distribution of loading between the two supporting tissues, and is rarely necessary in the bounded saddle situation.

When deciding on the secondary classification of free-end saddles, it should be noted that, ideally they should be mucosa supported. This avoids the risk of overloading of the abutment tooth, and uneven loading of the soft and hard tissues in the saddle area, which tooth-and-mucosa support may cause. The ideal situation may, though, only be attainable by the introduction of undue complexity into the design. In such cases, the compromise approach of using combined tooth-and-mucosa support may be selected. This should only be considered if the periodontal condition of the abutment tooth is satisfactory.

Factor 2

In the mandibular denture, it is desirable that bounded saddles be made tooth supported. This is necessitated by the very limited area of mucosa which is available in the mandible to provide support. If bounded saddles in the mandible are made mucosa supported, they are liable to be traumatic to the underlying tissues. Where the abutment teeth of the mandibular bounded saddle are judged to be unable to carry the load that will be transferred to them by the saddle, it may be necessary to extract one or more of the teeth until tooth support becomes feasible.

In the maxilla, different conditions prevail, since here the hard palate provides a sizeable area of mucosa which can be used to help support the denture. Hence, either tooth support or mucosa support is acceptable for bounded saddles in the maxilla.

Factor 3

Where long bounded saddles are present on a maxillary denture, they are often better made mucosa supported, to avoid the risk of overloading of the abutment teeth.

Factor 4

The presence of multiple bounded saddles in a maxillary denture often indicates the desirability for them to be made mucosa supported, to avoid over-complexity in denture design.

On completion of the classification of the saddles, they should then be outlined. In the case of saddles of the mucosa-supported or tooth-and-mucosa-supported class, the outline developed should be that which will provide coverage of the maximum possible area of mucosa. Labially, buccally and lingually, flanges should be extended to lie at the base of the sulcus defined by a functionally moulded impression. This ensures that the load applied to each unit area of covered mucosa will be of minimal value. The risk of evoking a pathological response in the covered tissues is thereby reduced.

With tooth-supported saddles, the need for maximal mucosal coverage to spread the applied load over the mucosa does not apply. Here, saddle outline is dictated by aesthetic needs. The extension developed is that necessary to provide restoration of alveolar form, and will be proportional to the degree of alveolar resorption that has occurred in the area.

In the case of all classes of saddle, the outline decided by application of the above considerations may need to be modified by two further criteria:

1. Aesthetics. Aesthetic considerations may necessitate the use of an open-face structure in the anterior maxillary area of a denture, even where other factors indicate the use of a labial flange.

2. Undercuts. Note must be made of the presence and extent of undercuts in areas where flange extensions of saddles are to be positioned. The flange outline developed must allow free insertion and withdrawal of the denture.

Provide support

To be successful, a partial denture must be satisfactory at the time of insertion, and must maintain that condition throughout its normal period of life expectancy. Providing proper allowance for support during the designing of a partial denture is essential if this requirement is to be met. Within a year or two of the insertion of a partial denture, it is usual to find that some degree of alveolar resorption has occurred under the saddles. Unless proper provision has been made for support, this may allow the fitting position of the saddles to change. When this occurs, the artificial teeth carried by the saddles may lose contact with the opposing dentition, so impairing masticatory efficiency. A further serious consequence of a change in the position of the saddles is that it may be accompanied by a change in position of other denture components (e.g. connectors or clasp arms). Because of this, these other components may become traumatic to the soft and hard tissues which they contact. Improperly supported dentures, which give rise to this phenomenon, have rightly been termed 'gum strippers'. To avoid the risk of such consequences occurring, the following procedures should be applied.

Provision of support for bounded saddles

Where bounded saddles are to be mucosa supported, the whole denture — including the saddles

— should cover the maximum possible area of mucosa compatible with other requirements. It should be remembered that it is normally only in the maxilla (via use of the hard palate) that a sufficient area of mucosa will be available to allow bounded saddles to be made mucosa supported, without risk of undue trauma to the mucosa arising.

Where tooth support of bounded saddles is required, this is achieved by the placement of a rest on each of the abutment teeth. To ensure that the load borne by the saddle will be transferred fully to the abutment teeth, the rests must provide a rigid attachment between the saddle and the teeth. This requirement is met by placing each rest on the portion of the abutment tooth immediately adjacent to the saddle, as illustrated in Figure 15.1.

The form and positioning of the various types of rests that may be used to achieve tooth support on both anterior and posterior teeth are considered in Chapter 14. By their correct use, tooth support of the saddles of a partial denture can be achieved where this is desired.

Additional support for the denture may arise from components other than rests. For example, this will occur where connectors are placed on the hard palate or on the anterior teeth. Used alone, such auxiliary supportive devices will not ensure that the saddles are tooth supported. They should be regarded as an addition to, and not a substitute for, the use of rests to achieve tooth support in the saddles.

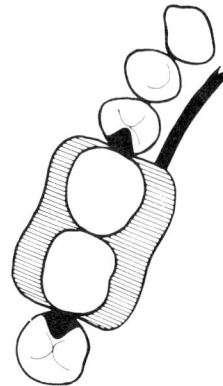

Fig. 15.1   Tooth support in the bounded saddle of a mandibular partial denture replacing 36 and 37, achieved by placing occlusal rests on the disto-occlusal fossa of 35 and the mesio-occlusal fossa of 38.

Provision of support for free-end saddles

Irrespective of whether the saddle is to be made mucosa supported, or tooth-and-mucosa supported, it must cover the maximum possible area of mucosa. In the case of a maxillary denture, buccal flanges should extend to the full depth of the sulci, the tuberosities should be fully covered and the posterior extension lie in the pterygomaxillary fissures. With a mandibular denture, buccal and lingual flanges should extend to the full depth of the sulci, with emphasis on achieving full engagement of the posterolingual areas. Posteriorly, the saddles should extend over at least the anterior one-third of the retromolar pads.

With a saddle which is to be tooth-and-mucosa supported, there is an additional requirement for a rest to be placed on the single abutment tooth. It is usually desirable that this rest should be placed on the mesial aspect of the abutment tooth. This applies unless the design includes the use of a stress-breaker, interposed between the rest and the saddle. In that case, the placement of the rest on the distal aspect of the abutment tooth is permissable.

Further information on the rationale for rest placement, and the types of stress-breakers that may be used in this situation, appear in Chapter 14. Reference should also be made to Chapter 22, which deals with the specific problems presented by partial dentures which carry free-end saddles.

Provide direct retention

Direct retention is one of the means by which a partial denture is provided with resistance to displacement. When a patient who is wearing a partial denture chews foods, especially those of a sticky consistency, forces arise which tend to cause a bodily translation of the denture away from the supportive tissues. Forces giving rise to translation may also be developed by the action of the oral and facial musculature during activities such as speech and laughter.

If translatory displacement occurs, it can clearly be a source of embarrassment to the patient. In addition, the repetitive unseating and reseating of the denture which occurs can cause trauma to both the soft and hard tissues contacted by the denture.

The function of direct retention is to develop forces which oppose those tending to cause translatory displacement. Where the sum of the retentive forces equals or exceeds that of the displacing forces, translation of the denture will be inhibited. The development of direct retention to the level where this is achieved is an essential feature of partial denture design. The methods available for achieving direct retention are as follows:

1. Utilisation of the forces responsible for achieving retention in complete dentures.

2. Frictional resistance to displacement, arising from the development of tight contacts between the artificial teeth and the natural abutment teeth.

3. Placement of direct retainers on the abutment teeth.

It should be noted that in a given denture it is sometimes possible to achieve adequate direct retention by the use of only one of these methods. Most dentures, though, will require the use of a combination of two or more of the available methods.

Method 1 of providing direct retention

Included here are:

1. Use of the physical forces arising from the presence of a saliva film between the denture and the underlying soft tissues.

2. The engagement of undercuts in the tissues underlying the saddles.

3. Shaping of the denture so that the environmental musculature will provide a positive retentive force.

4. Utilisation of the force of gravity in the mandibular denture.

The level to which these forces can be developed in a partial denture is often quite low, relative to that achievable in a complete denture. This applies particularly to the development of the physical forces, which will be limited by the decreased area of tissue coverage in a partial denture, and by the presence of the natural teeth which interfere with the development of a full peripheral seal. Thus, in only a very limited number of cases will this method, used alone, provide adequate retention in a partial denture. It may be considered in the case of a maxillary denture which carries only mucosa-supported free-end saddles. In the case of all partial dentures, though, this method will contribute to the overall retention which is achieved.

Method 2 of providing direct retention

This method can assist the development of direct retention where the partial denture carries one or more bounded saddles. Maintenance of the force will be assisted by the use of porcelain artificial teeth in preference to the use of acrylic teeth, since this will reduce the degree of wear which occurs at the contact points.

Methods 1 and 2, used in combination, will provide adequate retention for many maxillary partial dentures which carry only mucosa-supported saddles. Success will be aided by the presence of multiple bounded saddles.

Method 3 of providing direct retention

The direct retainers which are used may take the form of either preformed (precision) attachments or clasp units. The various types which can be used are considered in Chapter 14.

Their use will prove to be necessary in nearly all instances where a partial denture carries tooth-supported or tooth-and-mucosa-supported saddles. As previously noted, this will apply to nearly all mandibular dentures, and to a proportion of maxillary dentures.

When considering the placement of tooth-borne direct retainers, it should be borne in mind that each saddle needs to be provided with adequate direct retention. That requirement can best be met by placing a direct retainer on each abutment tooth, and this is done wherever possible. Certain conditions may be encountered, though, where departure from that principle is indicated. These are as follows:

1. Where the abutment tooth concerned is a central or lateral incisor, the placement of a clasp unit on the tooth as a direct retainer would generally prove to be unacceptable on aesthetic grounds.

2. Where it would involve the placement of a clasp unit as a direct retainer on an abutment tooth which possesses no usable undercuts. In that case, an adjacent tooth may offer more favourable condi-

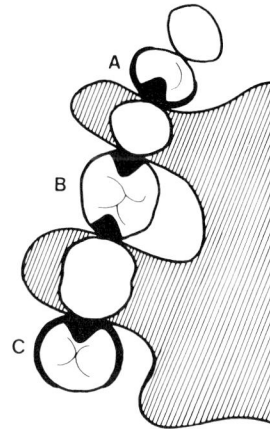

Fig. 15.2 An example of a case in which adequate retention for two short saddles may be obtained by placing direct retainers on only the terminal abutment teeth (A and C). Abutment tooth B carries rests to aid the development of tooth support in both saddles, but carries no direct retainer.

tions for placement of the clasp unit.

3. Where it would involve the introduction of unnecessary complexity into the design of the partial denture, with associated increased risk of causing caries or periodontal breakdown of the abutment tooth. This arises where two short tooth-supported saddles are separated by a single abutment tooth (Fig. 15.2).

In all instances, an attempt should be made to keep the distance between a saddle and its direct retainers to a minimum. This is necessary since the principles of the action of levers shows that the more remote a retainer is placed relative to the saddle, the less effective it will be in providing retention for that saddle.

Provide, where necessary, indirect retention

Indirect retainers are used to assist direct retainers in resisting displacement of partial dentures in function. As noted above (see p. 134), when a patient who is wearing a partial denture chews sticky foodstuffs, forces arise which tend to cause the saddles to be displaced away from the underlying tissues. Direct retention is provided to prevent this translatory displacement. Where the denture has been provided with rests to develop the necessary support in the second stage of design, it will, however, be found that a second method of displacement is possible. This is by rotation of the

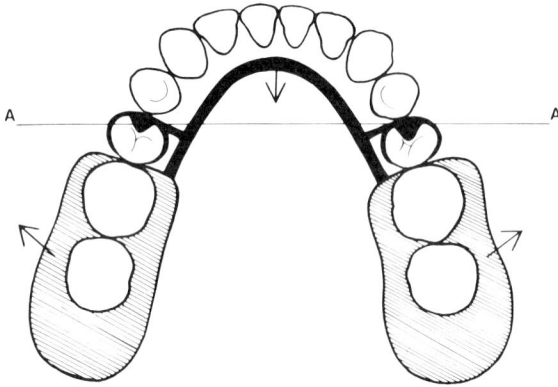

Fig. 15.3 Plan view of a mandibular partial denture carrying saddles replacing 47, 46, 36 and 37. Clasp units have been placed on 45 and 35 and a lingual bar used as the major connector. Rotation of the denture may occur about axis AA in the directions indicated by the arrows.

denture about one or more axes developed by the supporting rests, in the manner of a see-saw. The portion of the denture which lies on the saddle side of the axis will move away from the supporting tissues. At the same time, the portion of the denture which lies on the opposite side of the axis to that of the saddle will be depressed tissuewards. This situation is depicted in Figure 15.3, which presents a plan view of a mandibular partial denture being provided for a dentition of the Kennedy class I type.

In the opening movement of the masticatory cycle, a force may arise which will cause the saddles to move away from the underlying tissues. The denture may then rotate about an axis passing through the rests on 45 and 35, and the portion of the lingual bar which lies anterior to this axis will correspondingly be depressed tissuewards.

If such rotatory displacement is able to occur, it will clearly be a source of embarrassment to the patient. In addition, it may well give rise to severe tissue trauma. It is to prevent such rotation that indirect retainers are used.

The procedures involved in this stage of partial denture design are as follows.

Procedure 1

Examine the cast and note the elements already provided in the preceding design stages. Where rests have been provided in stage 2 of design,

potential axes of rotation will exist which may be defined as follows:

1. A line joining any two rests which have been provided for support of the denture.

2. Where a tooth-and-mucosa-supported free-end saddle is present, a line passing along the crest of the ridge underlying the saddle and passing through the rest on the abutment tooth.

The above definitions of potential axes of rotation do, however, require a degree of qualification. This is necessary because, in some circumstances, an axis may pass through the tip of a clasp arm (when one is present), instead of passing through the associated rest on a tooth.

Whether a rest, or the free end of a clasp arm, serves to generate an axis of rotation depends on which of these elements is positioned the greatest distance from the saddle which is subject to rotatory displacement.

In order to simplify the consideration of indirect retainer placement, an assumption will be made that in all cases the potential axes of rotation pass through rests. Since the positioning of clasp arm tips and their associated rests are in close apposition relative to the overall dimensions of a removable partial denture, the above assumption would not seem to be unreasonable.

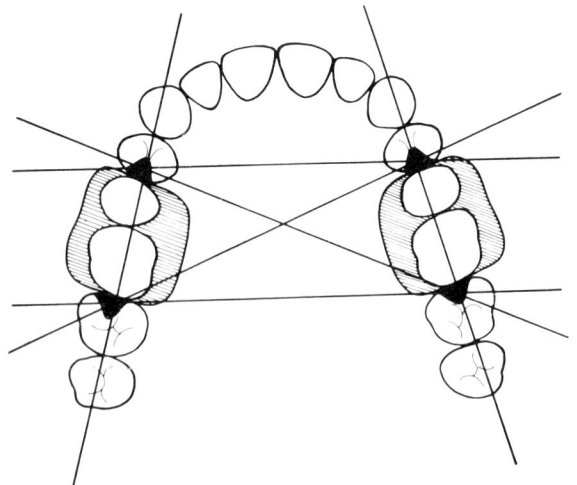

Fig. 15.4 The six potential axes of rotation present in a maxillary partial denture with two tooth-supported bounded saddles replacing 16, 15, 25 and 26. Occlusal rests have been place on 17, 14, 24 and 27.

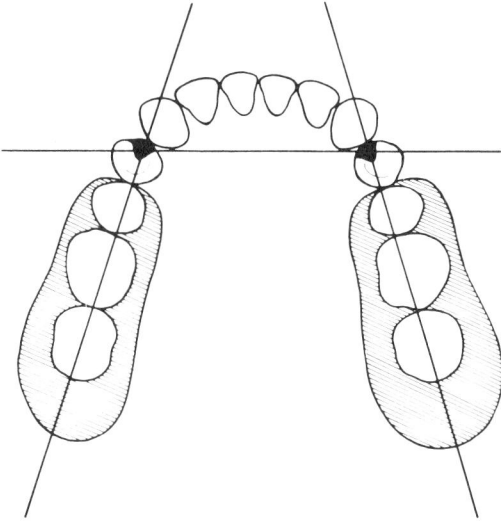

Fig. 15.5 The three potential axes of rotation present in a mandibular partial denture with two tooth-and-mucosa supported free-end saddles replacing 47, 46, 45, 35, 36 and 37. Occlusal rests have been placed on 44 and 34.

The number and disposition of the potential axes of rotation must, then, be noted. Examples of the application of this procedure are shown in Figures 15.4 and 15.5. The direction in which rotation can occur about a potential axis of rotation should also be noted (i.e. clockwise or anticlockwise).Where more than one saddle is present on a partial denture, the combined action of the saddles can lead to two-way rotation being possible about a given axis of rotation. For example, if reference is made to the diagonal axis passing through 14 and 27 in Figure 15.4, it will be seen that, where forces arise which tend to cause the anterior end of the saddle carrying 25 and 26 to move away from the underlying tissues, the denture will rotate in an anticlockwise direction about this axis. If, instead, forces arise which tend to cause the posterior end of the saddle carrying 16 and 15 to move away from the underlying tissues, the denture will now rotate in a clockwise direction about the axis.

Procedure 2

Examine the disposition of rests provided in stage 2 of design and of any tooth-borne direct retainers provided in stage 3 of design, in relation to the axes of rotation.

Decide whether or not these elements will provide resistance to rotation about all the existing axes. In reaching that decision, it should be noted that resistance to rotation can be provided by:

1. A rest placed on the opposite side of the axis of rotation to that on which the displacing saddle is situated. For example, in Figure 15.4, clockwise rotation of the denture about the axis passing through 14 and 27 will be resisted by the rest placed on 24. Likewise, anticlockwise rotation about that axis is resisted by the rest on 17.

2. A tooth-bearing direct retainer placed on the same side of the axis of rotation as that on which the displacing saddle is situated. Referring again to the axis passing through 14 and 27 shown in Figure 15.4, a direct retainer on 17 will resist clockwise rotation, and a direct retainer on 24 will resist anticlockwise rotation, about the axis.

When procedure 2 is applied to dentures which are being designed for dentitions of the Kennedy class II and class III types, it is usual to find that the elements already provided render the denture resistant to rotation about any potential axes of rotation. In that case, no further action is necessary in stage 4 of design.

With dentitions of the Kennedy class I or IV type, though, application of procedure 2 will usually demonstrate the existence of one or more axes where resistance to rotation will not be provided by the elements already placed. As an example of this finding, consider a dentition of the Kennedy class I type as depicted in Figure 15.6.

When the three axes are examined in turn, it will be found that the elements already present provide resistance to rotation about each of the antero-posterior axes. This does not apply, though, to the lateral axis passing through the rests on 44 and 34. Clockwise rotation of the denture about this axis is possible. The direct retainers on 44 and 34 will resist the tendency for rotation to some extent, but may be unable to prevent it fully because of their proximity to the axis of rotation.

In all such cases, where residual potential axes of rotation are found to be present, the provision of indirect retainers is necessary to provide resistance to rotation about these axes. This is effected in procedure 3.

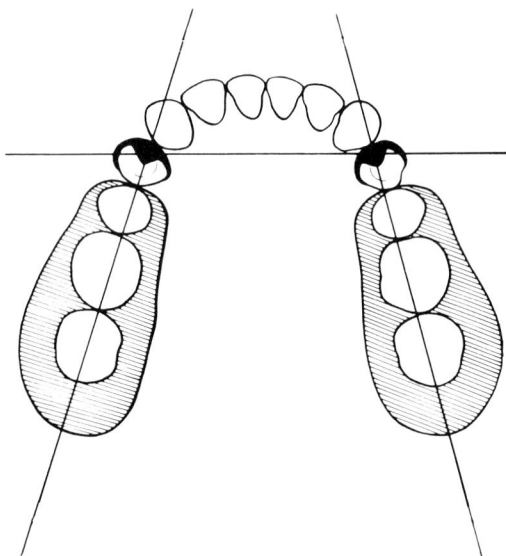

Fig. 15.6 Potential axes of rotation in a mandibular partial denture with two tooth-and-mucosa supported free-end saddles replacing 47, 46, 45, 35, 36 and 37. Clasp units to provide support and direct retention have been placed on 44 and 34.

Procedure 3

Where a need for the addition of indirect retainers has been demonstrated in procedure 2, a decision must now be made on:

1. The type or types to be used
2. Where they should be placed.

Decision 1. As previously noted, resistance to rotation about potential axes may be achieved by the use of either tooth-borne direct retainers or rests. Where the former are to be used, they are conventional in form. Where indirect retention is to be achieved by rests, then this action can be obtained by placement of conventional rests of the occlusal, cingulum or incisal type. Alternatively, certain other elements can be used to achieve the necessary resting action. For example, certain types of connectors, when positioned on the hard palate, will serve as indirect retainers of the rest type. The necessary resting effect can also be obtained by the use of elements designed specifically to act as indirect retainers, e.g. continuous clasps or the Cummer arm. These find application particularly where placement on the anterior teeth is required.

Reference should be made to Chapter 14 for details of the form and positioning of the various types.

Decision 2. In all instances, indirect retainers should be positioned the maximum possible distance from the potential axis of rotation. This will ensure by lever action that they obtain maximal mechanical advantage. In the case of a maxillary denture, indirect retainers may be placed on either the hard palate or the teeth. With a mandibular denture, only tooth-bearing indirect retainers should be used.

When dealing with a potential axis of rotation developed by the placement of two rests, the best position for placement of an indirect retainer may be found as follows: Determine the mid-point of the axis between the two rests. From that point, draw a line at right angles to the axis until the line intersects the dentition. The point of intersection represents the best position for placement of an indirect retainer.

If this procedure is applied to the case previously illustrated in Figure 15.6, it will be found that the point of intersection lies in the vicinity of 41 and 31 (Fig. 15.7).

Where this procedure is applied to dentitions of the Kennedy class IV types, it may be found that the line drawn from the mid-point of the axis will fail to intersect the dentition. In such a case, the indication is for the placement of bilateral indirect retainers, situated as posteriorly as possible (Fig. 15.8).

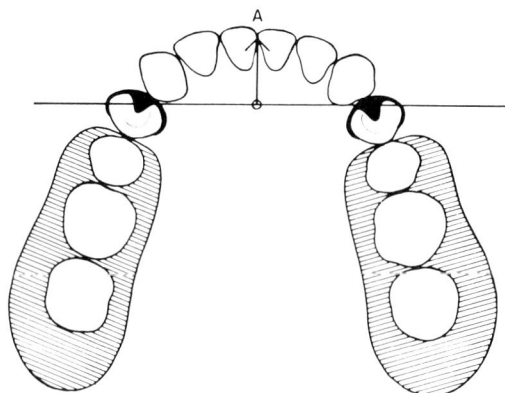

Fig. 15.7 Optimum position for the placement of an indirect retainer in the denture illustrated in Figure 15.6 is indicated by the arrow at point A.

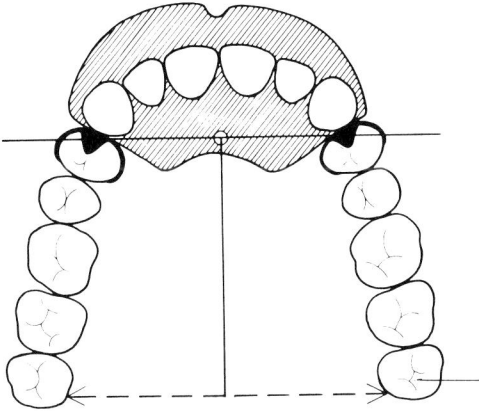

Fig. 15.8 Optimum positions for the placement of indirect retainers in a maxillary partial denture replacing 13, 12, 11, 21, 22 and 23 are indicated by the arrows. Clasp units to provide support and direct retention have been placed on 14 and 24.

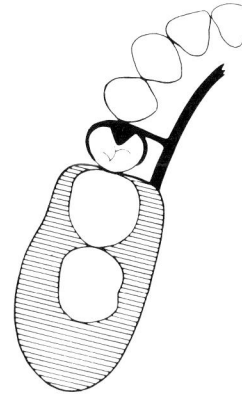

Fig. 15.9 An example of the use of a minor connector. A clasp unit on 35 is being joined to a major connector (lingual bar) in a mandibular partial denture.

Unite the various components of the denture with connectors

At the conclusion of the fourth stage of partial denture design, the placement of a series of isolated components will have been planned. In all cases, the saddle areas will have been outlined. In some cases, rests will have been placed on teeth to provide support for the denture, along with the possible placement of direct and indirect retainers. The final stage in denture design involves the placement of connectors to unite these isolated components into a single entity.

Connectors are classified as being either major or minor according to their length or the area of tissue which they cover. Major connectors include those used to join saddles, and they are always rigid in nature. Minor connectors have an auxiliary connecting role, as where a support/retention unit on a tooth needs to be joined to a major connector (Fig. 15.9). They are also usually made to be rigid but, occasionally, an intentional degree of flexibility is introduced into their structure by the inclusion of a stress-breaker. The form and function of stress-breakers is considered in Chapters 14 and 22. In the present section, further consideration will be limited to rigid connectors. The normal requirement that connectors should be rigid, stems from the need for a partial denture to be able to function as a single unit. When forces are applied to any part of the denture, it is usually deemed desirable that the

denture should be able to transfer the forces to all the soft and hard tissues which it contacts. That aim can best be achieved by the use of rigid connectors.

The various types of major connectors which can be used to join saddles are considered in Chapter 14. The choice lies between four connectors which can be used in a maxillary denture and four which can be used in a mandibular denture:

Maxillary connectors:

1. Posterior palatal bar
2. Middle palatal bar
3. Anterior palatal bar
4. Palatal plate.

Mandibular connectors:

1. Lingual bar
2. Lingual plate
3. Labial or buccal bar
4. Modified continuous clasp.

It should be noted that, in some cases, the use of two or more of the available range of connectors may be desirable in a single denture.

The factors that should be taken into consideration when selecting the appropriate connector or connectors to use in a denture are as follows:

1. The patient's history of partial denture wearing (if any).
2. Biological features related to the area of tissue which will be covered by the connector.

3. The material of construction which is to be used.

4. Whether the denture is to be provided for the maxilla or for the mandible.

Factor 1

Where the history reveals that a particular form of connector has been successful, both in terms of patient tolerance and tissue reaction, it is usually desirable for the same form of connector to be used in the replacement denture. Where the converse is true, change to an alternative form of connector should be considered.

Factor 2

The use of a bar type of connector relative to the use of a plate will normally result in an appreciable decrease in the area of tissue covered by the connector. Since tissue coverage is always accompanied by the risk of evoking a pathological response in the area concerned, reducing the area of coverage can be beneficial to tissue health. In the case of a maxillary denture, reduced coverage of the palate may also reduce impairment of the patient's taste sensation. These features favour the choice of a bar connector where possible. Against this must be weighed the fact that plate connectors, by virtue of their greater tissue coverage, offer superior support to the denture than that achievable by the use of bar connectors. The auxiliary support offered by plate connectors may be an essential feature of some denture designs, as where all the saddles in a maxillary denture are to be made mucosa supported.

Factor 3

Choice of the material of construction is closely linked to that of the type of connector to be used. To achieve the necessary rigidity in a bar type of connector, it must be made in metal. It may be cast in a gold alloy or cobalt–chromium alloy, or be fabricated by wrought work using a gold alloy or stainless steel. Plate connectors can also be made in metal but, here, because of the greater area of coverage, it may also be possible to achieve the necessary rigidity by use of a plastic such as acrylic resin. The use of a plastic in place of a metal for the construction of a plate connector offers a clear economic advantage. In addition, it will decrease the weight of the denture and thus favour retention in the case of a maxillary denture.

In terms of the preservation of tissue health, however, the use of metal for the construction of plates is to be preferred. Tissues which are covered by a metal plate usually maintain a healthier state with less pathological reaction than that seen where a plastic plate is used. In part, this may be due to a different response by the tissues to the chemical nature of the overlying materials. The much greater value for the coefficient of thermal conductivity of metals, relative to that of plastics, may also play a part in the observed difference. Yet another factor which may help to explain the difference in tissue response is the comparative rigidity of the two structures. The modulus of elasticity of cobalt–chromium alloy, for example, is approximately 60 times that of acrylic resin. Even a thin lingual plate constructed in cobalt–chromium alloy will be more rigid than the thickest tolerable form of acrylic lingual plate. During the normal functioning of the denture, far less flexing of a metal plate will occur than is the case with a plastic plate and consequently, less mechanical irritation of the tissues is likely to arise.

Where bar connectors are to be used, selection of the appropriate connector system will be influenced by the modulus of elasticity of the metal to be used in their construction. The modulus of elasticity of cobalt–chromium alloys is approximately twice that of gold alloys. As a consequence, where a maxillary denture carries only two short, laterally-positioned bounded saddles, adequate rigidity can often be achieved by the use of a posterior palatal bar as sole connector if cobalt-chromium alloy is used. Where, instead, the same denture is to be constructed in a gold alloy, the use of a combination of anterior and posterior palatal bars will usually be necessary to achieve the same rigidity.

Factor 4

The general preference for use of bar connectors rather than plate connectors, wherever possible, has already been noted. It applies equally to dentures being provided for the maxilla or for the mandible.

Where a plate connector is to be used in a maxillary denture, it is desirable that it should be constructed on the principles advocated by Every. Important amongst these principles is that of developing a self-cleansing gap of approximately 4 mm between the palatal plate and the palatal aspects of the gingival margins of the standing teeth. This helps towards the maintenance of the health of the periodontal tissues of the teeth. Alternative designs, which involve colleting of the palatal plate around the standing teeth, carry a greater risk of producing an inflammatory reaction in the gingival tissues.

A simplified version of the 'Every' palatal plate connector is seen in the 'spoon' form. This can be used where a maxillary partial denture is being constructed for a Kennedy class IV dentition and not more than two adjacent teeth are to be replaced. As a 'spoon' connector avoids contact with any of the standing teeth, it has biological merit, but it suffers the disadvantage of achieving only limited retention and stability. The development of an acceptable level of retention will be favoured by the presence of a 'U'-shaped palate, relative to that of a 'V'-shaped palate. It is more successful in children and adolescents than in adult patients, probably because younger patients find it easier to develop control of the denture by tongue action.

When selecting the connector to be used to join saddles in a mandibular denture, the biological superiority of the lingual bar should always be borne in mind. Against this must be weighed the fact that it may give rise to tongue irritation in some patients. The risk of this occurring can be reduced by positioning the bar as low as possible in relation to the floor of the mouth. The adoption of a sublingual position for the bar may also aid its acceptance. The lingual plate is usually well tolerated by patients, especially when made in metal and carefully contoured to simulate the form of the natural teeth which it covers. However, the lingual plate crosses the gingival margins of the teeth it covers, and this always carries the risk of producing periodontal damage.

The buccal or labial bar is poorly tolerated by many patients on both aesthetic and functional grounds, and its use should be restricted to those cases where there is no alternative. This is usually due to the presence of a retroclined dentition.

The modified continuous clasp is rarely selected for use. It is indicated where the teeth upon which it is to be positioned have long clinical crowns, where the health of the gingivae of those teeth contraindicate their being covered, and yet inadequate space is available for use of a lingual bar.

FURTHER READING

Barbenel JC 1971 Design of partial denture components. J Dent Res 50: 586

Bates JF 1968 Studies in the retention of cobalt–chromium partial dentures. Brit Dent J 125: 97

Davenport JC, Basker RM, Heath JR, Ralph JP 1989 A colour atlas of removable partial dentures. Wolfe, London.

Dyer MRY 1972 The 'Every' type acrylic partial denture. Dent Pract Dent Rec 22: 339

Feingold GM, Grant AA, Johnson W 1986 The effect of partial denture design on abutment tooth and saddle movement. J Oral Rehab 13: 549

Feingold GM, Grant AA, Johnson W 1988 Abutment tooth and base movement with attachment retained removable partial dentures. J Dent 16: 264.

Firtell DN 1968 Effect of clasp design upon retention of removable partial dentures. J Prosthet Dent 20: 43

Krogh-Poulsen W 1954 Partial denture design in relation to occlusal trauma and periodontal breakdown. Int Dent J 4: 847

Lammie GA, Laird WRE 1986 Osborne and Lammie's partial dentures, 5th Edn. Blackwell Scientific, Oxford

McGivney GA, Castleberry DJ 1989 McCracken's partial prosthodontics, 8th Edn. Mosby, St Louis

Scally VL 1988 The 'Every' partial denture system: the mandibular partial denture. NZ Dent Ass Prosthodont J 7: 19

Wilson JH 1949 Partial denture construction — some aspects of diagnosis and design. Dent J Aus 21: 347

16. The impression stage of treatment

PRIMARY IMPRESSIONS

Introduction

Primary impressions are used in the preparation of study casts, which play a vital role in the planning and construction of a removable partial denture. After a record has been made of the patient's jaw relationship, the casts will be mounted on an anatomical type of articulator, and the occlusion and articulation of the dentition will be examined. The casts will also be surveyed as an essential preliminary to denture design. These procedures are considered in Chapter 5, which deals with the examination of the patient.

When diagnostic uses of the study casts have been completed, they will then be utilised in the construction of special trays.

To perform the above functions satisfactorily, it is essential that study casts provide an exact copy of the oral tissues. This will only be possible if the primary impressions meet the required level of accuracy. It will, for instance, be impossible to obtain an accurate picture of the occlusal relationship of the teeth if imperfections are present on the occlusal surface because air inclusions were present in the impressions. Primary impression taking should thus be approached with an appreciation of the care and attention to detail which is necessary for success.

Choice of trays

Stock trays of the 'box' form are normally used to obtain primary impressions of a partially dentate patient. The trays are available made in either metal or a polymeric material, the preference being for metal trays because of their greater rigidity.

Where a choice is available of trays with or without perforations, the former are to be preferred as the perforations aid the retention in the trays of certain impression materials, such as alginate.

Stock trays are available in a range of sizes. Selection of the size to use should be based on finding trays which provide a spacing which is as even as possible from the tissues to be recorded in the impression, and which cover the required tissue area to an optimal extent. Where doubt exists as to which tray to use, it is suggested that a better result will usually be obtained by selecting a tray which is slightly oversize, in preference to one which is undersize.

Preparation of trays

It is rare to find a stock tray which fully meets with the size requirements noted above. This helps to explain why it is usually necessary to use a two-stage impression procedure, the construction of a special tray being interposed between the primary and secondary impression stages. Even so, every effort should be made to obtain accuracy in the primary impression stage. This aim can often be helped by modifying stock trays prior to their use. Where, as is commonly the case, a hydrocolloidal or elastomeric impression material is to be used to take the primary impression, tray modification can be made by the use of impression compound. Additions of impression compound may be made to the tray to increase peripheral extension in any area where the tray itself fails to provide the required tissue coverage. This need will often be found to arise in the upper labial sulcus region, and posteriorly in both upper and lower trays.

Where long edentulous regions are to be recorded in the impression, especially where free-end saddles are involved, it is beneficial to place softened impression compound in the tray in the areas concerned. The tray is then inserted and border moulding is carried out. The compound impression is examined and any areas where compound has flowed into regions of standing teeth are trimmed back, to leave only the impression of the edentulous regions. The compound should also be trimmed to remove any undercuts which have developed.

Impression compound may also be applied to any areas of the trays where an excessive spacing is seen to be present between the tray and the underlying tissues. The area where this form of modification is most commonly required is in the palatal region of an upper tray.

To avoid the risk of distortion of an impression occurring during and subsequent to the impression-taking procedure, steps must be taken to ensure that an adequate bond is developed between stock trays and the impression material which is used. This is especially important where hydrocolloidal or elastomeric impression materials are being used, as such materials do not themselves bond to trays. The required bonding is achieved in two ways. Firstly, by the use of perforations in the trays, which offer a mechanical lock for the impression material. Secondly, an adhesive may be applied to the tray surface before the tray is filled with the impression material. The adhesive used should be of a type specifically intended for use with the chosen impression material. Studies have shown that perforations in a tray provide an effective means of resisting the shear stresses which arise during removal of an impression, but are poor in resisting tensile stresses. The latter deficiency can be overcome by the application of an appropriate adhesive to the tray. Thus, the combined use of perforations and an adhesive is advisable to provide full security of retention of the impression material in the tray.

Choice of impression material

Impressions of the oral tissues of partially dentate patients usually involve a need to reproduce a multitude of undercuts, particularly found in relation to the standing natural teeth. Reproduction of these undercuts will be facilitated if an impression material of the elastic type is used. Alternative impression materials of the plastic or brittle types can be used, but are rarely selected because of the difficulty in use they present in the multiple undercut situation.

Elastic impression materials can be divided into two main groups, each of which can be further subdivided:

1. Hydrocolloids
   a. Reversible — agar-agar
   b. Irreversible — alginate
2. Elastomers
   a. Polysulphides
   b. Silicones
   c. Polyethers.

Some of these materials are available in a range of viscosities. For example, polysulphides are available in light-, medium-, and heavy-bodied forms, the light form often being intended for application to the tissues by a syringe, the other forms being applied via a tray. Silicones are available in a putty form and a lower viscosity form.

Of the above materials, alginate is selected most frequently for use in primary impression taking. It is relatively cheap to purchase, easy to manipulate and, if used with the application of appropriate precautions, will, in most instances, produce excellent results. Alginate does, though, present two major disadvantages. Firstly, it is very liable to distort if abused, both during and subsequent to impression taking. Secondly, it shows a relatively low resistance to tearing when withdrawn from moderate to severe undercuts. Where the latter problem is encountered, improved resistance to tearing will be obtained if one of the elastomeric materials is used. Of the three types of elastomers which are available, the preference is usually for the use of silicones in obtaining primary impressions.

Impression-taking procedure

As alginate is commonly selected as the material to be used in primary impression taking, the procedure for using this material will be discussed in some detail. Where alternative materials are being used, some modification in the procedure will be necessary, particularly in relation to the preparation of the impression material for use.

The procedure for alginate should be applied in a step-by-step manner, as summarised below:

1. Read carefully the instructions provided by the manufacturer of the brand of alginate being used. Note in particular features such as powder/water ratio and the temperature of the water to use.

2. Ensure the bowl and spatula to be used are clean and free of any extraneous matter. Place the measured amount of powder in the bowl and add the correspondingly measured amount of water. Start mixing slowly and then, when the powder particles have been wetted, mix more vigorously. Avoid a beating action which may incorporate air. Mix for the period indicated by the manufacturer (commonly of the order of 30 seconds). Some brands of alginate incorporate a coloured indicator and show by colour change of the material the point where mixing is complete.

3. Use the spatula to place the mixed alginate into the impression tray. Bare areas of the tray should be filled to the level of the margins, and any areas where additions of impression compound have been applied should be covered by at least a 3 mm deep layer of alginate.

4. An optional procedure is now to apply some of the excess mix over areas of the tissue surfaces where trapping of air is liable to occur. Such areas include the occlusal surfaces of the teeth, the palate and any grossly undercut regions labially, bucally or lingually. Speed is essential where this procedure is used, as oral temperature accelerates setting of the alginate and the main mass of alginate within the tray must be positioned before setting commences, or distortion of the impression is likely to occur.

5. Adopt the correct stance relative to the patient for the impression concerned (upper or lower), as described in Chapter 9. Rotate the tray into the correct position over the oral tissues and apply pressure until excess material is observable all round the periphery. Apply border-moulding movements of cheeks, lips and tongue as required by the impression concerned. Await the expiration of the setting time indicated by the manufacturer. During the setting period, support the upper tray in position by light pressure to counter gravity. The lower tray only requires downward pressure to resist displacement by the tongue, but support for the mandible should be provided by placement of the operator's thumbs under the lower border of the mandible, in about the premolar area on each side. It is very important that there should be no change in the pressure applied to either the upper or lower tray as setting of the alginate proceeds, otherwise distortion of the impression is liable to occur. Do not attempt to remove the impression until excess material around the periphery shows setting has occurred by the development of elastic solidity. Little, if any, harm will arise by leaving the impression in situ for a minute or so after setting. In contrast, if an attempt is made to remove the impression before setting and the development of elasticity has fully occurred, distortion of the impression will be inevitable.

6. Release the impression from its seating position by the application of a rapid pull away from the tissues. This is necessary since alginate has greater elasticity when subjected to a rapid displacing force than when a slow displacing force is applied. Once the impression has been released from undercuts, rotate it carefully out of the mouth.

7. Rinse the impression in cool running water to remove saliva and mucus from its surface. Use an air syringe to displace water from areas of the impression where natural teeth have been reproduced.

Examine the impression carefully for any imperfections such as the presence of air inclusions or inadequate coverage of the required tissue area. The margins of the impression, except posteriorly, should show a peripheral roll developed by border moulding.

Where any imperfections are found to be present, the impression must be repeated until a satisfactory result is obtained.

Impressions should be immersed in an antiseptic solution for the recommended period before cast production is carried out (see Ch. 8, p. 65).

Preparation of study casts

As the study casts will be used to analyse the occlusion and articulation of the natural dentition, and will also be surveyed, it is essential that they possess adequate surface hardness and abrasion resistance. This can best be achieved by the use of an artificial stone in their construction.

Where the primary impressions have been taken in alginate, the impressions should be cast up within half an hour of being taken. Otherwise, a dimensional inaccuracy is liable to develop as a consequence of syneresis or imbibition. Impressions should be protected from change in the interval between being taken and cast up by being covered with a damp napkin.

Appropriate precautions should be taken in the casting-up process to avoid errors such as air inclusions or distortion of the impression material.

Where alginate has been used, the impression material should be removed from the study casts in not less than half an hour nor more than one hour, after casting-up commenced. If removal of the impression material from the casts is attempted before the elapse of half an hour, there is a considerable risk that any teeth being reproduced will fracture. Where the impression material is left in contact with the cast for more than an hour, the alginate may absorb water from the cast and lead to the development of a weak, chalky surface on it. Also, developing rigidity and forcible contraction of the alginate increases the difficulty of removing the alginate from the cast, and the risk that tooth fracture will occur in this procedure.

Prescription writing

Two main requirements will arise at this stage:

Preparation of study casts

The material to be used in the casting-up of the impressions should be indicated. This will normally be an artificial stone.

Preparation of special trays

The information provided should include:

1. Extension. Lines should be marked on the study casts to indicate the required extension. The lines should be approximately 2 mm short of the sulcus buccally, labially and lingually, with appropriate allowance for frenae. The posterior border of an upper tray should be a straight line between the pterygomaxillary fissures, and the posterior border of the lower tray should extend approximately half way across the retromolar pads.

2. Spacing. The thickness of spacer to be used should be indicated. This will usually be two sheets of baseplate wax (approximately 3 mm) where alginate is to be used as secondary impression material. The spacer can be a little thinner than this where an elastomeric impression material is to be used.

3. Material of construction. It is essential that a special tray which is to be used to take a secondary impression should be rigid and resistant to warpage at oral temperatures. This can best be achieved by the use of a polymeric material such as acrylic resin. Either the self-curing or heat-curing types may be used.

4. Perforations. An indication should be given as to whether or not perforations are to be provided in the tray. Perforations are essential for alginate and desirable for elastomers.

SECONDARY IMPRESSIONS

Introduction

Secondary impressions are taken in order to prepare the casts on which denture construction will be carried out. This may include the construction of a cast or wrought metal framework, where dimensional accuracy is critical. It is, thus, essential that secondary impressions should provide an exact negative form of the oral tissues they record. The procedure followed should be based on the need to achieve this requirement.

Choice of trays

It is recommended that special trays be used to take secondary impressions in partial denture construction. The general advantages which arise from the use of trays of this type have been indicated in Chapter 9. In addition, in partial denture prosthodontics, certain design features demand a knowledge of the exact position of the functional sulcus relative to the gingival margins of the standing teeth. For example, a decision on the use of a lingual bar or a lingual plate as the connector for a lower partial denture will be influenced by knowledge on this point. It is only by the use of a special tray that such features can be reliably determined.

The special trays should be constructed using a material which can provide the required structural rigidity without necessitating undue bulk. The material used must also be resistant to warpage at oral temperatures and allow easy modification of peripheral form by trimming, should this prove to be necessary. As previously noted, acrylic resin in either the heat-curing or self-curing form provides a material which adequately meets these needs.

Choice of impression material

In recording the oral tissues of a partially dentate patient at the secondary impression stage, it is usual to apply a minimum-pressure impression procedure (considered in Chapter 9).

If digital pressure on the tray is kept to the minimal value necessary to ensure correct seating of the impression, the pressure applied to the tissues will be dependent on the viscosity of the impression material which is used. The materials chosen for use are normally taken from the 'elastic' range considered above (see p. 144).

Of these materials, the hydrocolloids are generally of low viscosity while the heavy-bodied polysulphides offer maximum viscosity, other materials providing intermediate values.

By selection of an appropriate impression material, the operator has a means of controlling the level of pressure which will be applied to the tissues in the impression taking procedure. This choice is of particular value when dealing with dentures carrying free-end saddles, and is considered further in Chapter 22. In these circumstances, it may also be decided that a true pressure or muco-displacive type of impression is indicated, which may be achieved by the use of impression composition. Special impression procedures such as this will be further considered in a later section (see p. 148).

In most instances, an 'elastic' type of impression material will be used, and of the available materials alginate will be prime choice, as at the primary impression stage. An alternative material may be chosen where relatively severe undercuts are to be reproduced, to avoid the problem of tearing of alginate. Silicones are chosen most commonly to meet this need, the preference being for use of the paste type rather than the combined use of a putty form, followed by use of a low-viscosity surface layer. The latter procedure has been subjected to criticism on the basis of possible development of internal stress, with consequential distortion of the impression.

Impression-taking procedures

The special trays to be used are first tried in and checked for satisfaction. They should cover the entire tissue areas to be reproduced in the impressions, and their margins should relate correctly to the levels of the functional sulci. If any areas of overextension are found to be present, the trays should be trimmed to the correct level. If any deficiencies of extension are noted, these can be corrected by the application of green-stick impression compound in the areas concerned. Where long edentulous tissue areas are present, especially when free-ended, the application of carefully positioned wax stops to the fitting surface of the tray, in a crest-of-ridge position, will aid correct location of the trays.

Where, as is usual, alginate is to be used as the secondary impression material, the impression-taking procedure should follow that outlined above (see p. 144). Where other materials are being used, the procedure followed will be similar, except for the preparation for use of the material. In all cases, the instructions for proportioning and mixing of the material provided by the manufacturer of the product concerned should be followed.

Cast production

Choice of the material to be used in the preparation of the working or master casts from secondary impressions is based on the constructional procedures to be used in denture construction. Where a polymeric denture base such as acrylic resin is to be used, the casts should be prepared using a prosthodontic grade of artificial stone. Where, though, the denture design involves the use of a metal framework, especially where this is to be prepared by casting, it is advisable to use, instead, a die grade of artificial stone. The additional surface hardness of the latter material reduces the risk of cast damage occurring in the procedures associated with the construction of a metal framework.

Where alginate has been used to take the secondary impressions, precautions must be taken in the casting-up procedure, as detailed on page 146.

Prescription writing

The requirements which may arise at this stage are as follows.

1. The design of a metal framework

Where the construction of a metal framework is required, detailed instructions must be given. This can best be provided by means of a diagram, accompanied by information on each of the component elements. Use of a prescription form such as that illustrated in Figure 16.1 will facilitate this process. It is also helpful to the technician if the required design for the framework is drawn on the study casts. This can provide more definitive information on the required position of elements such as palatal connectors than is afforded by a two-dimensional drawing on the prescription form.

2. Occlusal rims

These may be required in certain cases for use in the subsequent clinical stage of registration of the patient's jaw relationship. Whether or not they are required is dependent on the number and distribution of tooth contacts which are present, and this will be discussed further in Chapter 17.

Where occlusal rims are required, the prescription for them should indicate:

1. The material or materials to be used in baseplate construction, with required extension.
2. Whether placement of strengthening elements or retainers is required.
3. The material to be used in rim construction.

SPECIAL IMPRESSION PROCEDURES

Pressure or muco-displacive impressions

In certain circumstances a decision may be made to take an impression which records the tissues under loading conditions which simulate those arising in masticatory functioning of the appliance. The rationale for this procedure is considered in Chapter 22, where the problems presented by dentures carrying free-end saddles are discussed.

Two approaches are possible when obtaining pressure impressions in the partially dentate condition:

1. Pressure may be applied evenly over the whole area to be recorded by the impression. This can be achieved most readily by the use of impression composition as impression material. Since undercuts are likely to be associated with standing teeth, accuracy of reproduction of these undercuts will only be obtained if a sectional approach is used. The impression is built up in sections, each having a different path of insertion, allowing withdrawal from associated undercuts. As each section is added, it is positioned in relation to other sections by means of notches, which allow accurate re-assembly of the sections following withdrawal from the mouth. For more detailed information of this procedure, a specialist text should be consulted.

2. Pressure application may be concentrated on the edentulous areas to be recorded by the impression, a lower level of pressure being applied to the standing teeth. This procedure may be selected since it is the edentulous tissue areas which will be liable to show any gross level of displacement under pressure, displacement of the teeth being limited to the movement permitted by the periodontal attachment tissues. The advantage of this procedure is that the recording of the undercuts on the teeth is facilitated by the ability to use an elastic impression material in the tooth-bearing section of the impression.

A suitable combination of impression materials to use in this procedure is provided by impression compound in the edentulous areas, and alginate in the tooth-bearing areas. A special tray is used and compound applied initially in the edentulous regions. Any excess that has flowed into the tooth-bearing section is trimmed back and then, as a second stage, the tooth-bearing section is recorded in alginate. To avoid the problem of a parting line between the two impression materials, the alginate may be extended as a wash over the compound portion, if so desired.

At each of the stages of impression taking, manual pressure is applied to the tray to an extent which is felt will match that developed in the functioning of the appliance.

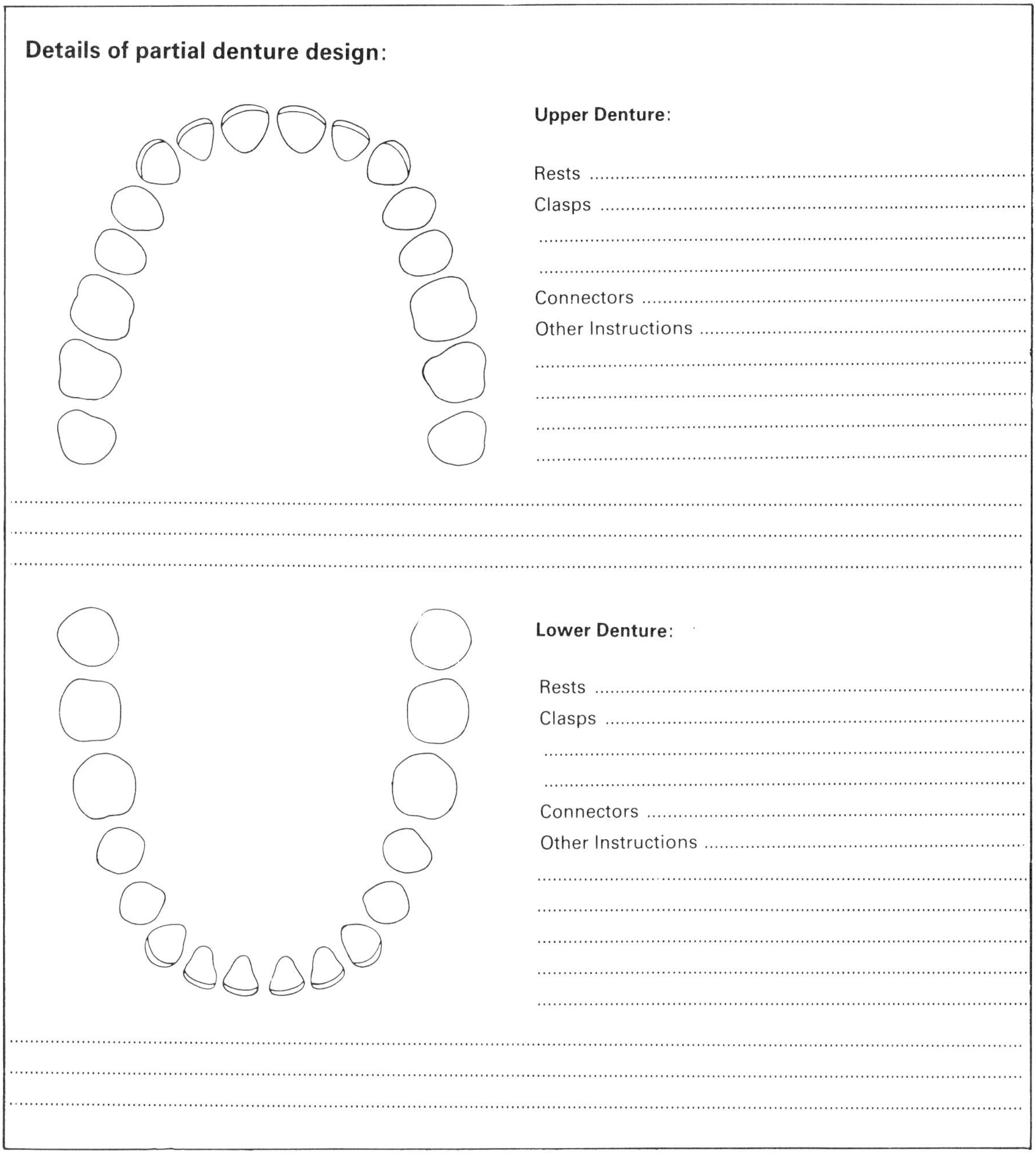

Details of partial denture design:

Upper Denture:

Rests ....

Clasps ....

....

....

Connectors ....

Other Instructions ....

....

....

....

....

....

....

....

Lower Denture:

Rests ....

Clasps ....

....

....

Connectors ....

Other Instructions ....

....

....

....

....

....

....

....

Fig. 16.1   Prescription form for partial dentures.

Impression procedures for relining partial dentures

The relining of mucosa-supported partial dentures is a rarely applied procedure, because of the technical difficulties which can arise. These are associated with the multiple undercuts which are usually present. In the original construction of the denture, interproximal undercuts will have been blocked out to allow insertion of the denture along the chosen path. If a reline impression is taken in the denture, the impression material will flow into any interproximal undercuts. Unless special steps are taken, this material entering the undercuts will be reproduced in the relined denture, and insertion will be impossible. For this reason, remaking rather than relining of mucosa-supported dentures is often advocated.

Although relining of mucosa-supported dentures may be deprecated, the same is not true of tooth-supported and especially, tooth-and-mucosa supported dentures.

Relining of removable partial dentures of the tooth-and-mucosa-supported type, which normally carry free-end saddles, is a frequent requirement. Where a metal base is included in the design, relining can only be applied to those saddles where the metal work has been relieved from direct contact with the tissues. The lack of adhesion between metals and polymeric materials such as acrylic resin debars the addition of a thin polymeric film on a metal base.

Where the relining of free-end saddles on a tooth-and-mucosa-supported partial denture is required, the following procedure may be used:

1. Examine the extension of the saddle areas and correct this if found to be necessary.
2. Remove any undercuts present on the fitting surface aspects of the saddles.
3. Take a reline impression in the saddle areas. Zinc oxide–eugenol impression paste is frequently used as the impression material at this stage. Alternatively, an available alternative to Kerr's Korecta Wax No. 4 may be used, with application of wax in stages until full surface coverage of the saddle area is achieved and excess wax appears all round the margins. In taking the impression it is important that pressure should only be applied to the anterior framework aspect of the denture, to ensure it seats correctly in a fully fitting position on the standing teeth. Manual pressure should not be applied to the saddle areas, nor should the patient be requested to apply biting pressure on the denture.

When the denture is reinserted following the completion of the laboratory procedure of relining of the saddles, it will usually be found that some degree of occlusal disharmony will be present, premature contact occurring on the posterior teeth. This must be corrected by selective grinding of the dentition until the required occlusion has been developed.

This procedure for relining the free-end saddles of a partial denture may be used in those instances where anteroposterior rocking of the denture is found to occur about an axis joining the occlusal rests, when pressure is applied in a tissueward direction on the free-end saddles. The circumstances which give rise to instability of this type are considered in Chapter 22.

Relining may be necessary for the 'completed' denture prior to it being worn by the patient, or the need may be found to arise at any or all of the subsequent 6-monthly review appointments of the patient.

An alternative procedure which may be used to overcome the problem of anteroposterior rocking of the denture is to use a technique based on that proposed by Applegate. This is termed the 'altered cast' technique and can only be used during the original construction of the denture. If relining is subsequently found to be necessary during the period of wear of the appliance, another procedure such as that described earlier will need to be used.

In the altered cast technique, a conventional metal framework for the denture is first prepared on a cast taken from an impression in which an impression material of a relatively low order of viscosity was used, such as alginate. Baseplates are now attached to the metalwork in the saddle areas to fully cover the required tissue areas of the saddles, and so that they are relieved from the tissue contact by a gap of approximately 2 mm.

Kerr's Korecta Wax No. 4, or an available alternative, is now painted on the fitting surface aspect of the baseplates to a depth of 2 mm. The denture is inserted with pressure applied only on the anterior tooth-bearing area of the metal framework. Wax additions and reinsertion are carried out until overall coverage of the tissues in the saddle regions has been achieved, and excess wax has flowed out around all the margins.

In the laboratory, the original cast is now sectioned to remove those portions of the cast which originally reproduced the tissues under the saddles. The section lines used for a lower cast are shown in plan view in Figure 16.2. The framework is then positioned on the remaining portion of the cast and new saddle areas are poured up in the saddle

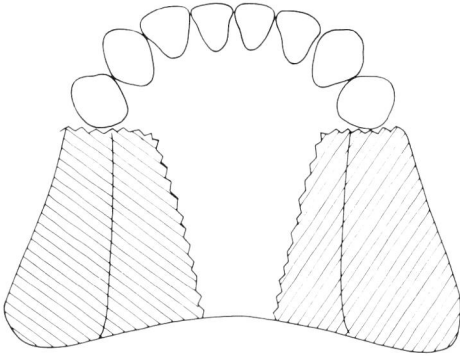

Fig. 16.2   Plan view of a lower cast showing the section lines used in the Applegate 'altered cast' technique.

impression zones to reform the cast. Setting up of the teeth and finishing of the denture are then carried out on the altered cast. A particular advantage of this procedure is that as the teeth are set up on the altered cast, no occlusal disruption arises. Against this must be considered the demanding nature of the procedure from both the clinical and laboratory aspects, which restrict its application.

FURTHER READING

Beckett LS 1955 Partial denture impressions. Dent J Aus 27: 135
Birnbach S 1984 Impression technique for maxillary removable partial dentures. J Prosthet Dent 51: 286
Henderson D 1966 Writing work authorizations for removable partial dentures. J Prosthet Dent 16: 696
Holmes, JB 1970 The altered cast impression procedure for the distal extension removable partial denture. Dent Clin North Am 14: 569
James JS 1985 A simplified alternative to the altered-cast impression technique for removable partial dentures. J Prosthet Dent 53: 598.
Jasim FA, Brudvik JS, Nicholls JI 1985 Impression distortion from abutment tooth inclination in removable partial dentures. J Prosthet Dent 54: 532
Kramer, HM 1961 Impression techniques for removable partial dentures. J Prosthet Dent 11: 84
McCrorie JW 1982 Corrective impression waxes. A simple formula. Br Dent J 152: 95
Mack PJ 1979 Inhalation of alginate powder during spatulation. Br Dent J 146: 141.
Rothwell PS, Dinsdale RCW 1988 Cross-infection control in dental practice Part 1. Br Dent J 165: 185
Shiloah J Schuman NJ, Covington JS, Turner JE 1988 Periodontal hazards of retained impression materials. Quintess. Int 19: 143
Storer R, McCabe JF 1981 An investigation of methods available for studying impressions. Br Dent J 151: 217
Wilson HJ, Smith DC 1963 Bonding of alginate impression materials to impression trays. Br Dent J 115: 291

17. The jaw registration stage of treatment

INTRODUCTION

In the provision of removable partial dentures, the jaw registration stage has to be applied at two treatment stages:

1. To allow the study casts to be mounted on an articulator in the correct relationship. This is an essential precursor to the stages of occlusal analysis and partial denture design.

2. To allow the working casts to be mounted on an articulator in the correct relationship, prior to the setting-up of the artificial teeth.

Often, the same or similar procedures will be used to effect jaw registration in both these stages. However, one essential difference is that where a cast metal framework has been prepared for a denture this will be used, where appropriate, as a baseplate for the registration procedure in the second stage.

In all cases, the jaw registration stage requires:

1. The correct vertical dimension
2. The correct horizontal relationship.

Additional records will be required where complex analysis of the dentition is indicated. These involve a face-bow and protrusive or lateral records of jaw relationship. In all cases, the procedures adopted should be based on the principles of registering jaw relationships considered in Chapter 10.

ESTABLISHING THE CORRECT VERTICAL DIMENSION

Three types of case may be encountered, each requiring a separate approach:

1. Cases in which natural tooth contact occurs at a vertical dimension providing an acceptable freeway space.

2. Cases in which natural tooth contact occurs at a vertical dimension providing an excessive freeway space.

3. Cases in which no natural tooth contact occurs.

Cases in which natural tooth contact occurs at a vertical dimension providing an acceptable freeway space

Where a stable contact of upper and lower natural teeth occurs at a vertical dimension at which an adequate and yet not excessive freeway space is present (normally 2–4 mm), the registration should be established at this contact height in the subsequent stage of establishing the horizontal relationship.

Cases in which natural tooth contact occurs at a vertical dimension providing an excessive freeway space

Here, the vertical dimensions should be established at a value increased on that of tooth contact by an amount necessary to bring the freeway space down to an appropriate value. This may be achieved by the use of a wax wafer interposed between the teeth, the thickness of the wax being varied until the required freeway space has been achieved. It is desirable that the wax wafer registration should include a metal plate, cut to lie within the arch of the teeth, and with the wax affixed to it peripherally. This considerably reduces the risk that distortion of the registration will occur in the interval preceding mounting of the casts. The use of a wax wafer registration is only feasible where the number and disposition of standing teeth are such that the wafer will locate precisely on the study casts. This normally necessitates the presence of contacting teeth in both the premolar and molar regions on each side of the arch. Where this condition is not met, the registration is carried out using occlusal rims, the height of rim/rim or rim/tooth contact being varied by addition or subtraction of wax until the required freeway space has been developed.

Cases in which no natural tooth contact occurs

Where no contact of natural teeth occurs on mandibular closure, the registration must be made via the use of occlusal rims in one or both jaws as necessary. The height of the occlusal surfaces of the rims is adjusted until contact of rim and teeth and/or rim and rim occurs at a vertical dimension providing the required freeway space. A particular type of case of this category which is frequently encountered is that where an edentulous maxilla opposes a partially dentate mandible, the standing natural teeth being the six lower anteriors. Establishing the vertical dimension in this type of case requires initially that the upper occlusal rim be developed as in a complete denture case. Wax is added or subtracted from the labial and buccal aspects of the rim until it is judged that correct lip, and cheek support has been developed. The occlusal surface of the rim is then developed so as to lie at the required level relative to the upper lip and so that it is parallel to the interpupillary and ala–tragal lines. The mandible is then closed to bring the standing anterior teeth in contact with the occlusal surface of the rim, and the freeway space (if any) which is present at this contact height is measured relative to the rest vertical dimension. The contact relationship between the upper rim and the lower standing teeth is then adjusted until the required freeway space has been achieved. This will usually necessitate softening the rim surface in the area where the teeth contact to allow the teeth to indent the rim, so developing an overbite. Occasionally, where excessive freeway space is found to be present, it will, instead, be necessary to increase the depth of the upper rim until contact occurs at an acceptable value of freeway space.

ESTABLISHING THE CORRECT HORIZONTAL RELATIONSHIP

Two methods may be used to establish the correct horizontal jaw relationship. Selection of the method to use in an individual case is based on an assessment of the intercuspal relationship of the dentition which is present.

1. Where the number and disposition of the standing teeth in both jaws are such that when the mandible closes in a retruded relation, a definitive and regular intercuspal relationship develops at the correct occlusal vertical dimension, this horizontal contact relationship should be the one which is registered.

2. In all other cases, the relationship which is registered should be that of retruded jaw relationship (centric jaw relationship), as utilised in complete denture construction.

Establishing horizontal jaw relationship by use of the intercuspal relationship of the natural dentition

The procedures that can be used to obtain the registration are as follows.

1. Hand occlusion of the casts

In a small number of cases it will be found that when upper and lower casts are placed into occlusion by hand they will locate in a constant and definite manner. A check should be made that the relationship of the casts so developed parallels that observed in the natural dentition in the closed relationship. Where this condition is satisfied, no further registration procedure need be applied. The method has the advantage that no registration material lies between the teeth; hence, the risk of the recording being made at an increased vertical dimension is avoided.

2. Use of a wax wafer registration. a zinc oxide–eugenol impression paste registration, or a buccal plaster record

Where an adequate number of teeth are present (which usually involves bilateral contact on premolars and molars), and yet the casts will not themselves locate in a definitive position, a wax wafer registration may be used. The wax wafer should be stabilised by incorporation of a metal plate, as previously noted in the consideration of the development of the vertical relationship. The wax horseshoe is thoroughly softened and then placed between the upper and lower teeth. The mandible is closed in a retruded position until the maximal intercuspal relationship of the teeth is achieved. The wafer is removed from the mouth, chilled in cold water, and then buccal excess wax is trimmed off until the remaining portion of the registration lies within the cuspal arch. The trimmed wafer is then replaced in position on the teeth and repeated mandibular closure is applied, to ensure that a consistent intercuspal relationship has been recorded. Removal of buccal excess wax facilitates observation of this relationship, and also aids correct positioning of the wafer on the casts in the subsequent procedure in which the casts are mounted on an articulator.

A disadvantage arising from the use of a wax wafer registration is that the wax always has a positive thickness — it is impossible to expel wax totally from between teeth which would, otherwise, come into full contact in the absence of the wafer. The registration is thus obtained at a slightly increased vertical dimension relative to that of tooth contact. Some operators prefer to use zinc oxide–eugenol impression paste instead of wax for the registration, since this may reduce the increase in vertical dimension which arises. Such a registration can best be obtained by using a wire carrier frame covered with gauze, to facilitate positioning of the paste between the arches. A low-viscosity type of zinc oxide–eugenol impression paste should be used in the procedure. The paste is mixed and a thin layer placed over the gauze. The frame is immediately placed around the lower teeth, and the mandible is closed until maximal intercuspal relationship is achieved. This position must be maintained until the paste is fully set.

Yet another alternative is the use of a buccal plaster record. Here, the patient is requested to close into the position of maximal intercuspal relationship. With maintenance of this jaw relationship, a mix of impression plaster at the 'putty' stage is massaged into the right and left buccal sulci, to lie over the contacting teeth. When the plaster has set, the right and left records are removed and may subsequently be positioned on the casts to provide the required location. In theory the method is excellent, in that no increase in vertical dimension should occur. Some difficulty may be encountered, though, in achieving full location of the plaster records on the casts, and this problem restricts the use of this procedure.

3. Use of occlusal rims

Where an insufficient number of teeth are present to allow the registration to be made by procedure 1 or 2, the use of occlusal rims will be necessary in one or both jaws. Where the occlusal surface of a rim opposes standing teeth, a layer of modelling wax, approximately 2 mm deep, is added to the occlusal surface of the rim, and the wax is thoroughly softened by use of a hot wax knife. The rim is seated in the mouth and mandibular closure applied until maximal intercuspal contact of opposing natural teeth occurs. Where the occlusal surface of a rim opposes that of another rim in the opposing jaw, the registration procedure used should follow that utilised in complete denture construction. A notch is cut in one rim surface (usually the upper one), and about 2 mm of wax is cut away in the opposing area of the lower rim, to provide an escape way for excess wax. A pillar of softened modelling wax is now built on to the lower rim opposite the notch, providing a volume of wax which is just a little more than that estimated as necessary to fill the notch and make up the cut away portion of the rim. The rim is inserted and mandibular closure applied, until maximal intercuspal contact of the opposing natural teeth occurs.

Where the registration is being carried out to allow mounting of working casts on an articulator, and the denture design includes use of a cast metal framework, the reader is reminded that the metal framework should be used as the baseplate on which any necessary occlusal rim areas are constructed. This will ensure that a baseplate of optimal retention and stability is used in the registration, and avoid the risk of one potential error — that of baseplate distortion — arising in the registration procedure.

Establishing horizontal law relationship at the position of mandibular retrusion

Where the contact of standing teeth does not provide adequate indication of horizontal jaw relationship at the required occlusal vertical dimension, the registration procedure should parallel that utilised in complete denture construction. This need will arise in cases of the second and third types considered on page 153 in relation to the establishment of the correct occlusal vertical dimension.

The registration is based on achieving retruded jaw relation (centric jaw relation) at the established vertical dimension of occlusion. A common procedure utilised to develop the required position of mandibular retrusion is to ask the patient to curl their tongue upwards and backwards until the tip lies in contact with the posterior palatal tissues. Other procedures may sometimes prove to be necessary (see Ch. 10). Repeated mandibular closure should be applied and a note made via rim marking or otherwise that a reproducible position of full retrusion is being achieved. Location of this position is then obtained, usually by use of softened modelling wax added to appropriate areas of a wax wafer or occlusal rim. A wax/tooth relationship or a rim/rim relationship (via use of notching) is recorded, as previously described. Care should be taken that the previously developed occlusal vertical dimension is not disrupted in this process.

Although modelling wax provides a satisfactory means of recording jaw relationships in most cases, alternative procedures are desirable where a free-end saddle is present in the lower jaw, especially where it extends to the premolar region. If, in the recording procedure, pressure is applied to the occlusal surface of a rim overlying a lower free-end edentulous span, the rim will descend tissuewards due to displacement of the underlying soft tissues. The registration will thus be recorded in a position of tissue displacement. No such displacement will occur when the registration is subsequently placed on the cast, and the position of upper and lower casts will be different than that present in the oral cavity at the time of registration. If the casts are mounted on an articulator using such a registration and the artificial teeth are set up, premature contact of the posterior teeth will be seen at the trial denture stage. To overcome this problem, it is necessary to record the relationship applying minimum load to the free-end saddle area of the rim. This can best be achieved by reducing the level of the free-end saddle rim until it is free of contact with the opposing teeth or opposing occlusal rim surface by about 2 mm. Notches are cut in the lower occlusal rim surface to provide location, and then impression plaster at the 'putty' stage is placed over the rim and mandibular closure applied to achieve retruded jaw relation. This position is maintained until the plaster has set. When the casts are assembled by use of such a record, their relationship will now coincide with that present intra-orally.

Whatever method of recording of the vertical and horizontal jaw relationships is selected for use, the casts should always be assembled via use of the record obtained, and a check made for coincidence between the relationship of the casts and that seen by examination of the oral tissues. This should be done while the patient is still in the chair, so that any errors noted can be corrected at that visit.

ADDITIONAL RECORDS FOR OCCLUSAL ANALYSIS

Where study casts are to be mounted on an adjustable articulator to allow full occlusal analysis, the following additional records will be required.

A face-bow record

In the partially dentate situation, the method used to locate the face-bow fork orally in relation to the maxilla will depend upon the number of standing teeth present in the maxilla. Where teeth are present in the anterior and both posterior segments, the link may be achieved by allowing the teeth to indent softened modelling wax wrapped around the face-bow fork. Where this condition is not satisfied, the fork will be attached to a maxillary occlusal rim.

Other features of the procedure for obtaining the record, and for using it to mount the maxillary cast, will be as described in Chapter 11.

A protrusive and/or right and left lateral records of jaw relationship

These will allow setting of the condylar inclinations of the articulator.

Where standing teeth are present in both jaws in the anterior and right and left posterior segments, the registration(s) may be obtained using a wax wafer alone. The wax should be about 3 mm thick initially, and be wide enough to allow upper and lower teeth to indent the wax in a position where the mandible is either about 4 mm anterior, or lateral, to the position of retruded jaw relation. Where insufficient standing teeth are present to meet this requirement, the registration(s) is made using a wax wafer placed between occlusal rims in one or both jaws as necessary. Location of the wafer on the occlusal surfaces of the rims is achieved via the cutting of notches in the rim surfaces.

The further procedure for obtaining the records, and for using them to set the condylar inclinations of the articulator, are as described in Chapter 11.

SELECTION OF TEETH

It is usual to select the artificial teeth for denture construction at the conclusion of the jaw registration stage of treatment. In partial denture prosthodontia, especially where natural teeth are present both anteriorly and posteriorly, selection of the artificial teeth can be a much simpler task than that which may face the operator in complete denture prosthesis. Examination of the standing teeth and of the edentulous spaces will provide guidance on the size, form, texture and colour of anterior teeth to be used and on the size, form and colour of posterior teeth to be used.

Where standing teeth are absent in either the anterior or posterior regions, it may be necessary to select appropriate teeth using the guiding principles considered in Chapter 12. In all cases, though, the colour of the standing teeth should be used as a guide to selection of the colour of the artificial teeth.

In relation to the selection of the material from which the artificial teeth are made, the choice rests between acrylic resin and porcelain. In partial denture prosthesis, there is much to be said in favour of the selection of porcelain teeth. When set in opposition to natural teeth, porcelain posterior teeth will resist occlusal wear much better than acrylic resin teeth.

Where a partial denture is to be mucosa supported, as in the use of maxillary dentures of the

'Every' form, the development and maintenance of good contacts between the natural and artificial teeth is essential to obtain adequate retention. Such contacts will be maintained better in the service life of the denture where porcelain teeth have been used, because of their better wear resistance. Unfortunately, the irregular nature of the occlusal surfaces of natural teeth, combined with the fact that there is often minimal space available between the occlusal surface of an artificial tooth and the underlying edentulous ridge, often necessitates considerable grinding of the artificial teeth in the setting-up process. The mechanical system of retention which is necessary in porcelain artificial teeth (normally, diatoric holes in posterior teeth and pins in anterior teeth) limits the degree of grinding which can be applied to such teeth without loss of retention occurring. Thus, despite the theoretical advantages offered by porcelain teeth, it is often necessary to use acrylic resin teeth in partial denture prosthodontia.

As part of the selection process, it is important that the patient should be questioned as to any special wishes they may have. For example, they may request the use of facsimile restorations to duplicate the original natural dentition. Any special requests which the patient may make in relation to tooth arrangement should also be noted at this stage.

PRESCRIPTION WRITING

The information necessary to allow the technician to proceed to the stage of preparing trial dentures is as follows:

1. The type of articulator to be used.
2. An indication that the maxillary cast should be mounted via use of a face-bow record, where one has been taken.
3. A request that the mandibular cast be mounted in relation to the maxillary cast, utilising the record of vertical and horizontal relationship provided.
4. Requirements in relation to the setting of the condylar inclinations, where an adjustable articulator is to be used, and protrusive and/or right and left lateral records of jaw relationship have been taken.

5. Details of the required setting of the angle of the incisal guidance table, where a fully adjustable or semi-adjustable articulator is to be used.

6. Full details of the artificial teeth which have been selected for use, along with any required modifications to the teeth (e.g. facsimile restorations).

7. Guidance on any special features of tooth arrangement not provided by occlusal rims (e.g. rotation or overlapping of individual teeth).

FURTHER READING

Beckett LS 1954 Accurate occlusal relations in partial denture construction. J Prosthet Dent 4: 487

Beyron HL 1954 Characteristics of functionally optimal occlusion and principles of occlusal rehabilitation. J Am Dent Assoc 48: 648

Boos RH 1962 Maxillomandibular relations, occlusion, and the temporomandibular joint. Dent Clin North Am 19

Braley BV 1972 Occlusal analysis and treatment planning for restorative dentistry. J Prosthet Dent 27: 168.

Lundquist DO, Fiebiger GE 1976 Registration for relating the mandibular cast to the maxillary cast based on Kennedy's classification system. J Prosthet Dent 35: 371.

McCracken WL 1958 Functional occlusion in removable partial denture construction. J Prosthet Dent. 8: 955

Silverman MM 1953 The speaking method in measuring vertical dimension. J Prosthet Dent 3: 193.

18. The principles of tooth arrangement

INTRODUCTION

Tooth arrangement should aim at aiding the achievement of the objectives of removable partial denture provision. As noted in Chapter 13, the objectives may be summarised as follows:

1. Restoration of appearance
2. Restoration of masticatory efficiency
3. Restoration of speech to a normal quality
4. Maintenance of the health and integrity of the soft and hard tissues of the oral cavity.

Achievement of the first of these objectives will mainly be influenced by the arrangement of any anterior teeth carried by the partial denture, while achievement of the second objective will mainly be dependent on the arrangement of any posterior teeth carried by the denture. Objectives 3 and 4 can be helped by appropriate placement of anterior teeth and/or posterior teeth.

For convenience, the principles of arranging the anterior teeth and the posterior teeth will be considered in separate sections. It should be realised, however, that many partial dentures replace both anterior teeth and posterior teeth. Where this applies, the arrangement of the anterior and posterior teeth should be integrated to create a harmonious unit with the standing natural dentition.

ARRANGEMENT OF THE ANTERIOR TEETH

Where some anterior teeth only are to be replaced

Here, the arrangement of the teeth to be replaced should simulate that of the standing natural anterior teeth in relation to length and axial inclination. In general, the development of a symmetrical arrangement about the midline is desirable. Special note should be made of any ageing features which are present in the natural dentition, such as incisal wear and gingival recession at the necks of the teeth. Where present, these features should be simulated in the setting of the replacement teeth.

Wherever possible, the development of tight contact points between the natural and replacement teeth should be obtained. In the case of mucosa-supported dentures, friction at contact points can play a significant role in the achievement of retention.

Often, it will be found that the natural standing teeth will not be all the same colour. The optimal aesthetic result will usually be achieved by selecting replacement teeth for the span concerned with a colour which presents a compromise between the colours of the abutment teeth.

Occasionally, colour matching from the available range of stock teeth is difficult, perhaps because of the presence of abnormally stained natural teeth. Where necessary, teeth of the required colour can be individually prepared in the laboratory using dentine-type acrylic resins of an appropriate shade. Alternatively, stock teeth may be modified by the application of surface stains.

Where all the anterior teeth are to be replaced

Here, the anterior teeth should be arranged in a manner similar to that used in complete denture construction. An upper occlusal rim should be available, the labial surface of which has been contoured to indicate the required setting of the teeth to achieve correct lip support. The occlusal

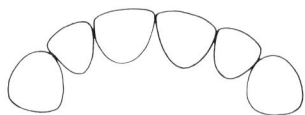

Fig. 18.1   Plan view of an arrangement for the upper anterior teeth appropriate for a female patient.

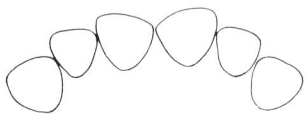

Fig. 18.2   Plan view of an arrangement of the upper anterior teeth designed to produce a heightened masculine effect.

plane of the rim should have been developed to indicate the required incisal edge level of the teeth, and the centre line should have been marked. The anterior teeth should then be arranged in conformity with the information provided by the occlusal rim. Tight contacts should be developed with the posterior abutment teeth which are present.

In Chapter 12, which dealt with the principles of tooth selection, reference was made to the work of Frusch and Fisher in the development of 'dentogenic restorations'. Their principles can also provide a useful guide at the stage of tooth arrangement. For a female patient, an appropriate arrangement may be achieved by setting the labial surfaces of the upper anterior teeth to lie on a smooth arc (Fig. 18.1). In contrast, masculinity may be signified by developing a more angular (cuboidal) tooth arrangement. For a male patient whose personality is judged to be at the vigorous end of the spectrum, the masculine effect may be heightened by setting the two upper central incisors so that they lie a little anterior to the lateral incisors, the labial surface of all four incisors facing anteriorly (Fig. 18.2).

ARRANGEMENT OF THE POSTERIOR TEETH

In the introduction to this chapter, reference was made to the role of the posterior teeth in developing masticatory efficiency in a removable partial denture. The level of masticatory efficiency which is achieved will depend mainly on the cuspal form of the posterior teeth which are used, and on arranging the teeth so that optimal stability is obtained.

Stability, in turn, will be influenced by three factors:

1. The positioning of the teeth relative to the underlying residual alveolar ridge.

2. The positioning of the teeth relative to the environmental musculature (the neutral zone concept).

3. The degree to which occlusal balance is attained.

Often, these factors present opposing needs in tooth placement. The interplay of the factors and the way in which a compromise setting is decided upon to achieve optimal stability is considered in some detail in Chapter 25, which deals with the parallel situation in complete denture construction.

It should be noted that occlusal balance is often more difficult to achieve in partial dentures than in complete dentures. This is due in part to the irregular nature of the occlusal surfaces presented by many natural teeth. In addition, guidance from the contact relationship of the natural teeth often results in a steeply inclined mandibular movement path. In all instances, though, every effort should be made to develop the highest possible level of occlusal balance. This can be helped by the use of replacement teeth with a cuspal form similar to that of any natural posterior teeth which are present.

When setting the replacement posterior teeth, it is important that the role they play in developing the aesthetics of the dentition should not be overlooked. Although of less importance than the anterior teeth in terms of direct display, the first premolars at least are often visible when the patient smiles. If an unnatural appearance is to be avoided, the first premolars should be set to present a balanced length relative to the adjacent canines. A sudden transition in length between the anterior and posterior teeth, especially in the maxilla, is rarely seen in the natural dentition, and should be avoided when setting the replacement teeth on a partial denture.

Further features of the arrangement of posterior teeth can best be considered according to the presence or absence of posterior natural teeth.

Where some posterior teeth only are to be replaced

Where the posterior teeth are to be set in a bounded saddle situation, they should normally be set to lie in a straight line drawn through the centres of the abutment teeth. Either a normal or cross-bite arrangement may be developed, as indicated by the situation of the opposing dentition. In all instances, an adequate buccal overjet should be developed to reduce the risk that cheek-biting will occur.

It should be noted that, in partial denture prosthodontia, substitution of teeth relative to the natural predecessors is permissable and, indeed, is often desirable. For example, where an upper first premolar is to be replaced, and the jaw relationship is such that little if any functional contact can be developed with the lower opposing teeth, a more aesthetic result will often be achieved by substituting an extra canine for the premolar. In many instances, it will be found that tilting and drifting of the natural teeth leaves less space for the positioning of the replacement teeth than the space originally occupied by their natural predecessors. In such instances, substitution may again be required. For example, the space originally occupied by two molars may only now present space for the placement of, say, a premolar and molar as the replacement teeth.

Where the posterior teeth are to be set on a free-end saddle, the procedures considered in the next section should be followed.

Where all the posterior teeth are to be replaced

The free-end saddle situation encountered here poses special problems in posterior teeth arrangement, especially in the case of a lower denture.

Basically, the teeth need to be arranged to achieve optimal stability, and this requires that they be set in a manner similar to that used in the posterior segments in complete denture construction (considered in Chapter 25). Where opposing natural posterior teeth are present, some departure from the 'ideal' arrangement may be necessary, in order to achieve a functionally acceptable occlusal relationship.

Modifications in tooth arrangement in the free-end saddle situation may also be necessary to reduce the load which is applied to the tissues underlying the saddle. The rationale for this move is considered in Chapter 22. Load reduction, where indicated, may be achieved by reducing the size of the occlusal table. This can be done by reducing the number of teeth which are set (for example, omitting the second molars) or by using smaller teeth than might otherwise have been used. Reducing the buccolingual width of the replacement teeth relative to that of the natural predecessors will help. It is, indeed, often advocated that such width reduction should be applied in all instances where posterior teeth are replaced, and not just in the free-end saddle situation.

FURTHER READING

Frush JP, Fisher RD 1958 The dynesthetic interpretation of the dentogenic concept. J Prosthet Dent 8: 558
Henderson D 1971 Occlusion in removable prosthodontics. J Prosthet Dent 27: 151
Weiner S, Krause AS, Nicholas W 1987 Esthetic modification of removable partial denture teeth with light cured composites. J Prosthet Dent 57: 381
Zarb GA, MacKay HF 1981 Cosmetics and removable partial dentures — the class IV partially edentulous patient. J Prosthet Dent 46: 360

19. The trial denture stage of treatment

INTRODUCTION

This stage of treatment may require action in two phases:

1. Trial of a cast metal framework, where one is included in the design of a partial denture.
2. Trial of the partial denture, with the replacement teeth arranged on a temporary or 'permanent' (metal) baseplate.

The examination procedure which should be carried out in each of these phases is considered in the following sections. Advice will also be given on the actions necessary where faults are detected in the course of the examination procedure.

TRIAL OF A CAST METAL FRAMEWORK

Checking fit

It is advisable generally for this to be carried out before any wax additions have been made to the metal framework. The absence of wax facilitates visual examination of the fit of the framework, and also makes it easier to carry out modification of the framework where this proves to be necessary.

The framework should be positioned correctly over the standing natural teeth, and gentle seating pressure applied along the path of insertion selected when the study cast was surveyed. It should be found to slide easily into the fully seated position, only moderate resistance being encountered, corresponding to the retentive value of any clasps which are present. If any undue resistance to movement is encountered in the seating process, excessive force should not be applied as this may cause discomfort, or make it difficult to remove the framework

subsequently without overstressing the periodontal attachment of the tooth or teeth concerned. By visual and tactile examination, an attempt should be made to determine where resistance to further movement is occurring. Location of the exact site of resistance can be assisted by the use of a disclosing wax. An even layer of the wax, approximately 1 mm thick, should be applied to the fitting surface of the framework in the area under investigation. The framework should then be inserted up to the point where resistance to further movement is encountered. The insertion path of the framework should be reversed carefully and the fitting surface then examined. The resistance area will be revealed as the area where the wax has thinned to display the underlying metal.

Often, resistance to movement will be found to arise at interproximal metal/tooth contact areas, or at the origin of clasp arms. If the thickness of metal at the resistance area is such that it is felt that the metal could be reduced without adversely affecting the strength of the framework, then grinding may be undertaken. Carborundum stones may be used for grinding a gold alloy framework, but special abrasion-resistant stones, usually based on aluminium oxide, should be used to trim a cobalt–chromium alloy casting. The procedure of trial insertion of the framework, location of resistance areas and grinding of the areas should be repeated until either satisfactory insertion is obtained, or it is judged that any further modification by grinding would endanger the strength of the denture. Where the latter applies, it will be necessary to take a further impression, prepare a new metal framework and repeat the examination procedure.

When satisfactory insertion of a framework has been obtained, the fit of all the component elements should be examined with the aid of a mouth mirror. A probe may also be used to check the closeness of fit of any elements contacting the teeth. Clasp arms should be checked for non-traumatic placement relative to the gingival margins of the teeth. The various component elements should also be checked for correct positioning relative to the soft tissues. For example, gingivally approaching clasp arms should not enter soft tissue undercuts. Palatal connectors on an upper framework should be in contact with the underlying tissues. Where a lingual bar has been used in the design of a lower framework it should be correctly positioned relative to the gingival margins of the standing teeth and the functional level of the lingual sulcus.

The patient should be questioned as to whether or not they feel any discomfort when the framework has been inserted. Where the patient can detect a pressure area, particularly in relation to covered soft tissues, it may be necessary to relieve pressure in the area concerned by grinding the fitting surface of the framework. Disclosing wax may be used, where necessary, to locate the site of pressure. Before grinding is applied, the framework should be carefully examined to check that the intended reduction in section will not unduly prejudice its strength.

Checking retention and stability

Retention should be checked by attempting to displace the framework from its fitted position in a direction reversing the path of insertion, noting the resistance that is encountered. Due allowance needs to be made for the fact that full retention may not be present at this stage. Where the design includes the use of wrought clasps, these are unlikely to be present at the stage of trial of the metal framework, but will be added later.

Stability of the framework should be checked by applying pressure on various elements — rests, saddles and palatal connectors in particular — and noting whether any rotational displacement occurs. Special attention is necessary when checking the stability of a framework carrying one or two free-end saddles. It is usual for the free-end saddle portion of a metal framework to have been relieved

from tissue contact in the constructional procedure, to enable the saddle to be relined where this is subsequently required. Before testing the stability of the free-end saddle element of a metal framework which has been relieved from tissue contact, it is advisable that a wax baseplate be positioned to bridge the gap between the metalwork and the underlying tissues.

Where the design of the partial denture includes the use of a stress-breaker, especially where this is of type 1, (Chapter 14, p. 128), an appreciable degree of rotational displacement should be observable when pressure is applied to the metalwork of the free-end saddle. Where no stress-breaker has been used, and yet an appreciable degree of rotational displacement of the free-end saddle occurs when this check is applied, there is a need for subsequent action to be taken to overcome this instability. This will usually involve relining of the free-end saddle at the insertion stage of treatment.

Checking aesthetics

The framework should be inserted and its appearance noted when the patients lips are at rest and when the patient is smiling. If any elements of the metalwork are visible when the patient smiles, it is advisable to point this out to the patient and show them what is involved with the aid of a hand mirror. If proper care has been applied in the stages of treatment planning and denture design, objections to the aesthetics of a metal framework should be rarely encountered. Where objections do arise, they usually relate to an unaesthetic display of clasp arms or incisal rests. Where this is due to an unnecessary thickening having occurred in the construction of the framework, it may be possible to overcome the objections by reducing the thickness of the element concerned by grinding.

Checking the occlusion

The framework should be inserted and the occlusal relationship of the teeth checked. In those cases where the natural teeth contact at the required occlusal vertical dimension, the relationship which occurs with the framework inserted should be the same as that which occurs when the framework has been removed. If the presence of the metal framework is seen to cause any disruption to the occlusal relationship of the natural teeth, articulating paper should be used to indicate where premature contact is occurring. Caution must be exercised when analysing the contact pattern produced by articulating paper, as its interpretation requires careful visual observation in order to ensure that markings arise from tooth contact. Correction may be applied by grinding either the metalwork or the natural tooth at the point of premature contact. The metal should be selected for grinding only where it is judged that this can be carried out without undue weakening of the framework. Often, a combination of grinding of both tooth and metal is used, to avoid undesirable disruption of either. The process of detection of points of premature contact and their reduction should be continued until occlusal harmony is re-established.

Where the natural dentition does not contact at the required occlusal vertical dimension, and the design of the framework includes onlays, a check should be made that, with the framework inserted, the opposing natural teeth and the metalwork contact evenly at a vertical dimension providing an acceptable freeway space. Where necessary, articulating paper can be used to detect the site of any premature contact areas. Where interference has been shown to be present, grinding of the natural teeth and/or of the metal framework should be applied, until an acceptable occlusal relationship has been established.

General observations

On completion of the above check procedures for a metal framework, it will be possible to develop an overall appraisal of its satisfaction or otherwise. In all cases, where one or more of the checks have revealed the presence of unsatisfactory features which cannot be corrected in the ways indicated, it will be necessary to take a new impression and prepare a new metal framework. This may repeat the original design, or may involve modifications where indicated. The check procedures listed above should be applied to the new framework. Only when a framework has been shown to be fully satisfactory should the next stage be undertaken — that of setting the replacement teeth to develop a trial denture.

It should be noted that it is inadvisable to attempt to rectify any faults which are present in a framework (for example, inadequate retention in clasp arms) by bending the framework. It is virtually impossible to apply bending without disrupting the essential passive placement of the elements relative to the oral tissues. A bent framework may well give rise to appreciable tissue damage.

TRIAL OF THE PARTIAL DENTURE

The procedures used in checking a partial denture at the trial stage are similar to those used at the corresponding stage of complete denture construction, and they should be applied in the same order. The procedures are as follows.

Checking extension, retention and stability

The extension of the baseplate on the master cast should be checked for conformity with the outline requested on the design prescription form. The denture should be inserted and the extension of any flanges which are present should be checked in relation to the levels of the functional sulci. Where appropriate, the position of the posterior border of an upper baseplate should be checked for correct relation to the vibrating line. Where extension faults are found to be present, they should be corrected by addition or subtraction to the baseplate as necessary.

The fit of the baseplate on the master cast should be noted. The denture should then be inserted and a check made that a similar fit is present on the hard or soft tissues covered by the baseplate. Where a discrepancy is evident between the fit of the baseplate on the master cast and the fit in the mouth, there is an indication that an error has occurred in the previous stages of impression taking or cast preparation. Before proceeding further, it will then be necessary to repeat these and other intermediate stages and to prepare a new partial denture for retrial.

When the fit of the baseplate has been shown to be satisfactory, the retention of the denture should be checked. This involves determination of the resistance to displacement which arises when a force is applied to the denture in a direction reversing the path of insertion. It should be noted that the retention present at this stage, except where a cast metal framework incorporating cast clasps forms the baseplate, is likely to be appreciably less than that achievable in the final (processed) denture. The presence of reasonable retention is, however, a prerequisite for being able to carry out satisfactorily subsequent check procedures and, when absent, consideration should again be given to the need to repeat the impression and subsequent stages before proceeding further.

Stability of the denture should be checked by applying pressure in a tissuewards direction to the replacement teeth at a series of points around the arch. If a rotatory displacement of the denture is seen to occur, the cause of this should be sought and an appropriate remedy should be applied. The most common finding will be that the replacement teeth have been positioned buccal or labial to the crest of the residual alveolar ridge to an excessive degree. Where this applies, the teeth should be reset to a position where stability is achieved.

Where a free-end saddle is present, it should be checked for the display of anteroposterior rotatory displacement when pressure is applied to the teeth on the saddle.

As previously noted in relation to the trial of a metal framework (p. 164), where such displacement arises it may be an intentional feature of the design of the denture, as where a type 1 stress-breaker has been used. Alternatively, where no stress-breaker has been used, subsequent action will be necessary to overcome the rotation. This will usually involve relining of the saddle at the insertion stage of treatment.

Checking aesthetics

The denture should be inserted and the appearance of the patient noted with the mouth closed, with the lips slightly parted and with the patient providing a full smile. The patient should also be given a hand mirror and invited to make similar observations.

Where the visible aspect of the occlusal plane and/or centre line of the dentition is developed by the replacement teeth, these features should be checked for compliance with the appropriate facial landmarks.

It should be borne in mind that the result will be influenced not only by the replacement teeth but also by the form of any buccal or labial flanges carried by the denture. Of particular importance will be any gingival contouring which is displayed when the patient smiles. This should harmonize with that of any natural teeth which are visible.

Where either the operator or the patient are unhappy about any of the aesthetic features of the denture, chairside modification should be carried out until a mutually acceptable result has been achieved. This may involve resetting of the replacement teeth and/or modification of the form of the flanges.

Checking the vertical component of the jaw relationship

Where the occlusal vertical dimension is defined by the contact of opposing natural teeth, the denture should be inserted and a check made that both the natural teeth and the replacement teeth on the denture meet evenly at this vertical dimension.

Where the natural standing teeth do not meet at the occlusal vertical dimension, the denture should be inserted and a check made that even contact of the artificial teeth and the natural teeth (including onlays where used) occurs at a vertical dimension which provides an acceptable value of freeway space.

The procedures that should be used to correct any errors found to be present at this check stage are considered in conjunction with those used to correct any errors found in relation to the horizontal component of jaw relationship, and appear below.

Checking the horizontal component of jaw relationship

Note should be made of the intercuspal relationship of the natural and artificial teeth as developed on the articulator. Where the number and relative positioning of the natural teeth provide a definite intercuspal relationship in the horizontal plane, the denture should be inserted and the patient persuaded to close into this relationship. In all other cases, the patient should be persuaded to close into the retruded jaw relationship. The intercuspal relationship which is present intra-orally should coincide with that previously observed on the articulator.

When this requirement is not satisfied, or where an error was found to be present at the previous stage of checking the vertical component of jaw relationship, a new registration must be taken.

Where an error was found to be present in the vertical component of jaw relationship, this should be corrected first. The artificial teeth should be removed from the denture and the corresponding areas replaced by wax occlusal rims. The height of the rims should be adjusted until contact occurs between the rims and opposing natural teeth, and/or between opposing rim surfaces, at the required occlusal vertical dimension.

A new registration should then be made of the horizontal component of jaw relationship. Where natural teeth oppose a rim surface, the registration should normally be obtained by adding softened modelling wax to the rim surface and registering the indentations of the teeth in this wax when the patient closes into retruded jaw relationship. Where the registration is to be made between opposing rim surfaces, a notch should be cut in the upper rim and about 2 mm should be removed from the surface of the lower rim in the area opposite the notch. Softened modelling wax should then be built up on the lower rim surface to an extent judged to be necessary to fill the notch in the upper rim. The previous step of reducing the depth of the lower rim provides an escape way for any excess wax which is present. The patient should then be persuaded to close into retruded jaw relationship until the rim surfaces contact. It should be noted that where a decision was made to use a low-pressure registration procedure when the original registration was made (usually because of the presence of a free-end saddle), this procedure should also be used in reregistration.

At the conclusion of reregistration of the horizontal component of jaw relationship, a check should be made that an acceptable freeway space is still present. Unless the procedures for registration of the horizontal component have been applied carefully there is a risk that the previously developed vertical component will be changed.

The casts should then be remounted on the articulator to the relationship given by the new registration, and new trial dentures developed by resetting of the replacement teeth. The checks listed for application at the trial denture stage should then be repeated at a subsequent visit of the patient. If necessary, the procedures for reregistration and redevelopment of a trial denture should be repeated until satisfaction is achieved. Authority for finishing the denture should never be given until both patient and operator are fully satisfied with the result at the trial denture stage.

When satisfaction has been achieved, two final observations should be made, where necessary, before the patient is dismissed:

1. Where an upper denture is being provided, and a palatal plate in a polymeric denture base material is to be used, if the plate is to extend to the vibrating line then the correct position for the posterior border of the denture should be clinically determined. Note should also be made of the displaceability of the tissues in this area, via the use of an instrument such as a ball-ended burnisher. A post-dam preparation should then be made on the cast in the manner used in complete denture construction (see Ch. 26).

2. The denture-bearing areas should be examined and a decision made as to whether any relief zones are required, where the denture will not come into contact with the underlying tissues. Where relief is required, the tissue areas concerned should be mapped out on the casts.

PRESCRIPTION WRITING

When a trial denture is returned to the laboratory for finishing, the following information should be provided:

1. The colour and nature of the denture base material to be used.

2. Details of position and depth of any peripheral seal lines required at the borders of palatal connectors in an upper denture.

3. Details of any areas which require relief. Information on the site and depth of relief areas should be given in the written prescription, supplemented by the mapping out of the required extent of relief areas on the casts. Sites which frequently require relief include a torus palatinus which is to be covered by an upper denture base, and the gingival areas of standing teeth, where these are to be covered by connectors.

FURTHER READING

Applegate OC 1965 Essentials of removable partial denture prosthodontics, 3rd edn. WB Saunders, Philadelphia

Culpepper WD 1970 A comparative study of shade matching procedures. J Prosthet Dent 24: 166

Fedi PF 1962 Cardinal differences in occlusion of natural teeth and that of artificial teeth. J Am Dent Assoc 62: 482

Lammie GA, Laird WRE 1986 Osborne and Lammie's partial dentures, 5th edn. Blackwell Scientific, Oxford

Silverman MM 1974 The comparative accuracy of the closest speaking space and the freeway space in measuring vertical dimension. J Acad Gen Dent 22: 34

Swoope CC 1970 The try-in — a time for communication. Dent Clin North Am 14: 479

Travalgini EA, Jannetto LB 1978 A work authorization format for removable partial dentures. J Am Dent Assoc 96: 429

20. The insertion stage of treatment

EXTRA-ORAL EXAMINATION

Before attempting to insert the finished partial denture, it should be checked carefully to ensure that no blemishes are present which could traumatise the oral tissues. Particular attention should be paid to the fitting surface of the denture. Where part, at least, of this has been constructed in a polymeric denture base material such as acrylic resin, the surface should be checked for the presence of any blebs arising from the presence of air cavities in the corresponding area of the cast on which the denture was processed. Where blebs are found to be present, they should be removed by the use of a sharp cutting instrument or by grinding, care being taken not to damage the surrounding surface of the denture.

Where metallic elements are present on the denture, they should be checked to ensure that no potentially traumatic features are present. For example, the free end of clasp arms should be rounded and not tapered to a sharp point.

Where connectors or other elements cross gingival margins, a check should be made that adequate relief has been provided.

The denture should be examined for the presence of any undercuts which might interfere with its insertion. Where undercuts are present, they may need to be modified in the course of the subsequent intra-oral examination procedure.

INTRA-ORAL EXAMINATION

The check stages which are used in the intra-oral examination of a finished partial denture are similar to those used at the trial denture stage, and they should be applied in the same order. If a regular routine is developed for checking dentures at both the trial and insertion stages of treatment, the risk that any individual stage will be overlooked will be reduced.

The following sections provide details of the checks that should be applied, along with advice on dealing with any problems that arise.

Checking fit

The denture should be positioned correctly in the oral cavity in relation to the standing natural teeth, and gentle pressure should be applied along the path of insertion. It should glide into a fully fitting position, the only resistance encountered corresponding to retentive features such as clasps which are present on the denture.

Where any appreciable degree of resistance to further movement is met in the course of attempted insertion of the denture, additional force should not be applied. Instead, an attempt should be made to determine the cause and site of the resistance. Providing that all unwanted undercuts on the standing teeth have been correctly blocked out in the course of denture construction, the resistance to movement will commonly be found to be arising from the presence of undercut flanges. These should have been noted during the extra-oral examination of the denture. The site where an undercut flange is becoming impacted on the underlying tissue as denture insertion is attempted is often made apparent by blanching of the tissues in the area concerned. The patient may also be able to provide evidence of the impaction area by indicating where pressure or pain is arising in the course of attempted insertion of the denture.

Any undercut flanges which are found to be

preventing denture insertion should be modified to reduce, or, where necessary, eliminate the undercut which is present. This may be achieved by reduction of flange extension or, where flange thickness permits, by the trimming of the fitting surface of the flange.

Modification of the denture should be continued until insertion into the fully fitting position has been achieved.

Checking extension, retention and stability

The extension of the inserted denture should be checked for compliance with the level of the functional sulci. Any peripheral over-extension which is found to be present should be removed by trimming of the area or areas concerned.

Retention should be checked by inserting the denture and applying a force in a direction away from the underlying tissues and along a path reversing that of insertion. A definite resistance to displacement should be observable, the value of which must be at least equal to the displacing forces which arise during mastication, if denture displacement in function is to be avoided. Because of its subjective nature, the retention check presents difficulty for the inexperienced operator.

Stability should be checked by inserting the denture and applying pressure in a tissueward direction to the replacement teeth at a series of points around the arch. No displacement of the denture should occur except, perhaps, where free-end saddles are present. The latter may show an anteroposterior rotatory displacement when pressure is applied to the teeth on the saddles. This may be an intentional feature of the design of the denture where a stress-breaker is present. In other cases, where no stress-breaker has been used, the finding implies a need for corrective procedures to be applied. These usually involve the relining of free-end saddles. The special impression procedures which are used in the relining of the saddles are considered in Chapter 16 (p. 149).

Checking aesthetics

The denture should be inserted and the appearance of the patient noted with the mouth closed, with the lips slightly parted and with the patient providing a full smile. The patient should also be given a hand mirror and invited to make similar observations.

The result should simulate that approved by both patient and operator at the trial denture stage. Occasionally, some modification of the depth or width of flanges may be necessary, to achieve the required degree of support for the facial tissues. This need should only arise where flange form has been accidentally modified in the course of denture finishing.

Checking the vertical component of the jaw relationship

Where the occlusal vertical dimension is defined by the contact of opposing natural teeth, the denture should be inserted and a check made that both the natural teeth and the replacement teeth on the denture meet evenly at this vertical dimension.

Where the natural standing teeth do not meet at the occlusal vertical dimension, the denture should be inserted and a check made that even contact of the artificial teeth and the natural teeth (including onlays where used) occurs at a vertical dimension which provides an acceptable value of freeway space.

If either of these conditions is not satisfied, a thin grade of articulating paper should be used to determine the point or points where premature contact is occurring. Premature contacts should be ground and this process repeated until full harmony between the natural and artificial dentition has been established at the required vertical dimension.

Checking the horizontal component of the jaw relationship

Where the intercuspation of the natural dentition provides a definitive position in the horizontal plane, the denture should be inserted and the patient persuaded to bring the teeth into contact in this relationship. In all other instances, the patient should be persuaded to bring the teeth into contact in retruded jaw relationship. The observed interdigitation of the natural and artificial teeth should be the same as that approved at the trial denture stage. If a minor error in the occlusal relationship of the teeth is apparent, the site of premature contact should be determined by the use of a thin grade of articulating paper. Selective grinding of premature contacts should be carried out until a harmonious relationship of the natural and artificial dentition has been established.

Where any major error in the occlusal relationship of the teeth is seen, remaking of the denture will usually be necessary.

It should be noted that procedures for remounting and selective grinding of dentures on an articulator are rarely used for partial dentures, because of the difficulties which arise from the presence of natural teeth.

INSTRUCTIONS TO THE PATIENT

When a partial denture has been found to be satisfactory by application of the check procedures detailed above, the patient should be given verbal instructions on the care and maintenance of the denture and the associated oral tissues. It is desirable that the verbal instructions should be reinforced by the provision also of written instructions. This is particularly important where the patient is either elderly or handicapped, since there is a risk that verbal instructions alone will be either misunderstood or forgotten.

The instructions should be designed to enable the patient to learn to use the denture as quickly as possible, and to get the greatest possible benefit from it. The points covered both verbally and in written form should be as follows.

1. Eating may be difficult at first. Food should be cut into small pieces and adequate time allowed for chewing. Tough and sticky foods are best avoided in the initial learning period.

2. Difficulty may be experienced in removing a new partial denture. Where the denture contains thin metal parts, these should not be used to lever out the denture. Instead, only the plastic parts of the denture should be held, both when removing and replacing the denture.

3. The denture should be removed from the mouth and cleaned after each meal. A soft brush, soap and cold water are satisfactory for cleaning.

Alternatively, a proprietary denture cleanser may be used, following the manufacturer's instructions. Household bleach solutions should not be used as they may damage the denture. Where metal parts are present on the denture, great care should be taken not to bend these during cleaning, or the denture could be ruined.

In addition to the denture, the natural teeth must also be cleaned thoroughly after each meal. With the denture removed, a toothbrush and toothpaste should be used in the usual way. This is very important since a partial denture can lead to food being trapped around the natural teeth, with associated increased risk of tooth decay or gum disease occurring.

4. The denture should be removed at night and stored in water, to prevent drying-out and warping.

5. Pain and soreness may occur when a new denture is first worn, and adjustment of the denture may be necessary to overcome this. If the pain becomes severe the denture should be left out, and an appointment arranged with the dental surgeon as soon as possible. The denture should be worn on the day of the appointment so that the sore area will be visible. The patient should not attempt to adjust the denture, or irreparable damage could arise.

FURTHER READING

Abelson DC 1985 Denture plaque and denture cleansers: a review of the literature. Gerodontics 5: 202
Bassiouny MA, Grant AA 1975 The toothbrush application of chlorhexidine. Br Dent J 139: 323
Bassiouny MA, Grant AA 1981 Oral hygiene for the partially edentulous. J Periodontal 52: 214
Bauman R 1979 Minimising post-insertion problems: a procedure for removable partial denture placement. J Prosthet Dent 42: 381
Blatterfein L 1958 Rebasing procedures for removable partial dentures. J Prosthet Dent 8: 441
Lawson WA 1965 Information and advice for patients wearing dentures. Dent Pract Rec 15: 402
Lawson WA, Bond EK 1969 Speech and its relation to dentistry. Dent Pract Dent Rec 19: 150
Neill DJ 1968 A study of materials and methods employed in cleaning dentures. Br Dent J 124: 107
Storer R 1962 Partial denture saddle correction. Br Dent J 112: 454

21. The review stage of treatment

INTRODUCTION

Following the insertion of a partial denture, an appointment for review in approximately 7 days should be made for the patient.

At the review visit, the patient should be questioned concerning any problems that have been experienced when wearing the denture. A detailed examination should then be carried out of the oral cavity and the denture, in the course of which signs of symptomless tissue damage may be noted. A diagnosis is then made of the cause of all the problems revealed in the history and examination procedures. Appropriate treatment should then be applied to overcome these problems.

HISTORY OF THE PATIENT'S EXPERIENCES

The patient should be asked to give an account, in his or her own words, of any difficulties that have occurred since the denture was inserted. The commonest complaint will be that of pain. Where this applies, the patient should be asked how long the pain has been present, and whether it is relieved by leaving out the denture. Note should also be made as to whether the pain is localised to one area of the oral tissues or is widespread, and whether any analgesics or other medication have been used to try to alleviate the pain. The operator should also establish whether the pain is present continually when the denture is being worn, or if it only arises at certain times, e.g. when eating.

The second most commonly encountered complaint is that the denture seems to be loose. Where this applies, the patient should be asked if the denture is loose all the time, or only when chewing food or speaking. The patient should also be asked to indicate whether displacement seems to initiate from a particular area of the denture, and, if so, where this is.

Less commonly, the patient will complain that the denture has caused problems with appearance or speech. Where the complaint relates to appearance, the patient should be asked to indicate the exact nature of the problem. For example, where anterior teeth are replaced by the denture, do the teeth seem to be too large or too small, or do they show too much or too little? Alternatively, are denture flanges producing exaggerated or deficient support for the lips and cheeks? In relation to complaints concerning speech, the patient should again be asked to indicate the exact nature of the problem. For example, does whistling or lisping arise during pronunciation of the 's' sound, or is difficulty being encountered with the 'plosive' sounds 'p' and 'b'?

A further complaint which is occasionally encountered is that of intolerance to the presence of the denture in the oral cavity. Where this problem arises, the patient should be asked how long the denture can be worn before it has to be removed. The patient should also be asked whether any special circumstances arise which necessitate removal of the denture. For example, does it make him or her feel sick, or produce actual retching? Alternatively, does it produce the sensation of an unpleasant taste in the mouth, or lead to a 'gripping' feeling in the mouth, which could be likened to the effect which the wearing of a new pair of shoes can produce on the feet?

EXAMINATION OF THE ORAL CAVITY AND THE DENTURES

The denture should be removed from the mouth and a thorough examination made of the oral tissues, with the help of a mouth mirror. Particular attention should be paid to any areas where the patient has experienced discomfort, but all the oral tissues should be examined, since symptomless changes may be observed which warrant treatment. The soft tissues should be checked for signs of injury or inflammation, which may vary in intensity from mild hyperaemia to frank ulceration. Where the patient has complained of discomfort in relation to the standing natural teeth, the crowns of the tooth or teeth concerned should be rechecked to exclude the presence of any disease process. The level of oral hygiene being maintained by the patient should be noted. The periodontal status of the tooth or teeth concerned should also be reassessed, including a test for the presence of tenderness to percussion. Radiographic examination should be carried out where thought to be necessary.

The denture should be examined extra-orally, to recheck that no irregularities are present on the fitting surface which could have caused tissue irritation. The denture should then be inserted and the peripheral form examined for the presence of any areas of overextension. Retention should be checked for adequacy, and stability checked by applying pressure in a tissuewards direction on tooth-bearing areas of the denture. The aesthetic effect of the denture should be observed, particularly in relation to any complaints of poor appearance raised by the patient. The occlusal vertical dimension should be checked to ensure that an acceptable value for freeway space is present. The dentition should also be checked to ensure that the natural and artificial teeth develop a harmonious relationship when closure occurs in retruded jaw relationship or, where appropriate, in the jaw relationship dictated by the intercuspal relationship of the natural dentition.

THE CAUSE AND MANAGEMENT OF PATIENTS' COMPLAINTS

The history of the patient's experiences when wearing a new partial denture, and the examination of the oral cavity and the denture, should enable a diagnosis to be made of the cause of the patient's complaints. A decision must then be made of the appropriate treatment, which may, for example, involve modification of the denture where this is indicated.

In this section, the common causes of patients' complaints will be considered and advice given on the necessary treatment. The subject will be discussed under a series of headings representing major patient complaints.

Pain

Where pain has arisen in a *localised* area of the soft denture-bearing tissues, the likely causes are one or more of the following:

1. Overextension of the periphery of the denture.
2. Excessive engagement of an undercut by a denture flange.
3. Inaccuracy in the denture fitting surface, e.g. the presence of an irregularity not paralleled in the corresponding area of the soft tissues.
4. The presence of a premature contact in the occlusal relationship of the dentition, arising in either a static occlusal relationship, or during dynamic movements of the dentition.
5. Accidental damage to the denture, e.g. a clasp arm having been bent during cleaning.
6. Attempts by the patient to remove or insert the denture along paths other than the ones intended for withdrawal and insertion.

The above causes will usually have produced clearly visible signs of inflammatory changes in the soft tissues in the areas concerned. Visual examination of the inserted denture will usually have provided an indication of the area of the denture responsible for the tissue change. Where necessary, though, disclosing wax or pressure relief cream may be used to indicate the causative area of the denture.

Treatment of causes 1, 2 and 3 will require modification of the denture by trimming of the area concerned, until painful symptoms have been relieved. Cause 4 will require adjustment of the occlusion by selective grinding, until the premature contact has been obliterated. Cause 5 will require replacement of the defective clasp unit where this is feasible, otherwise remaking of the denture will be necessary. Cause 6 will necessitate the patient receiving further instruction in the correct procedures for inserting and removing the denture.

Where the complaint of pain arises from a *diffuse* area of soft tissues covering most, if not all, of the denture-bearing zone, the likely cause will be the presence of an excessive occlusal vertical dimension. If examination of the denture reveals the absence of an acceptable value for freeway space, treatment of the condition will necessitate remaking of the denture at a reduced value of occlusal vertical dimension.

At other times, a complaint of diffuse pain may be restricted to only part of the denture-bearing tissues. Here, the cause often relates to anatomical abnormality in the tissues concerned. For example, a sharp mylohyoid ridge may be present or, where a lower partial denture carries an anterior saddle, the pain may relate to the presence of a sharp superior margin in the residual alveolar ridge, or may be due to atrophy in the overlying mucosa. In some instances, relief of pain arising from these causes may be obtained by judicious relief of the corresponding area of the fitting surface of the denture, to reduce the pressure which is applied on the tissue area concerned. Where this is unsuccessful, treatment may necessitate surgical intervention. For those patients for whom surgery is contraindicated, the placement of a resilient lining in the denture may be considered.

Where the complaint of pain is localised to one of the standing natural teeth, the cause is likely to be overstressing of the periodontium of the tooth. This may arise through the application of excessive vertical load to the tooth, as where an occlusal rest on the tooth is in premature contact with the opposing dentition. Where this applies, the appropriate treatment will be occlusal adjustment to remove the premature contact. Alternatively, the problem may arise through excessive force application to the tooth in the horizontal plane, as where a clasp arm has been accidentally bent by a patient so that it engages an excessive undercut. Treatment here will require the damaged clasp unit being replaced where this is feasible, otherwise remaking of the denture will be necessary.

In some instances, a complaint of pain will relate to oral soft tissues external to the denture-bearing zone. For example, tongue irritation may arise through the presence of a sharp superior margin on a metal plate. Both the tongue and the cheeks may be injured by oversharp ends on clasp arms. Any such traumatic features should be removed by smoothing the elements concerned.

More commonly, though, the complaint will be due to tongue or cheek biting. The usual cause of this problem is lack of buccal overjet on the posterior teeth or, in the case of tongue biting, narrowing of the arch leading to inadequate provision of space for the tongue.

Where a complaint of cheek biting of a relatively mild degree arises in a case in which a lower denture provides replacement of the posterior teeth, resolution of the complaint can often be effected by grinding the buccal aspects of the lower molar teeth and rounding over the bucco-occlusal margins, to develop an improved buccal overjet. If, in a similar type of case, the complaint is that of tongue biting of a relatively mild degree, grinding the lingual aspect of the lower posterior teeth may successfully resolve the condition, by increasing the space available for the tongue. Where either tongue or cheek biting have occurred to a severe degree, it will usually prove to be necessary to reset the teeth to achieve the arch form or buccal overjet necessary to overcome the complaint.

Looseness of the denture

If the patient complains that the denture is loose when he or she is talking and eating, and at other times when no definite function is being performed, the probable causes are:

1. Overextension of the periphery of the denture relative to the level of the functional sulcus. If examination shows overextension to be present, the area of the denture concerned should be reduced by peripheral trimming.

2. Incorrect shaping of the denture relative to the environmental musculature. This cause is particularly liable to affect a lower partial denture if inadequate space has been allowed for the tongue. In some cases, the problem can be overcome by grinding of the lingual aspect of the denture (including the teeth where necessary) to increase tongue space, but often remaking of the denture will prove to be necessary.

3. Inadequate retention. In mucosa-supported dentures this may arise due to inaccurate fit of the denture base, or inadequate development of contact points between the artificial and natural teeth. Alternatively, in a tooth-supported denture, where clasps have been placed on the abutment teeth to obtain retention, the clasps may be incorrectly positioned relative to available undercuts. Where this applies, treatment will usually necessitate re-making of the denture.

If the patient complains that the denture is only loose when he or she is masticating foods, the likely cause is a lack of occlusal balance in the artificial dentition. Thin articulating paper and visual examination should be used to detect cuspal interferences which arise during protrusive and lateral excursions of the mandible. Selective grinding should then be carried out until the maximum possible level of occlusal balance has been achieved.

Where a partial denture carries free-end saddles, a complaint by a patient may arise that the denture moves during mastication of food (and sometimes at other times too). Examination may reveal the presence of an anteroposterior rock of the free-end saddle when pressure is applied to it. Treatment of this condition will usually involve relining of the saddle.

Problems with the appearance of the denture

A complaint of unsatisfactory appearance should rarely arise if adequate care was taken at the trial denture stage. Where complaints concerning the appearance of the denture are brought out by the patient at the review stage, questioning will often reveal that they arise from comments provided by the patient's relatives and friends. As far as possible, an attempt should be made to overcome the complaints by modification of the denture. For example, flanges may be modified in depth or thickness to increase or reduce, as necessary, the support of the facial tissues. Changes in tooth colour or tooth arrangement, where called for, can usually only be effected by remaking the denture.

Speech problems

Many patients encounter a minor speech disruption when a new denture is first worn. They should be reassured that this is likely to go in a period of a month or so, as the oral tissues adapt to the presence of the denture.

In some instances, though, the speech disruption may be such as to warrant denture modification. One instance of this is where pronunciation of the letter 's' is affected. The sound 's' is most commonly produced by the tip of the tongue being placed close to the palatal aspects of the upper anterior teeth and the anterior palatal tissues, to develop a narrow air channel. Where an upper partial denture has been provided which replaces the anterior teeth, if the teeth have been set too far forward the air gap may be excessive, and the patient may 'whistle' when pronouncing the letter 's'. Alternatively, if the anterior teeth have been placed too far back, or the anterior palatal aspect of the denture is too thick, the air channel may be too narrow, and the patient may lisp when pronouncing the letter 's'. Treatment of a whistling effect will require the air channel being reduced by wax additions until the correct sound is produced, the added wax subsequently being converted into the appropriate polymeric denture base material. To correct lisping, the air channel should be increased by grinding the palatal aspects of the teeth and the denture base material in the anterior palatal area, until the correct 's' sound is produced.

Another condition which will require treatment is where the patient complains of difficulty with the 'plosive' sounds 'p' and 'b'. These sounds are formed by the lips being closed to allow intra-oral build-up of air pressure. The lips are then suddenly parted to allow escape of air and development of the required sound. If the patient complains of difficulty with these sounds, the problem may arise due to the presence of an excessive occlusal vertical dimension, which makes it difficult for the patient to effect the necessary lip seal. If the patient presents with this speech problem, the vertical dimension of the dentures should be carefully checked. If found to be excessive, treatment will require remaking of the dentures.

Intolerance to wearing a partial denture

Although uncommon, this problem is by no means rare and can be very distressing to a patient. Usually found in association with the wearing of an upper partial denture, the main cause is enhanced sensitivity in the posterior palatal tissues, producing an abnormal retching reflex action. Increased sensitivity in the dorsum of the tongue can also initiate retching, if the denture contacts the tongue.

Where the problem is of a severe nature, it will almost certainly have become evident in the early stages of treatment, particularly during impression taking. Appropriate steps should then be taken in denture design to minimise the problem. Where the sensitivity lies in the palate, the palatal connector of an upper partial denture should be shaped to avoid coverage of the posterior palatal tissues. Where the sensitive organ is the tongue, an upper partial denture should be designed to have maximum retention, and a lower partial denture should provide the greatest possible space for the tongue.

Where the problem has only become evident at the review stage, the treatment required will depend upon the length of time that the patient can wear the denture before it has to be removed. With an upper denture, if the time is short — a matter of seconds or minutes only — it will usually be necessary to reduce the extension of the denture in the posterior palatal region, until tolerance improves. A posterior palatal seal should then be added at the new level of connector extension. Where the onset of the problem is delayed for a longer period — perhaps 6–8 hours after insertion, the cause may lie in excessive bulk in the denture. In this case, the base should be thinned to the limit allowed by strength requirements. Otherwise, all that will usually be required is reassurance of the patient that with persistence the problems will be overcome.

Further aspects of the problem of intolerance to denture wearing appear in Chapter 28, which is devoted to a consideration of the review stage in complete denture treatment.

Other complaints

The patient may raise a number of complaints at the review stage not covered in the above list. Frequently, there will be a complaint of excessive salivation. Where the denture includes metallic elements there may be a complaint of a metallic taste in the mouth. Dentures with metallic elements that are fitted in a mouth in which metallic restorations are present in the natural teeth may also give rise to a complaint of occasional pain in the natural teeth through galvanic action.

Complaints of this nature are usually of a short life span, and the patient should be reassured that the problems will resolve in the fullness of time.

General note

In all instances where the periphery, teeth or polished surface of the denture have been modified at the review stage, the areas concerned must be carefully repolished before the denture is returned to the patient.

Where severe tissue damage was noted at the review stage, an appointment for further review in approximately 7 days should be made for the patient, to ensure that the treatment provided has effected resolution of the condition. Further reviews at intervals of approximately 6 months should be arranged in all cases, so that both the denture and the standing natural teeth can be re-examined and any necessary treatment carried out.

FURTHER READING

Farrell J 1968 Partial denture tolerance. Dent Pract Dent Rec 19: 162

Guckes AD, Smith DE, Swoope CC 1978 Counselling and related factors influencing satisfaction with dentures. J Prosthet Dent 39: 259

Helel KS, Graser GN, Featherstone JD 1984 Abrasion of enamel and composite resin by removable partial denture clasps. J Prosthet Dent 52: 389

Hoad-Reddick G 1986 Gagging — a chairside approach to control. Br Dent J 161: 174

Lawson WA, Bond EK 1969 Speech and its relation to dentistry. Dent Pract Dent Rec 19: 150

Lechner SK 1985 A longitudinal survey of removable partial dentures. I. Patent assessment of dentures. Aust Dent J 30: 104

Lechner SK 1985 A longitudinal survey of removable partial dentures. II. Clinical evaluation of dentures. Aust Dent J 30: 194

Lechner SK 1985 A longitudinal survey of removable partial dentures. III. Tissue reaction to various denture components. Aust Dent J 30: 291

Miller EC 1977 Clinical management of denture-induced inflammations. J Prosthet Dent 38: 362

Morstad AT, Peterson AD 1968 Post-insertion denture problems. J Prosthet Dent 19: 126

22. The free-end saddle partial denture

INTRODUCTION

In this chapter, some of the problems faced in the design and construction of removable partial dentures carrying free-end saddles will be discussed. Dentures of this type are used to provide replacement of missing teeth in Kennedy class I and class II dentitions. The reader is reminded of the need to satisfy the biological requirement in partial denture prosthodontia, which places the preservation of the remaining tissues as the first priority.

Reports of surveys which have appeared in the literature serve to illustrate the difficulties which can arise in meeting this aim in the free-end saddle situation.

For example, where such dentures have been designed to be of a simple, mainly mucosa-supported form, Anderson and Lamie reported a widespread tendency for the periodontal tissues of the standing teeth to be traumatised, involving gingival inflammation, retraction of the gingivae and increased mobility of the abutment teeth. In another survey on dentures of that form, Koivumaa reported the occurrence of inflammatory reactions of the mucosa supporting the denture base, as well as a hastening of the rate at which resorption occurred in the edentulous alveolar ridges.

Where, instead, the dentures had been designed to include support from the standing dentition, a somewhat improved picture of tissue response has been reported, although tissue damage still occurred. For example, Carlsson, Hedegärd and Koivumaa found that after only 12 months' wear of such dentures, many patients showed inflammatory changes in the tissues at the gingival margins of the abutment teeth, along with increased mobility of the teeth. These changes were particularly apparent where the pa-

tient had failed to maintain a high standard of oral hygiene.

Despite the difficulties which are highlighted by surveys such as those quoted above, the chance of achieving biological acceptability with a free-end saddle type of partial denture will be improved where the patient has been motivated to maintain a high standard of oral hygiene. The operator should also have an understanding of the design problems which are peculiar to this type of denture, so that other steps can be taken to minimise the risk of tissue damage occurring.

DESIGN PROBLEMS

These will be considered under two main headings:

1. The provision of support for the free-end saddle partial denture.

2. The provision of retention for the free-end saddle partial denture.

The provision of support for the free-end saddle partial denture

A free-end saddle may be either mucosa supported or tooth-and-mucosa supported. From the biological point of view, there is much to be said in favour of the saddle being made mucosa supported. This will ensure that when vertical masticatory forces are applied to the free-end saddle they will be spread relatively evenly over the whole of the mucosal surface underlying the saddle. The provision of mucosal support for the free-end saddle should also ensure that potentially damaging forces will not be transferred to the abutment tooth.

In the case of maxillary partial dentures, mucosal support for free-end saddles can be achieved by designing the whole denture to be mucosa supported. As noted in Chapter 15, mucosal support is a viable proposition for maxillary dentures, because of the availability of the hard palate which can be utilised to gain support. It is desirable that dentures of this type should be constructed following the principles advocated by Every, in order to help the maintenance of the health of the remaining periodontal tissues.

Where only one free-end saddle is present on a maxillary denture, the Every principles can often be successfully applied, especially if two or more bounded saddles are present in addition to the free-end saddle. Where two free-end saddles are present and no additional bounded saddles exist, the prognosis for success with the Every mucosa-supported denture is much decreased, due to the likely lack of the development of adequate retention and stability. To counter this problem, it will often prove to be necessary to place direct retainers on the abutment teeth. Where, as is usual, these take the form of retentive clasp arms, it will be necessary also to place rests on the abutment teeth, in order to ensure correct location of the clasp arms on the teeth. The desirable principle of the free-end saddles being mucosa supported is thereby lost, the saddles becoming tooth-and-mucosa supported.

In the case of mandibular partial dentures carrying free-end saddles, there is an almost universal need for rests to be placed on the abutment teeth to achieve an acceptable level of support. Here, there is no hard palate available to aid the support of the denture. If rests are omitted, the whole of the vertical masticatory load applied to the saddles will fall on the relatively small area of mucosa underlying the saddles, which may respond by showing pathological change. In addition, if bilateral free-end saddles on a mandibular partial denture are to be solely mucosa supported, it will be necessary to use a non-tooth-bearing connector such as a lingual bar. Although biologically satisfactory as far as the teeth are concerned, such a denture is likely to lack retention and stability to a level which will prove unacceptable to the majority of patients. To attempt to overcome this problem there is a temptation to replace the lingual bar with a lingual plate and to place retentive clasp arms, but no rests, on the

abutment teeth. This approach, however, creates conditions which can lead to severe damage in the periodontal tissues. Over a period of time, it is almost inevitable that alveolar resorption will occur in the tissues underlying the free-end saddles. Where resorption occurs, it will allow the denture to adopt a different seating position from that present at the time of insertion. As a consequence of the displacement of the denture the lingual plate may become traumatic to the gingival tissues of the covered teeth. Contact may also be lost between the lingual plate and the underlying teeth, increasing the potential for plaque retention, with the accompanying risk that tissue damage will arise.

Retentive clasp arms placed on the abutment teeth may descend to a level where they become traumatic to the gingival tissues. Dentures of this type have rightly been termed 'gum strippers', and their use should be avoided. To prevent such consequences, it is necessary to utilise the abutment teeth to provide support for the denture, usually achieved by the use of rests. Then, and only then, may retentive clasp arms be placed safely on the abutment teeth, the rests serving to correctly locate the clasps arms on the teeth.

Thus, in a proportion of maxillary dentures carrying free-end saddles, and in the majority of mandibular partial dentures carrying free-end saddles, it is necessary to place rests on the abutment teeth. This results in the free-end saddles becoming tooth-and-mucosa supported rather than mucosa supported, as ideally desired. The creation of a condition of tooth-and-mucosa support in a free-end saddle raises the need to develop an equitable distribution of load between the two supportive tissues. If either the abutment tooth or the tissues underlying the free-end saddle are overloaded, irreparable damage may arise.

However, achieving the desired equitable distribution of load between the abutment tooth and the tissues underlying the free-end saddle can be difficult. To illustrate this point, consider the position in a mandibular partial denture with a free-end saddle providing replacement of 35, 36 and 37. An occlusal rest, rigidly attached to the saddle, has been placed on the disto-occlusal fossa of the abutment tooth, and clasp arms, to provide bracing, retention and reciprocation, have also been placed on the abutment tooth.

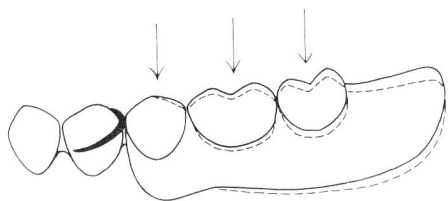

Fig. 22.1 Displacement of a free-end saddle under vertical load.

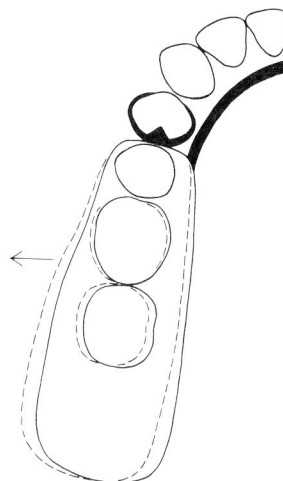

Fig. 22.2 Displacement of a free-end saddle under horizontal (lateral) load.

When vertical masticatory loads are applied to the free-end saddle they will be transferred both to the abutment tooth (via the rest) and to the mucosal tissues underlying the saddle. The anterior end of the saddle will be mainly tooth supported, the descent of the saddle under load being restricted by the fibres of the periodontal membrane of the abutment tooth. The posterior end of the saddle will be able to descend to a greater extent, lying as it does on the much more displaceable mucosa over lying the alveolar bone (Fig. 22.1). As a consequence, a rotatory torque will be applied to the abutment tooth in the sagittal plane.

Laterally directed forces in the horizontal plane will also be applied to the saddle, when masticatory movements of the saddle occur. At the anterior end of the saddle, movement will be restricted by the link between the saddle and the abutment tooth, via the occlusal rest and the clasp arms. Posteriorly, the saddle is freer to move, as the underlying displaceable mucosa offers less resistance (Fig. 22.2). A rotatory torque thereby arises on the abutment tooth in the horizontal plane.

Additional torque will be applied to the abutment tooth where posterior teeth of the anatomical form have been used. This torque force arises during protrusive mandibular movements where opposing cuspal surfaces meet in a protrusive position, and sliding then occurs to return the mandible into the maximal intercuspal contact position. By an inclined plane effect, a horizontal force component arises which is directed anteriorly in the maxilla and posteriorly in the mandible.

The combined effect of the above forces may well result in permanent damage to the periodontal tissues of the abutment tooth. If prolonged, exfoliation of the tooth can be the eventual outcome.

In addition to the effect on the abutment tooth, the effect on the supporting tissues underlying the saddle must also be considered. Here, the applied loads will be concentrated posteriorly, due to the lack of posterior tooth support. This may result in an accelerated degree of alveolar resorption occurring posteriorly. Once this has occurred, the descent of the posterior aspect of the saddle under vertical load will take on a dynamic quality, and a vicious circle of progressively increasing damage to both the abutment tooth, and the supporting tissues underlying the saddle, will be set in motion. It is clearly important that steps should be taken to reduce to a minimum the risk that such tissue damage will arise. The available procedures are considered in a subsequent section.

The provision of retention for the free-end saddle partial denture

There are two aspects of retention which need to be considered:

1. The provision of direct retention
2. The provision of indirect retention.

The provision of direct retention

The potential for achieving direct retention in a free-end saddle by placement of tooth-borne direct retainers is likely to be less than that of a bounded saddle, as retention can only be obtained at the mesial end of the saddle. Where it is desired to obtain direct retention by placement of a clasp unit on the single abutment tooth, the absence of usable undercuts on the tooth creates an additional problem.

Careful attention needs to be paid to the rigidity of a minor connector used to join a tooth-borne direct retainer on the abutment tooth to the free-end saddle. In general, the greater the rigidity of this connector, the greater will be the risk that potentially damaging torque forces will be applied to the abutment tooth, when masticatory forces are applied to the saddle.

The provision of indirect retention

The fact that partial dentures may show rotatory displacement in function has been noted in Chapter 15, (p. 135). The problem is encountered most commonly in partial dentures carrying bilateral free-end saddles and no bounded saddles (Kennedy class I dentition). When the patient is chewing sticky foodstuffs, the denture may rotate about an axis joining the rests placed on the abutment teeth on each side. The free-end saddles move away from the underlying tissues whilst, simultaneously, the anterior portion of the denture (forward of the axis of rotation) is depressed in a tissuewards direction. If rotatory displacement of this type occurs, it can be a source of embarrassment to the patient, and can also give rise to appreciable tissue damage anteriorly.

POSSIBLE SOLUTIONS TO THE DESIGN PROBLEMS

These will be considered under the same headings as used in the consideration of the design problems:

1. Possible solutions to the problem of providing support for the free-end saddle denture.
2. Possible solutions to the problem of providing retention for the free-end saddle denture.

Possible solutions to the problem of providing support for the free-end saddle partial denture

Four main procedures have been suggested for use. In a given case they may be used singly, or in any possible combination. They are as follows:

1. Selective load distribution between the supporting tissues
2. Reduction of the load applied to the saddle
3. Optimal spreading of load
4. Use of pressure impressions.

Selective load distribution between the supporting tissues

When load is applied to a free-end saddle which is tooth-and-mucosa supported, part of the load will be applied to the abutment tooth (via the support retention unit on the tooth), and part will be applied to the mucosa underlying the free-end saddle. The distribution of the applied load between these two supporting tissues can be altered by varying the rigidity of the connector used to join the support/retention unit on the abutment tooth to the saddle. If the rigidity of this connector is high, the proportion of the load applied to the abutment tooth will be at a maximum. Where, instead, a flexible connector is used, the proportion of load applied to the abutment tooth will decrease, and that applied to the mucous membrane under the saddle will increase. The more flexible the connector which is used, the greater will be the proportion of the load falling on the mucous membrane. Flexible connectors used for the purpose of achieving such selective load distribution are termed 'stress-breakers'. The various types of stress-breakers that may be used in association with either a precision attachment or a clasp unit on the abutment tooth are considered in Chapter 14 (p. 128).

The decision as to whether or not a stress-breaker is to be used and, where indicated, the type of stress-breaker to be chosen for use is based on a clinical assessment of the load-bearing potential of the two supporting tissues. Where it is judged that the abutment tooth can safely bear the brunt of the applied load, the use of rigid connection between the saddle and the support/retention unit on the abutment tooth is indicated. At the opposite end of the scale, where the periodontal status of the abutment tooth is suspect and the trabecular structure of the alveolar bone underlying the free-end saddle indicates that a favourable response to load bearing by the bone is likely, the use of a flexible type of stress-breaker would seem to be indicated. Intermediate clinical findings may indicate the use of a stress-breaker of moderate flexibility. It should, however, be pointed out that the period for which flexible stress-breakers remain functionally active in service can be disappointingly short. Doubts have also been expressed as to whether their theoretical benefits are fully achieved in the clinical situation.

Reduction of the load applied to the saddle

If the load which is applied to a free-end saddle during the mastication of food is reduced, the risk that the load will cause damage to the supporting tissues will be correspondingly reduced. It has been found that load reduction can be achieved by reducing the size of the occlusal table of the free-end saddle.

To explain this load reduction, it has been suggested that during the mastication of food the masticatory muscles only apply the level of force which is needed to crush the amount of food placed on the occlusal table by tongue and cheek action. If the size of the occlusal table is reduced, the volume of food placed on the table will normally be proportionally reduced, correspondingly reducing the load applied to the free-end saddle by the masticatory muscles.

An alternative explanation for the load reduction which occurs when the size of the occlusal table is reduced is based on the fact that, for a given applied load, higher pressures will develop between opposing teeth. As a corollary to this, the level of pressure necessary to achieve efficient mastication can be achieved at a lower level of applied force than that necessary where a larger occlusal table is present.

There are three main ways by which reduction in the size of the occlusal table may be obtained:

1. By reducing the number of teeth set on the saddle. For example, on a saddle which would normally replace the premolars and first and second molars, the second molars may be omitted.
2. By reducing the occlusal size of the teeth which are set on the saddle, relative to the size of their natural predecessors. This is most commonly achieved by reducing the buccolingual dimension of the replacement teeth.

3. By substitution of the teeth. For example, a canine may replace a first premolar, or a premolar may replace a molar.

There is a limit to which this procedure can be applied, dictated by the need to maintain a reasonable level of masticatory efficiency in the replacement dentition. Some reduction in the occlusal table is, however, nearly always indicated in the free-end saddle situation, relative to the size of the occlusal table in the original natural dentition.

Optimal spreading of load

The more widely spread the applied load, the less will be the load per unit area which the supporting tissues have to bear. Load spreading can benefit both the abutment tooth and the mucous membrane and alveolar bone underlying the free-end saddle. The support obtained by placement of a rest on the abutment tooth may be aided by positioning an additional rest on an adjacent tooth. In some cases other teeth may also be used to provide auxiliary support. For example, where the design of a lower partial denture includes the use of a lingual plate, part of the load borne by the free-end saddle will be transferred to all the teeth covered by the lingual plate. A continuous clasp, when present, will perform the same function.

Useful though it is, the principle of optimal spreading of load on the natural teeth must be applied with caution in partial denture design. The desirability of keeping the design of a partial denture as simple as possible should always be borne in mind. All coverage of tooth substance, especially when associated with coverage of the gingival margins, increases the risk that caries or periodontal problems will arise.

No such caution is necessary in the application of the principle of optimal load spreading to the tissues underlying the free-end saddle. In all cases, the saddle should extend to the limit defined by a functionally trimmed impression, bucally and lingually. Posteriorly, an upper free-end saddle should extend to the pterygomaxillary fissure (hamular notch), and a lower free-end saddle should extend over the anterior third of the retromolar pad.

Use of pressure impressions

On p. 180, attention was drawn to the tissue damage which can arise where tooth-and-mucosa support is used in a free-end saddle. When load is applied to the saddle, the risk that rotatory displacement of the saddle will occur will be at a maximum when the impression of the denture-bearing tissues has been recorded using a minimal pressure technique. This condition will be approached when, as is common in partial denture prosthesis, alginate has been used as the impression material.

If, instead, a pressure impression was taken, the problem of rotatory displacement of the saddle under load would be reduced. Both the teeth and the tissues underlying the free-end saddle would be recorded under pressure. Only minimal displacement of the teeth would occur, to the extent permitted by the fibres of the periodontal membranes. A greater degree of displacement would occur in the tissues underlying the free-end saddle, the extent to which this occurs depending upon the value of the applied pressure. In theory, when a denture which has been made on a cast prepared from a pressure impression is inserted, it will fit in position with the tissues underlying the free-end saddle in a condition of displacement corresponding to that present when the pressure impression was taken. There is thus less scope left for displacement of the tissues to occur when masticatory or other loads are applied to the saddle, thereby lessening rotatory displacement under applied load.

As noted in Chapter 16, a pressure impression of a partially dentate dentition may be obtained by the use of a sectional compound impression. An alternative approach is to limit pressure to the edentulous area of the impression, using alginate in the tooth-bearing portion of the impression and compound or compound plus alginate wash in the edentulous area. Unfortunately, it is difficult to control the level of pressure which will be developed by such impression procedures. If the pressure reaches an excessive level it may give rise to highly undesirable conditions when the denture is inserted.

Since the denture, when seated in position, causes displacement of the tissues under the free-end saddle, the tissues will react by producing an upward force on the saddle as they endeavour to return to their resting state. If the direct retention of the denture is such that the denture stays in the fitted position, the tissues under the saddle will be under constant pressure. If this is excessive, the soft tissues may show a pathological reaction varying from hyperaemia to necrosis. Alternatively, if the direct retention of the denture is inadequate to maintain it in its fitted position, the recoil of the displaced tissues will cause the denture to move away from the tissues and, except when under biting load, the denture will no longer attain its correct position in the oral cavity.

Because of the problems which may arise where pressure impressions are taken at the impression stage of treatment they are rarely used. A safer alternative is considered to be that in which the denture is constructed on a cast prepared from a minimum pressure impression, but a saddle relining procedure is then applied, either during or at the end of denture construction. By this means, a more controlled level of displacement of the tissues underlying the free-end saddle can be achieved. This serves to reduce the level to which rotatory displacement occurs when load is applied to the free-end saddle, but does not reach the level where the problems associated with the use of pressure impressions arise.

The procedures that may be used include the Applegate 'altered cast' technique, and relining the free-end saddle of a completed denture prior to insertion. The necessary clinical and laboratory procedures are considered in Chapter 16 (p. 149).

Possible solutions to the problem of providing retention for the free-end saddle denture

These will be considered under the headings used in the discussion of the problems:

1. Possible solutions to the problem of providing direct retention.

2. Possible solutions to the problem of providing indirect retention.

Possible solutions to the problem of providing direct retention

Where it is desired to obtain direct retention for a free-end saddle by placement of a clasp unit on the single abutment tooth, and yet the tooth possesses no useable undercuts, it will be necessary to seek alternative means of obtaining retention. The available alternatives are considered in Chapter 14 (p. 114). For example, they include the placement of a crown on the tooth to develop undercuts artificially, or alteration of tooth contour by the application of acid etch composite to a suitable surface.

Where the direct retention developed by the placement of a clasp unit on the abutment tooth is judged to be inadequate to meet the retentive needs of a free-end saddle, additional retention can be obtained by positioning a second clasp unit on the contiguous tooth.

When designing a clasp unit to be used to obtain direct retention on the abutment tooth, it should be remembered that in the absence of a posterior abutment tooth the saddle will possess a wide zone of possible translatory paths (Fig. 22.3). Often, the only usable undercut area on the abutment tooth will be found to be present on the distobuccal surface near the gingival margin. If a gingivally-approaching arm of the Roach 'L' form is used to engage this undercut (Fig. 22.4), it will not prevent posterior displacement of the saddle. If posterior displacement of the saddle arises in function, the clasp arm will correspondingly move posteriorly and it will cease to have a retentive action.

To avoid the risk of this happening, if it is desired to use a gingivally approaching retentive clasp arm, the portion of the clasp contacting the tooth should be extended to enter the interproximal embrasure on the mesial aspect of the tooth (Fig. 22.5). Alternatively, resistance to posterior displacement of the saddle can be provided by the use of an occlusally approaching clasp arm (Fig. 22.6).

Where the survey line on the abutment tooth permits the use of either an occlusally approaching or gingivally approaching retentive arm, the preference is often for use of the gingivally approaching type, in that its inherent greater flexibility results in less risk of damaging torque forces being applied to the abutment tooth during masticatory function. This will particularly apply where a decision has been made not to incorporate a stress-breaker in the denture design.

Where direct retention on the abutment tooth of a free-end saddle is to be obtained by use of a

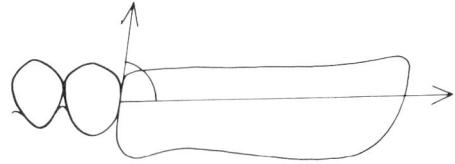

Fig. 22.3 Zone of translation of a free-end saddle (limits indicated by arrows).

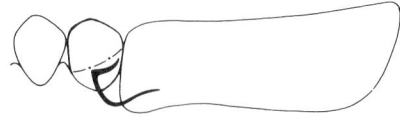

Fig. 22.4 A gingivally approaching clasp arm of the Roach 'L' form on the abutment tooth of a free-end saddle.

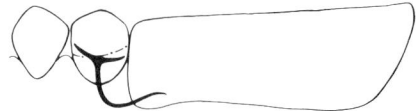

Fig. 22.5 A gingivally approaching clasp arm on the abutment tooth of a free-end saddle, designed to resist posterior displacement of the saddle.

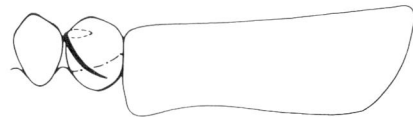

Fig. 22.6 An occlusally approaching clasp arm on the abutment tooth of a free-end saddle, designed to resist posterior displacement of the saddle.

precision attachment, the selection of a type of attachment incorporating a stress-breaker may be preferable, to avoid undue torque being applied to the abutment tooth. Suitable attachments are considered in Chapter 14 (p. 128).

Possible solutions to the problem of providing indirect retention

As noted previously, the need to provide indirect retainers to obtain resistance to rotatory displacement of a free-end saddle will be encountered most commonly where bilateral free-end saddles are present (Kennedy class I dentition). The various types of indirect retainers that may be used are considered in Chapter 14 (p. 119).

The type most commonly selected for use, because of its mechanical advantage, is the continuous clasp. Alternatives include Cummer arms, anterior placement of occlusal rests and, in the case of an upper denture only, the use of anterior palatal bars, palatal arms or anterior extensions of a palatal plate.

The improved stability which can be achieved in a partial denture by placement of indirect retainers needs to be weighed against their possible disadvantages. The latter include the biological disadvantages arising from increased coverage of soft or hard tissues of the mouth, and the fact that they may give rise to irritation of the tongue or other oral tissues. Their use is particularly indicated where long free-end saddles are present.

FURTHER READING

Anderson JN, Lammie GA 1952 A clinical survey of partial dentures. Br Dent J 92: 59

Carlsson GE, Hedegard B, Koivumaa KK 1961 Studies in partial denture prosthetics. II. An investigation of mandibular partial dentures with double extension saddles. Acta Odont Scand 19: 215

Frank RP 1986 Direct retainers for distal extension removable partial dentures. J Prosthet Dent 56: 562

Grady RD 1983 Objective criteria for relining distal-extension removable partial dentures: a preliminary report. J Prosthet Dent 49: 178

Hansen CA, Campbell DJ 1985 Clinical comparison of two mandibular major connector designs: the sublingual bar and lingual plate. J Prosthet Dent 54: 805

Jemt T Hedegard B, Wickberg K 1983 Chewing patterns before and after treatment with complete maxillary and bilateral distal-extension mandibular removable partial dentures. J Prosthet Dent 50: 566

Kroll AJ 1973 Clasp designs for extension base removable partial dentures. J Prosthet Dent 29: 408

Nairn RI 1966 The problem of free-end denture bases. J Prosthet Dent 16: 522

Neill DJ 1958 The problem of the lower free-end removable partial denture. J Prosthet Dent 8: 623

Preiskel HW 1977 The distal extension prosthesis reappraised. J Dent 5: 227

Spiekermann H 1986 Prosthetic and periodontal consideration of free-end removable partial dentures. Int J Periodont Rest Dent 6: 148

PART III

Special aspects relating to complete denture treatment

23. The impression stage of treatment

INTRODUCTION

As pointed out in Chapter 9, to enable accurate impressions of the oral tissues to be obtained it is mandatory that a two-stage impression procedure is used. Pressure impression methods can produce uncertain results, particularly when a closed-mouth technique is used, and it is not recommended that they be attempted by the inexperienced operator.

It is proposed to consider minimal-pressure and selective-pressure impression procedures for complete dentures. The choice of impression methods and materials for a patient under treatment is dependent on the clinical conditions present. Using the procedures to be described, a wide range of clinical conditions can be satisfied.

PRIMARY IMPRESSIONS

Impression compound is a thermoplastic material which is suitable for use in obtaining primary impressions of edentulous mouths. It is incapable of reproducing undercuts, but has very useful properties which enable an impression to be modified by trimming with a sharp knife to reduce excessive bulk, or additions to be made where underextensions exist, and for the impression to be reseated in the mouth as part of the modification procedure.

Impression compound is supplied in flat sheets of some 4 mm thickness. To prepare the material for use, it is placed in a water bath at 60–65°C, when it softens to form a plastic mass. Kneading of the softened compound helps to incorporate water into the mass, which acts as a plasticiser and also ensures that the material is softened uniformly throughout and is free of any lumps. When fully softened and kneaded, the compound is returned to the water bath to await its use.

Selection of stock trays

For the edentulous patient, stock trays having a curved form to the body of the tray are selected (see Fig. 9.1). The trays should be oversize to the extent of providing some 3 mm of space between the inner surface of the tray and the tissues to be impressed, and the flanges should not impinge on the frenal attachments.

The upper tray must extend posteriorly to cover the maxillary tuberosity and hamular notch regions, while being supported in correct relationship to the residual alveolar ridge in the anterior part of the mouth. The lower stock tray is selected to ensure coverage of the retromolar pads, while the tray is maintained in its correct relationship to the anterior aspect of the residual alveolar ridge.

Where the patient has existing dentures, tray selection is facilitated by observing the denture outline in relation to the stock tray. This is simply effected by resting the denture in the tray. The tray is unlikely to be of exactly the same form as the denture or the mouth to be impressed, and some form of compromise will almost certainly be required.

While generous dimensions of the trays have been recommended, gross overextension should be avoided, as this will cause distortion of the peripheral regions of the impression as a result of stretching of the tissues.

The upper primary compound impression

The selected stock tray is carefully warmed and dried by passing it above the flame of a Bunsen burner. Kneaded compound is removed from the water bath and moulded into the form of a ball, which is placed in the centre of the palatal region of the tray. Using the thumbs while supporting the tray with the fingers, the compound is spread across the inner aspect of the tray, being careful to avoid creases or folds forming on the surface. At the same time, a shallow trough form is developed in the surface of the compound, approximately corresponding to the form of the residual alveolar ridge. During this procedure, the temperature of the surface of the compound will have fallen, thus reducing its flow properties. To increase the flow properties, and thereby the ability of the material to record surface detail without the application of high pressures, it will be necessary to heat the exposed surface of the compound. This is conveniently carried out by flaming the surface of the impression material. Flaming consists of rapidly passing the exposed compound surface several times over the flame of a Bunsen burner, when the surface will appear very smooth and shiny. Burning or sizzling of the compound must be avoided.

The temperature of the compound surface will, at this stage, be too high to place in the mouth of a patient without the tissues being damaged, and the compound must be tempered before proceeding. Tempering the compound consists of immersing the loaded tray into the water bath in which the compound was originally softened. The temperature of the compound should now be tested gently with the wet palm of the hand. When satisfied that no tissue damage will occur in the mouth, the tray is inserted into the patient's mouth in the manner described in Chapter 9. The tray is centred over the crest of the residual alveolar ridge and pressure in an upwards and backwards direction is applied to the tray. Excess material will be observed to flow into the labial and buccal sulci and onto the soft palate. The patient should be advised to breathe through the nose during the impression procedure, so that the oral cavity will be sealed from the nasopharynx, thus reducing any tendency to gag or retch on the part of the patient.

While the compound is cooling, the tray should be maintained steadily in position using one hand, while the other hand is used to carry out border-moulding procedures around the periphery of the labial and buccal sulci. These procedures require

tissue movements with traction on the tissues in the general direction in which muscle activity would affect the form of the sulci. Particular attention should be paid to the region of labial and buccal frenae.

When the compound has hardened, the impression is removed by requesting the patient to partly close the mouth, when the cheek may be reflected on one side using the forefinger of the unoccupied hand to break the peripheral seal, and at the same time applying downward pressure. After removal from the mouth, the impression is washed in cold running water and examined. There should be no folds, creases or breaks in the continuity of the surface of the compound, and the anatomical landmarks of the denture-bearing surface should be readily distinguishable (Fig. 23.1).

The tray flange should not be visible through the compound. Where a minor deficiency, e.g. in the region of the tuberosity, is present, the compound should be dried and some fresh material softened and added to the impression in the region of the deficiency. After flaming and tempering of the added compound, the impression may be reseated into position in the mouth and border moulding reapplied. Where gross deficiencies are apparent, the impression must be repeated.

When a satisfactory impression has been obtained, steps must be taken to reduce the possibility of cross-contamination between the surgery and the

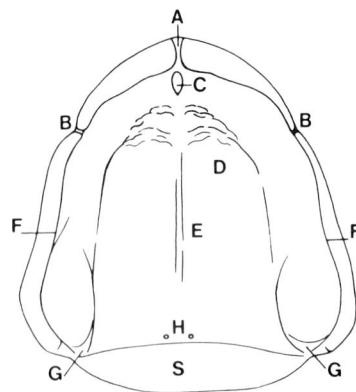

Fig. 23.1 Anatomical landmarks which should be apparent in the maxillary primary impression. A, labial frenum; B, buccal frenum; C, incisive papilla; D, rugae; E, median raphe; F, depression produced by the zygomatic process; G, hamular notch; H, fovea palatinae; S, soft palate.

laboratory. A satisfactory method of achieving this is to immerse the impression for 10 minutes in a suitable antiseptic solution, e.g. an aqueous solution containing 1000 p.p.m. of free chlorine, after which it may be transported to the laboratory for casting.

The lower primary compound impression

Following kneading, the compound is rolled into a cylindrical form approximately 1.5 cm in diameter and sufficiently long to cover the tray, which is then prepared in a similar manner to that described for the upper primary compound impression.

The loaded tray is rotated into the mouth, which should not be opened to the maximum extent, as this restricts the oral opening in the lateral dimension, making placement of the tray in the mouth difficult. The patient should be instructed to partly close the mouth and raise the tongue when the tray is in the mouth. The tray is centred over the residual ridge and the cheeks are reflected outwards to reduce the possibility of tissue entrapment. The patient is then instructed to relax the tongue as the tray is seated firmly downwards over the ridge, while the mandible is supported by the operator's thumbs.

Border moulding is then carried out. Lingually, the border is moulded by requesting the patient to protrude and elevate the tongue and move it to the left- and right-hand sides of the mouth, while the tray is held firmly in position. Labial and buccal border moulding requires the tray to be supported by one hand — the thumb under the chin and with the fingers in the premolar region of the tray — while the free hand provides the necessary traction and simulated activity of the buccal and labial tissues. After the compound has hardened, the tray is removed from the mouth by means of the handle, after reflecting the tissues in the buccal sulcus to break the seal. The patient is requested to maintain the mouth only partly open during removal, to ensure that the temporomandibular joint is protected from possible damage. The impression is washed in cold water and then examined. Landmarks which should be present on the impression are shown in Figure 23.2.

No folds, wrinkles or breaks in the continuity of the surface of the impression should be present, and the border of the tray should not be visible.

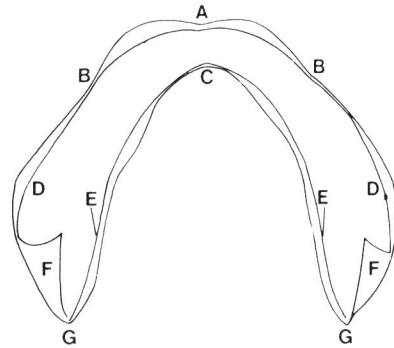

Fig. 23.2 Anatomical landmarks which should be apparent in the mandibular primary impression. A, labial frenum; B, buccal frenum; C, lingual frenum; D, groove produced by the external oblique line; E, groove produced by the mylohyoid line; F, retromolar pad; G, extension into the retromylohyoid fossa.

Additions or repetitions of the procedure are carried out where necessary and, when satisfactory, precautions against cross-contamination between the clinic and the laboratory are carried out as described for the upper impression.

Prescription writing

The instructions to the laboratory should include a request to cast the impression in dental plaster, being careful to preserve all margins. The material of which the special tray is to be made and the space to be provided for the secondary impression material should be noted, and also whether the tray is to be perforated (see Table 9.1). The form of the handle required should also be specified.

In respect of the extensions to be provided for the special tray, under ideal circumstances the cast produced from the primary impression should be made available, and the required extensions be scribed thereon by the operator, in accordance with the anatomical requirements of the patient. When this is not possible, an alternative method is for the operator to draw an outline on the compound impression using a wax pencil, and the outline will then be transferred to the cast during the casting procedure.

Other primary impressions

1. Where bony undercuts exist in the mouth of

the patient, alginate may be the material of choice for the primary impression. A perforated stock tray of suitable dimensions is selected and an alginate adhesive applied to the tray. The alginate is mixed in accordance with the manufacturer's instructions, the tray loaded and inserted into the mouth as described in Chapter 16 for partial denture impressions. Alginates cannot be modified where deficiencies may exist in an impression and where faults are present, the impression must be repeated. Before passing the impression to the laboratory for casting, anti-cross-contamination measures should be observed as described above.

2. Alginate may also be used as a primary impression material when a selective pressure impression technique is to be used at the secondary impression stage (see p. 195).

3. Where the residual alveolar ridge is so readily displaceable to the extent that severe distortion of the tissue form would result from the use of compound, a fluid type of alginate may be used for the primary impression. This situation most commonly arises in the upper anterior aspect of the residual ridge. Alternatively, where these conditions exist, a primary impression may be obtained using impression plaster in a stock non-perforated tray. The method of use of impression plaster is described below.

SECONDARY IMPRESSIONS

Several methods are described below in relation to their application to either the upper or lower jaw. It should be appreciated that they may be equally suitable to either jaw, where dictated by the clinical conditions.

The following methods are considered:

1. Plaster impression for the upper jaw
2. Alginate impression for the upper jaw
3. Zinc oxide and eugenol paste impression for the lower jaw
4. Selective-pressure impression for the lower jaw
5. Impression to define the form of the lower denture.

It has been our experience that the first three of the above methods produce satisfactory results for a wide range of patients, where no special problems related to the oral conditions exist. The other lower methods to be described have been proved to be useful in dealing with less commonly occurring clinical situations.

Plaster impression for the upper jaw

Modified plaster of Paris, when used in a special tray, is a very accurate impression material which produces minimal tissue displacement when used in the method to be described. It is less satisfactory for use as a material for obtaining impressions of the lower jaw, being slightly soluble in water, and therefore the risk of loss of surface details from a lower impression is present because of its accessibility to saliva.

Plaster being a brittle material allows reassembly following fracture and, provided this is carried out with care, the resultant impression will retain the accuracy which was present before fracture occurred. The special tray for impression plaster impressions is constructed to provide for a uniform layer of 2 mm thickness of material, and to allow 2 mm of freedom from the reflected tissues of the sulcus. The handle of the special tray must not interfere with the actions of the lip, so that a simple stub handle is required, or one where a sufficiently long vertical section is provided before it passes between the lips, to minimise any manipulative obstruction. Self-curing acrylic resin or shellac baseplate material may be used to construct the tray.

On delivery from the laboratory, the special tray should be placed in an antiseptic solution to provide a barrier against cross-contamination. Any cast brought to the clinic from the laboratory must be clean and free of any adherent debris.

As the tray was constructed with a spacer of 2 mm thickness, stops of this dimension must be placed in the tray to enable it to be maintained in correct relationship to the tissues during its use. It is convenient to place one stop in the posterior palatal region of the tray, as this will help to control the flow of the impression material and reduce discomfort to the patient. Anterior stops of small diameter may be provided in the premolar region, as shown in Figure 23.3. A region of minimum displaceability of the soft tissues should be chosen for the stops, so that possible distortion of the impressed surface resulting from localised pressure may be avoided. The stops may be incorporated in

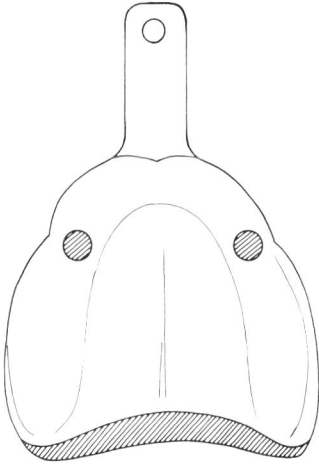

Fig. 23.3 The hatched areas indicate suitable sites for positioning stops in a tray.

the material from which the tray is constructed, or may be added using carding wax. With the stops in position, the tray is tried in the mouth and careful observation of the relationship of the tissues to the tray made. Posteriorly, the tray should cover the vibrating line and the hamular notches and, peripherally, the tray should be clear of the reflected tissues of the sulcus by 2 mm. Where over extension is present, the tray should be reduced and, where underextensions exist, tracing stick compound should be added to correct the extension.

When the tray is satisfactory, the patient is instructed to rinse the mouth to remove adherent mucous. Impression plaster is mixed in accordance with the manufacturer's instructions and placed on the special tray when a creamy consistency is achieved. Sufficient plaster to cover the palatal aspect of the tray and fill that part corresponding to the ridge form is required. When the mix just fails to fall from the tray on its inversion, it is ready for insertion in the mouth. Where the palate has a high vault, some of the excess material in the mixing bowl may be placed directly on the palate of the patient before insertion of the tray. Similarly, some mixed plaster may be placed lateral to the tuberosities before the loaded tray is inserted. These are areas in which air entrapment may prevent ready flow of material during impression taking. The tray is rotated into the mouth and carried tissuewards with a slight vibratory motion, until

resistance of the stops indicates that the correct tray/tissue relationship has been achieved. The tray is gently supported in position while border moulding procedures are carried out. Commercial impression plasters are formulated to prolong the initial setting stage to allow time for border-moulding to take place. The setting of the plaster is tested using some of the excess material remaining in the mixing bowl. When a clean break of the plaster sample accompanied by a snapping sound can be produced, the impression is ready for removal from the mouth.

Removal is effected by requesting the patient to partially close the mouth. The lips are then parted and the forefinger of one hand passed along the side of the tray so that the pad of the finger lies between the zygomatic process and the border of the tray. Wedging the finger in this position, while lifting the lip, should break the seal about the impression and allow its removal. The seal posteriorly can be broken by asking the patient to cough. This causes the soft palate to elevate away from the set impression. If difficulty in breaking the seal is encountered, a few drops of water from the water syringe should be placed at the periphery of the impression and the removal procedure repeated. Immediately on removal of the impression from the mouth, it should be placed on the bracket table and the mouth inspected for any fragments which may be remaining. Common sites from which a portion of the flange of the impression has fractured are the labial border and the tuberosity region. Any broken fragments should be removed from the mouth using dressing tweezers and placed carefully on the bracket table. The patient may then be invited to rinse the mouth.

After thorough drying, the broken pieces are fitted into place in the impression. As each piece is seen to fit accurately to place, it is held in position using molten sticky wax, which is applied to the outer aspects of the impression — not, of course, to the fitting surface. In the completed impression, the surface should be intact and free of defects. The tray should not be visible through the plaster, and all of the anatomical landmarks previously described for the upper denture-bearing surface should be clearly visible. The impression is then ready for the cross-contamination prevention procedure to be carried out prior to casting.

Alginate impression for the upper jaw

Where bony undercuts exist and alginate material has been selected, a tray is produced of similar form to that described for use with impression plaster, except that perforations and a 3 mm spacer are required. After coating with an alginate adhesive, the tray should be loaded with alginate mixed in accordance with the manufacturer's instructions. Only sufficient material to obtain the impression is required — gross excess must be avoided as this will result in distortion of the peripheral tissues. Alginate material may be placed directly in the mouth as described for the plaster impression. When set, the tray is removed from tissue contact using a rapid action, following breaking of the peripheral seal by elevating the lip. After removal from the mouth, the impression is washed in running water and inspected. When satisfied that the impression is acceptable, it is inserted into an antiseptic solution before removal to the laboratory for casting. No additions can be made to set alginate and where an impression is deficient, it should be removed from the tray and the impression repeated.

Zinc oxide and eugenol paste impression for the lower jaw

For this method, a close-fitting acrylic resin tray is required. When tried in the mouth, the peripheral extensions should be clear of the reflection of the soft tissues by some 3 mm. A short, stub handle which does not interfere with lip or tongue activity should be provided.

Zinc oxide and eugenol paste is an accurate impression material provided that it is fully supported, so that it is necessary to use an impression tray which covers the whole of the usable denture-supporting tissue. To achieve this, the periphery of the special tray is accurately border moulded using tracing stick compound. It is not possible to border mould the entire periphery in a single operation, and the procedure is carried out in conveniently manageable sections until the border is complete.

It is suggested that some eight sections might be used, as shown in Figure 23.4. Having checked in the mouth that the special tray is underextended to the extent of some 3 mm around the periphery, the section to be moulded is dried. Tracing stick

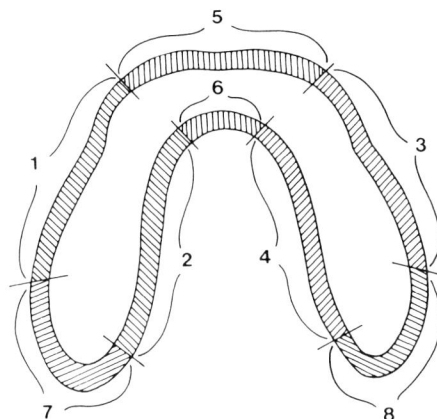

Fig. 23.4 Suggested sections about the periphery of a lower special tray which are manageable for border moulding, using tracing stick compound.

compound is carefully heated above a Bunsen burner flame and then attached to the margin of the impression tray in the chosen section. This should be done neatly, avoiding coverage of the fitting surface of the tray. After tempering in the water bath at 65 °C, the tray is inserted in the mouth and border moulding is carried out as described for the primary impression procedure. When satisfactory, the procedure is repeated for each section of the margin until border moulding is complete. There should be no visible joins between each section. The special tray is now ready for a wash impression to be taken using zinc oxide and eugenol paste. The paste is mixed in accordance with the manufacturer's instructions and a thin, complete layer of the material is spread over the fitting surface of the tray. This is inserted into the mouth and seated to contact the mucoperiosteum covering the residual alveolar ridge, taking care to avoid trapping the lingual and buccal tissues during seating. Border moulding procedures are carried out and the impression is removed from the mouth after setting, as indicated by the development of a firm, non-sticky surface of the excess material. After gentle washing in running cold water, the impression is examined for defects. There should be a thin covering of paste over the border-moulding compound, and a defect-free continuous covering of paste over the whole surface of the impression. The impression is now ready for immersion in an antiseptic solution, prior to its removal to the laboratory for casting in dental stone.

Selective-pressure impression for the lower jaw

In some circumstances, a selective-pressure impression may be indicated for the mandibular residual ridge. For example, the mucoperiosteum covering the crest of the ridge may not appear to be able to tolerate the forces transmitted to it during normal mastication without the patient experiencing considerable pain and discomfort, and the peripheral tissues may be considered better able to tolerate the major thrust of the forces developed during chewing. The first stage of the selective-pressure impression for such a patient is to obtain a primary impression of the lower ridge and the peripheral tissues, using an alginate impression material in a stock tray. It may be necessary to modify the stock tray using impression compound, as described for partial denture impressions in Chapter 16. The objective of this impression is to obtain a cast of the lower ridge where the mucosa has not been subjected to the displacing forces which would be applied using a more viscous material such as compound.

The impression is cast in laboratory plaster and a perforated special tray is produced in acrylic resin using a 2 mm spacer, and with the periphery some 3 mm short of the reflection of the tissues in the sulci. Three short stub handles should be provided – one in the midline anteriorly, and one on each side in the first molar region. Using impression compound, an impression of the primary cast is obtained in the special tray. This compound impression purports to represent the form of the undisplaced tissues overlying the ridge. The compound lined special tray is then tried in the mouth of the patient and border moulding procedures are carried out around the entire periphery of the tray.

On completion of the border moulding, all the impression compound overlying the crest of the ridge is cut and scraped away, exposing the perforations in the special tray, but leaving the moulded border intact. The tray should then be tried back in the mouth, when the patient should confirm that the tray is not in contact with the crestal mucoperiosteum. A freely flowing mix of zinc oxide–eugenol paste is then loaded into the tray, which is then inserted into the mouth and pressed firmly to contact the underlying tissues. The fingers should be located on the posterior stub handles to apply constant pressure, while the mandible is supported by the thumbs. The perforations will allow free escape of the excess impression paste over the crestal tissues without the development of high pressures, while the peripheral tissues will be displaced under the effects of the forces applied by the fingers. Border-moulding procedures are required during setting of the paste, to avoid overextension developing. The impression, when satisfactory, should be cast in dental stone after taking the usual cross-contamination prevention measures.

Impression to define the form of the lower denture

Because of the difficulties experienced by some patients in the management of a complete lower denture produced using conventional methods, special methods have been developed which aim to determine the form of an appliance in relation to the immediate environmental tissues during certain muscular activities. These methods delineate the space available for the lower denture within the large opposing muscle groups associated with the tongue and cheeks.

The method to be described assumes that a satisfactory upper denture can be produced or is already available. Where both upper and lower dentures are to be produced, the conventional procedures for complete dentures are carried out up to the stage of registration of the retruded jaw relationship, and allowing for an increased freeway space of up to 1 mm, in addition to the average value of 2–4 mm. The upper denture is then set up to meet the aesthetic requirements of the patient within the limits permitted by the available anatomical form of the tissues. A further special tray is then constructed. The body of this tray is of the form which would be used for an alginate impression, i.e. of acrylic resin which is spaced and perforated. The special tray carries a vertical diaphragm which is constructed to contact the occlusal surfaces of the upper posterior teeth, and anteriorly to contact lightly the lingual aspects of the upper teeth near the incisal edges. The diaphragm is thin to provide minimum interference with the tissues, and broadens out on the superior aspect to occlude with the upper teeth in the retruded jaw relationship (Fig. 23.5).

The diaphragm is perforated, as well as the body

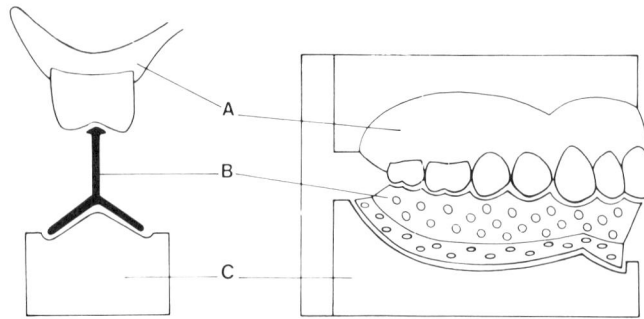

Fig. 23.5   Denture form impression technique. Left: coronal section through the molar region of a suitable tray for the denture form impression. Right: lateral view of the upper denture and prepared tray. A, upper denture; B, perforated special tray; C, cast of the lower residual alveolar ridge.

of the special tray, and stops are required to locate the tray in its correct relationship to the patient's tissues.

To obtain the impression, the patient is first instructed in the muscular activity to be used in forming the impression material. The activities include grimacing, sucking and swallowing, and the patient is required to carry these out three times with the tray and upper denture in the mouth, while closed into the retruded contact position. The tray is then removed from the mouth and dried, after which it is coated on all surfaces with alginate adhesive. Mixed alginate is then coated on all surfaces of the tray, which is returned to the mouth and the patient requested to carry out the rehearsed activities. Because of the time required for the impression to be moulded adequately, it is necessary to select a slowly setting alginate. When set, the alginate impression is removed from the mouth and carefully inspected. While such an impression is not likely to have a conventional appearance, careful inspection will indicate any absence of surface continuity or badly formed borders. Incorrect positioning of the vertical diaphragm will be indicated by its exposure through the alginate. In such a case, the impression should be repeated after relocating the diaphragm. It must be borne in mind that in addition to the conventional 'fitting' surface, the denture form impression utilises all surfaces as fitting surfaces.

The usual precautions are taken in respect of protection against cross-contamination and the impression is then forwarded to the laboratory for casting. All surfaces of the denture form impression must be recorded in the cast, so that sectional casting is required. The casting can be dismantled for removal of the impression and subsequently reassembled. The production of the various sections of such a cast requires a high degree of technical skill.

The reassembled cast will delineate the space formerly occupied by the impression and this represents the space available for, and the form which, the lower denture should take. Its location in relationship to the upper denture will also have been registered in the impression, as the swallowing action used in obtaining the impression will cause the mandible to assume the retruded contact relationship.

This brief description is only one of several methods available for defining the form of the lower denture. It has been included as an illustration of a way in which the denture space may be delineated. The upper denture form can be similarly delineated and the student is referred to the literature for more comprehensive information on this aspect of complete denture treatment.

IMPRESSIONS FOR RELINING AND REBASING COMPLETE DENTURES

Dentures which have been in use for a prolonged period often become ill-fitting because of changes such as continuing bone resorption which have taken place. In these circumstances, rather than produce new dentures, relining or rebasing the existing denture might be considered as an alternative. Relining consists of adding denture base material to the fitting surface of a denture, to improve its adaptation to the tissues. Rebasing is the process of providing a new denture base to an existing denture. Both procedures require an impression to be obtained using the existing denture as an impression tray.

Apart from improving the fit of an existing denture, a relining or rebasing impression may be required where a soft lining is to be incorporated in a denture.

Only the impression stage will be described in this section. The reader is referred to the literature for the indications and contraindications for the procedures and for the technical aspects of the processes used.

A careful examination of the mouth and of the existing dentures is required before commencement. Where there has been a loss of vertical dimension, for example, the procedure may be contraindicated, although some increase in vertical dimension can be produced in certain cases.

In general, the impression for both procedures is similar and involves using the existing denture as a special impression tray. For an upper denture, where the tissues are traumatised, a period of use of tissue-conditioning material may be required to produce a healthy tissue base for the new impression. When taking the impression, all undercuts are removed from the existing denture, and the denture flanges shortened to ensure clearance from interference with the reflected tissues about the periphery of the denture-seating area. As the impression will be obtained using zinc oxide and eugenol paste, accurate support of this material is required, and border moulding of the denture base using tracing stick compound may be required wherever deficiencies in extensions are present. Once the denture has been prepared to the form of a special, close-fitting impression tray having border-moulded flanges, it is ready for use. Zinc oxide and eugenol impression paste is mixed in accordance with the manufacturer's instructions and spread over the fitting surface of the denture. Where displaceable tissue is present, the palate of the denture may be perforated, prior to loading with the mixed paste, in order to prevent the development of high pressures during the impression procedure. The denture is then carried firmly to contact with the oral tissues, and the patient asked to close into the retruded contact position so that a check on the occlusal relationship with the opposing dentition can be made. If satisfactory, the patient is asked to open the mouth and the denture is supported in position while border moulding is carried out. A similar procedure, but using stops of the required thickness formed with impression compound, can be used where an increase in the occlusal vertical dimension is required as part of the rebasing procedure. This is not a recommended procedure to be attempted by the inexperienced operator, because of the difficulties likely to be encountered in respect of possible gross changes in the retruded contact position between opposing dentures.

For the lower denture, the preparation for the relining impression is similar. All undercut areas are eliminated by grinding, and the peripheral form of the denture is corrected wherever necessary by border moulding using tracing stick compound. A zinc oxide and eugenol impression paste impression is then taken using an open mouth method, as described above for the complete lower denture impression.

FURTHER READING

Boucher CO 1973 The relining of complete dentures. J Prosthet Dent 30: 521

Christensen FT 1971 Relining techniques for complete dentures. J Prosthet Dent 26: 373

Devlin H 1985 A method for recording an impression for a patient with a fibrous maxillary alveolar ridge. Quintess Int 6: 395

Ellinger CW 1973 Minimising problems in making a complete lower impression. J Prosthet Dent 30: 553

Kwok WM, Ralph WJ 1984 The use of chemical disinfectants in dental prosthetics. Aust Dent J 29: 180

Lawson WA 1978 Current concepts and practice in complete dentures. Impressions: principles and practice. J Dent 6: 43

Levin B 1984 Impressions for complete dentures. Quintessence, Chicago

Matthews E McIntyre H Wain EA, Bates JF 1961 The full denture problem. Br Dent J 111: 401

Osborne J 1964 Two impression methods for mobile fibrous ridges. Br Dent J 117: 392

Rudd KD, Morrow RM, Bange AA 1969 Accurate casts. J Prosthet Dent 21: 545

Shaffer FW, Filler WH 1971 Relining complete dentures with minimum occlusal error. J Prosthet Dent 25: 366

Watt DM, MacGregor AR 1986 Designing complete dentures, 2nd edn. Wright, Bristol

Young JM 1975 Surface characteristics of dental stone. Impression orientation. J Prosthet Dent 33: 336

24. The jaw registration stage of treatment

INTRODUCTION

To the inexperienced operator, this is likely to prove to be the longest and most difficult of the stages involved in complete denture construction. The length of the stage is due to the need to carry out in sequence a series of procedures, each of which can be quite time-consuming. The difficulty arises firstly from the fact that the stage calls for an element of judgement on the part of the operator, which, at times, can present problems to even the most experienced of operators. Secondly, the stage requires the exercise of controlled tongue and jaw movements by the patient. Some patients seem to lack the necessary neurophysiological control to be able to produce at will the required movements.

The keystone to success at this stage is achieving a state of full relaxation in the patient. If a satisfactory rapport has been developed between patient and operator, the patient will be confident of the ability of the operator and will be more able to relax, both mentally and physically.

The jaw registration stage is carried out using upper and lower occlusal rims. The sequence of procedures which is applied is as follows:

1. Checking extension, retention and stability of upper and lower occlusal rims.
2. Shaping the upper occlusal rim to provide a guide to the setting of the artificial teeth.
3. Registering the vertical component of jaw relationship.
4. Registering the horizontal component of jaw relationship (retruded jaw relationship).
5. Registering protrusive and/or lateral jaw relationships.
6. Obtaining a face-bow registration.

7. Selecting the teeth.
8. Preparing a written prescription.

All the above procedures, excepting procedures 5 and 6, need to be applied for all patients. Procedures 5 and 6 are optional, and are selected for use where special needs apply.

CHECKING THE EXTENSION, RETENTION AND STABILITY OF THE UPPER AND LOWER OCCLUSAL RIMS

The upper occlusal rim should be inserted and the peripheral extension of the baseplate checked labially and buccally for conformity with the level of the functional sulcus. Adequate allowance should be present for any frenal attachments. Posteriorly, the baseplate should extend to the vibrating line of the palate.

Retention should be tested by attempting to pull the baseplate away from the underlying tissues by the application of force bilaterally at right angles to the alveolar ridge.

Stability should be tested by applying pressure in a tissuewards direction to the occlusal surface of the rim on each side in the premolar area, and noting whether any rocking of the baseplate occurs. A similar series of checks should then be applied to the lower occlusal rim. Here, the check on extension will include an examination of the lingual extension of the baseplate. Posteriorly, the lower baseplate should be seen to extend onto the anterior third of the retromolar pads.

If the extension, retention or stability of either rim is found to be unsatisfactory, and yet the baseplates are correctly adapted to the master casts, there is an indication that a fault has occurred in the secondary impression stage, or subsequently in the preparation of the master casts. These stages should be repeated before proceeding further.

SHAPING THE UPPER OCCLUSAL RIM TO PROVIDE A GUIDE TO THE SETTING OF THE ARTIFICIAL TEETH

The upper occlusal rim should be inserted and the patient observed in front face and profile views to determine the degree of support for the facial tissues provided by the rim and baseplate. Wax should be added or trimmed from the labial and buccal aspects of the occlusal rim until it is judged that the correct level of support for the facial tissues has been achieved.

Where the patient is already wearing dentures and has indicated what aesthetic change, if any, he or she would like to be provided in the new dentures, useful guidance will be provided for the required form of the occlusal rim. Where the patient expresses satisfaction with the appearance of their present dentures, the labial and buccal form of the upper occlusal rim should duplicate the denture form. Alternatively, where the patient requests an increase or decrease in lip or cheek support relative to that provided by the present dentures, appropriate modifications should be made to the contour of the occlusal rim.

The occlusal plane should then be developed by modifying, as necessary, the occlusal surface of the rim. Correct placement of the occlusal plane is obtained by relating it to certain anatomical landmarks on the face. These are as follows:

1. In front face view, the occlusal plane is set parallel to a line joining the pupils of the eyes.
2. In lateral view, the occlusal plane is set parallel to the ala–tragal line.
3. The occlusal plane is set to lie approximately 2 mm below the lip at rest.

Choice of these landmarks is based on observations that they bear a fairly constant relationship to the occlusal plane of most natural dentitions. By using them to guide the development of the occlusal plane on the upper occlusal rim there is a reasonable assurance that the artificial teeth will be set in a position that will provide both acceptable aesthetics and satisfactory masticatory and phonetic functioning.

Setting the occlusal plane of the rim parallel to the indicated facial landmarks in front face and lateral views can be assisted by use of the Fox occlusal plane guide (Fig. 24.1A). This is made in either metal or plastic, and has intra-oral and

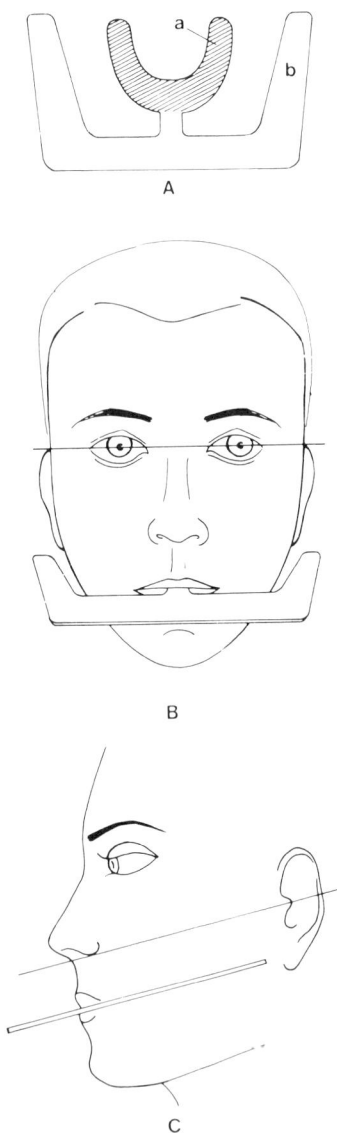

Fig. 24.1 **A** The Fox occlusal plane guide: a, intra-oral portion; b, extra-oral portion. **B** illustrating use of the Fox occlusal plane guide to set the occlusal plane parallel to the interpupillary line. **C** illustrating use of the Fox occlusal plane guide to set the occlusal plane parallel to the ala–tragal line.

extra-oral portions. The intra-oral portion is positioned to lie on the occlusal surface of the rim. The extra-oral portion serves to provide a magnified view of the inclination of the occlusal surface, facilitating observation of the rim inclination relative to that of the appropriate facial landmarks. Its use is illustrated in Figure 24.1B and C.

In developing the level of the occlusal plane relative to that of the lip at rest (action 3), setting the plane approximately 2 mm below the lip at rest is normally satisfactory for young and middle-aged patients. For elderly patients, setting the occlusal plane nearer to the level of the lip at rest may be indicated, to take account of the loss of lip tonus and attrition of the incisal edges of the natural teeth that would usually have resulted in decreased display of the natural dentition, were it still present. Note should also be taken of the level of the occlusal plane in the present upper denture, where one is being worn. If the patient expresses satisfaction with the appearance of the denture, it is usually desirable to duplicate the level in the occlusal rim, even where this may differ from the 'normal' level.

Following completion of the development of the occlusal plane on the upper occlusal rim, certain guidelines should then be scribed on the labial surface of the rim. These lines can provide guidance in the later stage of selecting the size of the anterior teeth to be used on the upper denture, and can also assist in achieving optimal aesthetics when the teeth are set up to develop a trial denture. The lines used are as follows:

1. Centre line
2. Canine lines
3. High lip line.

Centre line

A central vertical line should be scribed on the labial surface of the upper occlusal rim to the level of the occlusal plane. When setting up the upper anterior teeth, the centre line on the occlusal rim will be used to indicate the contact point of the central incisors. To achieve a symmetrical display of the dentition, it is thus necessary for the centre line to mark the median line of the face, with special reference to the lips. The position of the philtrum of the upper lip has a major but not exclusive role

in deciding the most appropriate position for the centre line — deviations of the nose from the midline, and any other asymmetry of the face, must also be taken into consideration.

Canine lines

Vertical lines should be scribed on each side of the labial surface of the upper occlusal rim to the level of the occlusal plane, to indicate the position of the canines. As noted in Chapter 12 (p. 89), these may be developed to indicate either the cusp tips of the canines or their distal surfaces. Marking of canine lines at the distal surfaces is generally selected, as it provides information which is more readily usable at the stage of selecting the overall width of the upper anterior teeth.

High lip line

A horizontal line may be marked on the labial surface of the upper occlusal rim to indicate the position of maximum elevation of the upper lip when the patient is smiling. This line can assist in selecting the length of the upper anterior teeth to be used. Teeth should be chosen whose length is equal to or exceeds that of the distance between the high lip line and the occlusal plane. This will ensure that an unaesthetic display of the labial flange of the denture does not occur when the patient is smiling.

REGISTERING THE VERTICAL COMPONENT OF JAW RELATIONSHIP

The importance of developing the correct occlusal vertical dimension in denture construction has been emphasised in Chapter 10. The serious consequences which can arise from the use of either an excessive or deficient vertical dimension are listed on page 74 of that chapter.

A method that may be used to determine the occlusal vertical dimension is presented in some detail on page 73 of Chapter 10, and may be summarised as follows. The patient should be seated comfortably in a dental chair in an upright posture with the head erect. Every effort should be made to obtain a state of full relaxation in the patient. Markers (e.g. self-adhesive paper dots) are attached to the nose and chin of the patient in the midline of the face, choosing sites which do not appear to move independently of the skeleton.

An initial measurement should be made of the distance between the markers when the mandible is in rest jaw relationship with the maxilla, using an instrument such as a Willis gauge. The lower occlusal rim only should be inserted when this measurement is made. The presence of the lower occlusal rim is desirable since, by providing support for the lower lip, it can influence the position of the chin marker. Also, the weight of the lower occlusal rim may influence the resting position adopted by the mandible. In distinction, the presence or absence of the upper occlusal rim has little effect on the nose marker because of the more remote position of the latter. Both rims must not be inserted at this stage, since if their combined vertical height exceeded that necessary for the mandible to be at rest vertical dimension, measurement of the latter would be impossible.

To persuade the patient to adopt the rest jaw relationship, he or she should be asked to moisten the lips and then close the mouth until light lip contact is obtained. Alternatively, the patient should be asked to swallow and then relax the jaws, or to pronounce the letter 'm'. For the experienced operator, observation of the state of relaxation of the patient's facial tissues also provides guidance on when the position of rest jaw relationship has been achieved.

The initial measurement of the distance between the markers with the mandible in rest jaw relationship should be repeated several times. A consistent value over several readings is essential if reliance is to be placed on the measurement.

The upper occlusal rim should then be inserted and the patient persuaded to close up to bring the occlusal surfaces of the upper and lower rims into contact in retruded jaw relationship. If uneven contact of the occlusal surfaces of the rims is seen to occur, the occlusal surface of the lower rim should be adjusted until even contact over the whole surface is achieved. A reading of the distance between the markers should then be made with the rims in contact. The difference between this reading, and the initial reading made at the rest vertical dimension, will show whether any freeway space is present. Modifications to the occlusal surface of the

lower rim should be made by trimming or addition of wax as necessary, until an acceptable value of freeway space has been achieved (normally in the range 2–4 mm). The value of the freeway space selected for use in the new dentures must, however, take into account any previous denture-wearing experience of the patient. If the patient is wearing dentures which have a deficient, absent or even negative value for freeway space, it is nearly always desirable for the new dentures to be made using a value of freeway space in the range 2–4 mm. Where, though, a patient has worn one set of dentures for many years and, as a consequence of alveolar resorption and/or tooth wear, an increased value of freeway space has developed, e.g. to 8 mm, the use of a greater than normal freeway space in the new dentures is often indicated. A compromise value about half-way between the 'normal' value and the freeway space of the old dentures may be selected, which would be of the order of 5 mm in the above example. Over the years, it is likely that the patient's musculature will have gradually adapted to the change in freeway space, and a gross change in value in the new dentures may make it very difficult for the muscles to be able to readapt in the short term, leading to possible rejection of the dentures by the patient. This problem is particularly liable to occur in elderly patients.

Where adjustment of the depth of the lower occlusal rim is necessary to achieve the required value of freeway space, note should be made of the relative depths of the upper and lower rims as the modification proceeds. The aim should be to achieve a reasonable balance between the two rims, which serve as prototypes for the eventual upper and lower dentures. Excessive depth or deficient depth in the lower occlusal rim in particular should be avoided. The former can result in instability of the lower denture by 'walling-in' of the tongue, while the latter can produce a denture which is both prone to fracture and provides unsatisfactory aesthetics. Although the position of the occlusal plane of the upper occlusal rim has been developed to provide optimal aesthetics in the denture, and hence should be unmodified if possible, instances arise where it may be necessary to change the initially selected level of the occlusal plane. Under these circumstances it is permissible for the occlusal plane to be raised or lowered as necessary, to avoid the development of an unsatisfactory depth in the lower denture.

REGISTERING THE HORIZONTAL COMPONENT OF JAW RELATIONSHIP (RETRUDED JAW RELATIONSHIP)

The retruded jaw relationship is the jaw relationship in the horizontal plane at which the location of the occlusal rims will be registered. The reasons for acceptance of this jaw relationship in complete denture construction are presented in Chapter 10 (p. 75).

When the occlusal rims have been trimmed to the occlusal vertical dimension, the rims should be inserted and the patient persuaded to bring the occlusal surfaces of the rims into contact, with the mandible in the retruded jaw relationship. Achieving this may be helped by asking the patient to curl the tip of the tongue upwards and backwards to touch the posterior border of the baseplate of the upper occlusal rim. Alternative methods which may be used to obtain retruded jaw relationship are usually based on tiring the muscles responsible for protrusion of the mandible. Reference should be made to a more advanced text for details of these methods.

With the mandible positioned in what is believed to be retruded jaw relationship, vertical lines should be scribed on the labial or buccal surfaces of both occlusal rims to indicate their location in the horizontal plane. This may be achieved by extending the previously marked centre and canine lines on the upper occlusal rim downwards onto the lower occlusal rim. Alternatively or additionally, new lines may be scribed on the buccal aspects of both rims in about the second premolar position on each side.

The patient should then be persuaded to open and then close the mouth alternatively to bring the rims into contact in retruded jaw relationship on four or five occasions. The relative position of the lines on the upper and lower occlusal rims should be observed each time closure occurs. If, on any occasion, the lines on the lower rim are seen to develop a position posterior to the corresponding lines on the upper rim, new lines should be marked in this position and the check procedure should then be repeated. Only when a consistent pattern of

coincidence of the lines is seen to occur on repeated closure should the developed position be accepted as that of retruded jaw relationship. When this has been achieved, registration of the rims in this position should be established.

To obtain the registration, 'V'-shaped notches, approximately 5 mm deep, should be cut in the occlusal surface of the upper rim in about the second premolar position on each side. The posterior segments of the lower occlusal rim should then be reduced in height by about 2 mm. This reduction should be carried out from the first premolar area of the rim on each side to the posterior extremities of the rim. This is necessary to provide space for the wax which will be built up on the lower occlusal rim at a later stage. It also provides an escape way for any excess wax which is present. The unreduced anterior segment of the lower rim serves to preserve the previously developed contact position of the rims in the vertical plane at the occlusal vertical dimension.

Softened modelling wax should then be added to the posterior segments of the lower rim to a height considered to be just a little in excess of that needed to restore the original height of the rim, with some heaping up of the wax in the regions opposing the notches cut in the upper rim. The occlusal rims should be inserted and the patient persuaded to close in retruded jaw relationship until the anterior segments of the rims come into contact. The lines previously scribed on the rims to denote the position of retruded jaw relationship should again be seen to coincide. If not, the registration must be repeated until this condition is satisfied. The assembled upper and lower occlusal rims should then be removed from the mouth, cooled under running cold water and the rims then separated. The upper and lower occlusal rims should then be reinserted and tested by repeated closure to ensure that a consistent position of full mandibular retrusion has been registered. The patient should also be asked to indicate if even contact of the rims is occurring.

The rims should then be fitted on the casts and a check made that no distortion of the baseplates has occurred in the registration procedure. Via use of the registration notches, the rims should then be located in the registration position and a check made that neither the baseplates nor the land areas of the casts are interfering with rim location. Where any interference is seen to occur, the baseplates and/or the land areas of the casts should be trimmed until location of the casts is provided only by the contacting occlusal surfaces of the rims.

The casts may then be mounted on an articulator in the position registered by the occlusal rims, in preparation for the development of the trial dentures.

Registration of the horizontal component of jaw relationship using the procedure described above will prove to be successful for the majority of patients requiring the provision of complete dentures. In the treatment of a minority of patients, considerable difficulty may be experienced, though, in achieving a consistent position of mandibular retrusion. These patients often give a history of having been edentulous for a number of years but of never having worn any dentures. The need to chew on edentulous ridges over a prolonged period often leads to the development of a habit of mandibular protrusion, which may be difficult to break in the above registration procedure. Habitual protrusive posturing of the mandible may also occur where the patient has worn one set of dentures for a prolonged period and an excessive freeway space has developed as a consequence of alveolar resorption and/or tooth wear.

Where the problem of achieving a consistent position of mandibular retrusion is encountered, the use of an alternative method of recording the horizontal component of jaw relationship may be considered. This is by the method of Gothic arch tracing. The tracing may be carried out extra-orally or intra-orally, a range of apparatus of varying design being available for use in each method. As an example of the use of Gothic arch tracing, a procedure involving intra-oral tracing using one of the available range of apparatus will be considered. Reference should be made to a more advanced text for details of the alternative procedures.

The apparatus used consists of two trapezoidal-shaped metal plates, each having a maximum width of approximately 4 cm, a depth of 2 cm and a thickness of 1 mm. One of the plates has a 3 mm diameter hole at its centre, the hole being provided with a screw thread which allows a pointed screw to be raised and lowered relative to the plate. A locknut is provided to allow the screw to be set at any required position.

The apparatus is used in association with upper and lower occlusal rims, the upper occlusal rim first being shaped as described above (see p. 200). The lower occlusal rim should then be trimmed to provide an exaggerated freeway space of about 5 mm. The two metal plates should then be attached securely to the upper and lower occlusal rims, spanning the central region of each, the plate carrying the screw normally being attached to the upper rim. A plan view of the metal plates in position on the occlusal rims is shown in Figure 24.2.

The rims should then be inserted and the vertical positioning of the screw carried on the upper metal plate adjusted until the tip of the screw contacts the lower metal plate at the occlusal vertical dimension. The locknut on the screw should then be tightened to maintain this position. An anterior view of the occlusal rims and tracing apparatus is shown in Figure 24.3.

The patient should be persuaded to make a range of horizontal jaw movements, during which a check should be made that the point of the screw remains in contact with the lower metal plate, and that

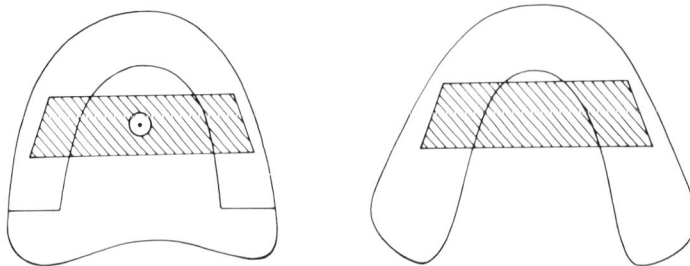

Fig. 24.2 Plan view of the apparatus for intra-oral Gothic arch tracing in position on upper and lower occlusal rims.

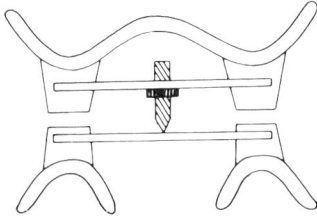

Fig. 24.3 Anterior view of the occlusal rims and the apparatus for intra-oral Gothic arch tracing.

contact does not occur between the rims or baseplates. Where contact between rims and/or baseplates is seen to occur, they should be trimmed to remove the obstruction.

A coating should then be applied to the upper surface of the lower metal plate to allow a tracing to be developed. This may be achieved by the use of engineer's marking ink, a wax pencil or carbon from a candle flame. The upper and lower rims with the attached tracing apparatus should be inserted and the patient persuaded again to make a series of mandibular movements in the horizontal plane. A tracing of the form shown in Figure 24.4 should be produced, the apex of the Gothic arch form marking the position of maximum mandibular retrusion (retruded jaw relationship). To enable the rims to be sealed together in the indicated position of retruded jaw relation, a small disc with a central perforation should be fixed to the lower metal plate, with the perforation overlying the apex of the Gothic arch tracing. The rims and tracing apparatus should be inserted and the patient persuaded to adopt the position of the mandible in which the tip of the screw enters the central perforation of the disc fixed to the lower plate. Location of upper and

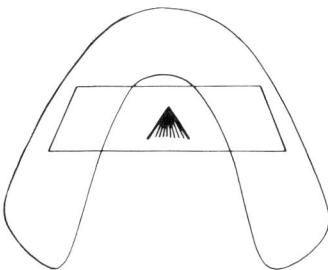

Fig. 24.4 Plan view of a Gothic arch tracing on the lower metal plate.

lower rims in this position should then be achieved by placing a mix of impression plaster between the rims in the premolar and molar areas on each side. The assemblage of occlusal rims and tracing apparatus should then be positioned on the casts in preparation for the mounting of the casts.

Certain clinical conditions contraindicate the use of Gothic arch tracing for the registration of the horizontal component of jaw relationship. For example, the method is difficult to apply where gross class II and class III skeletal jaw relationships are present. To allow tracing to occur, the upper and lower tracing plates need to be positioned on the rims so that they lie approximately one above the other. Such a setting can be difficult to achieve where there is a gross discrepancy in the antero-posterior relationship of the upper and lower jaws. The method is also not recommended for use where the mucosa of the denture-bearing areas shows marked variation in displaceability, as this can give rise to tilting of the baseplates as tracing proceeds.

REGISTERING PROTRUSIVE AND/OR LATERAL JAW RELATIONSHIPS

These relationships are recorded where it is desired to provide individual adjustment of the condylar guidance mechanism of an articulator. Theoretical aspects of their use are considered in Chapter 10 (p. 75 onwards).

It is usual practice to obtain records of protrusive and/or lateral jaw relationships by the utilisation of the occlusal rims which are also being used to obtain a record of retruded jaw relationship. Where multiple recordings of jaw relationship are to be undertaken using one set of occlusal rims, it is essential that the rims should posses a high level of resistance to distortion at oral temperatures. This can best be provided by the use of rims constructed in impression compound. Because of the greater difficulty likely to be encountered in the shaping of impression compound rims relative to those in wax, it is helpful if an initial registration is taken using wax occlusal rims, following the procedures described above. The casts can then be mounted on a simple hinge articulator in the position provided by this registration. Upper and lower impression compound rims can then be constructed on the casts to duplicate the form of the wax rims. Only minimum modification of the impression compound rims should then be necessary in their subsequent clinical application.

The upper and lower impression compound rims should be inserted and the occlusal surface of the lower rim adjusted until even contact of the rim surfaces occurs when the patient closes into retruded jaw relationship. Contact should also be established at a vertical height which provides approximately 2 mm more freeway space than that required to be present in the dentures. 'V'-shaped notches, approximately 5 mm deep, should then be cut in the occlusal surfaces of both the upper and lower occlusal rims in the second premolar region on each side of the arches. A thin coating of petroleum jelly should be applied to the occlusal surfaces of both rims and in the prepared notches, to act as a separator.

A wafer of softened modelling wax, approximately 3 mm thick, should then be placed between the inserted upper and lower occlusal rims and the patient persuaded to close in retruded jaw relationship until it is judged that a vertical dimension providing the required value of freeway space has been achieved. This should then be checked by measuring the occlusal vertical dimension relative to the rest vertical dimension. Where necessary, the registration should be repeated with an increase or decrease in the thickness of the wax wafer until the correct value of the occlusal vertical dimension has been established. Repeated closures should also be applied to ensure, by observation of consistency of rim markings, that the retruded jaw relationship has been recorded.

The wax wafer registration should then be removed from the rims and stored in cold water to reduce the risk of distortion occurring. Labelling of the record (e.g. with the letter 'R') is advisable to facilitate subsequent identification.

To obtain a record of a protrusive jaw relationship, the occlusal rims should be inserted and a wax wafer of softened modelling wax should be prepared. The wafer should be a little thicker than that used to record the retruded jaw relationship and a value of approximately 5 mm is desirable. The wafer should be placed between the upper and lower rim surfaces and the patient persuaded to close into a position providing approximately 5 mm of mandibular protrusion. It is important that the

position recorded is one of true protrusion, involving an equal level of translation in both condyles. As closure on the wax wafer occurs, careful note should be made of the centre line markings on the upper and lower rims, the mandible being guided by the operator into a position of line coincidence, indicating that no lateral deviation of the mandible has occurred. The vertical dimension of the recorded relationship in protrusion is not critical, although ensuring that the wafer is at least 2 mm thick after the record has been taken will help to reduce the risk of distortion occurring subsequently. No attempt should be made to check the record by repeated closure, or distortion of the wax in the notches is liable to occur. The record should be stored in cold water after suitable labelling has been carried out (e.g. by scribing on the letter 'P').

To obtain records of right and left lateral jaw relationships, the occlusal rims should be reinserted and further wax wafers in softened modelling wax placed between their occlusal surfaces — one to record the right lateral relationship and a second one to record the left lateral relationship. These wafers should be of a similar form to that used to obtain the record of a protrusive jaw relationship. With one of the wafers in position between the rims, the patient should be persuaded to close into a position providing approximately 10 mm of lateral deviation of the mandible to the right side, measured in the incisor region. The degree of vertical closure that occurs in this record is not critical, but it is desirable that the wafer should again not be reduced to less than 2 mm in thickness, to reduce the risk of distortion of the record occurring. Once closure to the required thickness of wafer has occurred, the mouth should be opened and the record removed from the rims. As with the record of a protrusive jaw relationship, no attempt should be made to check the position by repeated closure. The record should be stored in cold water after labelling (e.g. by scribing on the record the letters 'RL').

The procedure should then be repeated to obtain a corresponding wax wafer record of the left lateral jaw relationship.

Before wax wafers are used to obtain protrusive and/or lateral records of jaw relationship, it is desirable that the patient be rehearsed in the required degree of mandibular movement.

In using the records, the wax wafer registration of the retruded jaw relationship will first be used in association with the upper and lower impression compound occlusal rims to locate correctly the upper and lower casts for mounting on an adjustable articulator. Location of the wafer on the rims is provided by the wax extensions from the wafer engaging the notches in the occlusal surfaces of the rims.

The wax wafer records of the other jaw relationships may then be placed between the rims on the mounted casts and used to set the condylar inclinations of the articulator. Where right and left lateral records have been taken, these are used in turn to set the contralateral condylar inclination (i.e. a right lateral record is used to set the left condylar inclination and vice versa). A protrusive record may be used as a sole method of setting both condylar angulations simultaneously, or may be used as a check method in association with lateral records.

OBTAINING A FACE-BOW REGISTRATION

In complete denture construction, a face-bow is used to record the relationship between the intercondylar axis and the maxillary denture-bearing area of a patient. The relationship can then be transferred to either an average value or adjustable articulator, so that the casts of the patient's jaws will assume the same relationship to the hinge axis of the articulator as that of the upper or lower jaws of the patient bear to the intercondylar axis.

The use of a face-bow provides one link in a chain of procedures designed to ensure that an articulator will simulate as closely as possible the mandibular movements of a patient. It helps in meeting the aim that the level of occlusal balance developed when trial dentures are set up on the articulator will also be seen to be present when they are inserted in the mouth of the patient.

The registration is usually obtained using a simple face-bow.

A detailed description of the use of this instrument appears in Chapter 11 (p. 82). For convenience, this will be summarised below.

Markers should be placed on the skin of the face of the patient overlying the condyles. The fork of the face-bow should then be securely attached to the upper occlusal rim. This should be achieved by warming the prongs of the fork in a Bunsen burner flame and then gently pressing the fork into the labial and buccal aspects of the rim, about 5 mm above the level of the occlusal plane. Care should be taken that the prongs of the fork do not perforate the fitting surface of the rim and that molten wax is not allowed to run on to the occlusal surface. The occlusal rim should then be inserted, leaving the rod of the fork protruding from the mouth. The joint on the body of the face-bow for the fork is then slipped over the rod of the fork and the condylar indicators positioned over the skin markers. The indicators are adjusted until an equal number of graduations appear on each side and the universal joint is then tightened.

Where an orbital pointer is used, the tip of the pointer should be positioned on the lowest part of the orbit and the appropriate joint tightened. After slackening of the condyle indicators, the face-bow record should then be removed from the patient.

Mounting of the maxillary cast on the articulator may then be carried out using the face-bow record.

SELECTING THE TEETH

The principles of tooth selection are presented in detail in Chapter 12. A suggested application of these principles to the selection of teeth in complete denture construction follows.

Selection of the anterior teeth

The overall width of the six upper anterior teeth is commonly determined by reference to canine lines marked on the upper occlusal rim. Where the lines indicate the distal surfaces of the canines, a flexible ruler should be used to measure the distance between the lines around the lower border of the labial surface of the rim. A manufacturer's mould chart should then be consulted to determine the available moulds of teeth of the required width. An indication of the required length of the upper anterior teeth may be obtained by noting the distance between the occlusal plane and the upper lip line scribed on the labial surface of the upper occlusal rim. Alternatively, the length/width ratio of the patient's face may be determined and tooth length calculated by use of the formula

$$\frac{\text{Length of face}}{\text{Width of face}} = \frac{\text{Length of teeth}}{\text{Width of teeth}}.$$

In selecting the size of the lower anterior teeth, reference should be made to the manufacturer's mould chart, which may indicate moulds of lower teeth that match the size of the chosen upper anterior teeth. This provides a useful basis for selection where the patient has a class I skeletal jaw relationship. Where class II or class III skeletal jaw relationships are encountered, a limited change in the size of lower anterior teeth selected may be indicated. For a class II skeletal jaw relationship, slightly narrower teeth may be selected than those indicated by the manufacturer's mould chart, to take account of the decrease in area available for accommodation of the lower dentition. The opposite applies in the case of a class III skeletal jaw relationship. Gross change in the size of the lower anterior teeth selected should be avoided as the mismatch in the relative size of the upper and lower anterior teeth will be detrimental to aesthetics. Changing the number of teeth which are set provides a more acceptable solution than varying the width of lower anterior teeth, where gross class II or class III skeletal jaw relationships are present (see Ch. 25, p. 212).

In the absence of more positive information, the form of the anterior teeth is generally selected by the use of Leon Williams typal theory, which indicates that the shape of the crowns of the upper central incisors correspond to the inverted outline form of the face. Where the form of the teeth is being selected by that method, note should be made of the outline form of the patient's face — square, tapering or ovoid — and teeth of a corresponding form should be selected by reference to the manufacturer's mould chart.

Alternatively, form may be selected on the basis of the sex, personality and age of the patient, following the principles developed by Frusch and Fisher.

The texture of the teeth selected should be such as to harmonise with the texture of the patient's facial tissues. Particularly where plastic teeth are to be used, the texture of the labial surfaces may be modified by grinding to develop features such as imbrication lines and surface facets where this is thought to be indicated.

Selection of the colour of the teeth is based on the patient's age and sex and the colour of the patient's facial tissues. A preliminary selection should be made from the manufacturer's shade guide after consideration of the above factors. The chosen tooth should then be tested extra-orally in relation to the colour of the patient's skin, eyes and hair and also observed intra-orally when moistened and held under the lip. Similar tests should then be applied using lighter and darker teeth, until the most appropriate colour has been selected.

In relation to choice of material, either porcelain or plastic teeth may be selected. The relative merits of the two materials are presented in Table 12.1. The choice of which to use should be based on weighing up the advantages and disadvantages of each relative to the requirements of the individual patient. For example, if the patient shows a history of marked attrition of plastic anterior teeth, the use of porcelain anterior teeth may be considered to be desirable.

Selection of the posterior teeth

When choosing the size of the posterior teeth, three dimensions must be considered. These are the mesiodistal dimension, occlusogingival dimension and buccolingual dimension. Guidance on appropriate values of the first two of these dimensions may be obtained by examination of the occlusal rims and casts, following the completion of the jaw registration procedure. Posterior teeth should be chosen with a mesiodistal dimension such that the lower teeth will just fill the space available between distal surfaces of the canines and the mesial surfaces of the retromolar pads. Selection of the occlusogingival dimension should be based on an observation of the space available between the occlusal plane and the alveolar ridges. To obtain optimal aesthetics, the length of the premolars should harmonise with that of the canines, and this point should be borne in mind when selecting the occlusogingival dimension of the posterior teeth.

In selecting an appropriate buccolingual dimension for posterior teeth, the need to position the teeth in the neutral zone must be considered. This can often be helped by choosing teeth whose buccolingual dimension is less than that of their natural predecessors. A further benefit which may arise from a reduction of buccolingual width is that the load applied to the denture-bearing tissues may also be reduced.

Selection of the form of the posterior teeth requires a decision to be made on the appropriate cuspal angle. Although many different forms of posterior teeth are available, they fall into two main classes:

1. Anatomical posterior teeth, with a cuspal form approximately corresponding to that of unworn natural teeth and having a cuspal angle in the range $20°-30°$.

2. Non-anatomical or flat-cusped posterior teeth, with a cuspal angle of $0°$. Teeth of this type have grooves present below the level of the flat occlusal surface, to allow food to be expressed from between the occlusal surfaces in the course of mastication.

Teeth of form 1 are commonly selected for use in complete denture construction as a means of achieving an acceptable level of masticatory efficiency. Where teeth of form 2 are used, poorer aesthetics and possibly a decrease in masticatory efficiency may arise. To compensate, teeth of form 2 will transmit less lateral stress to the denture bases and hence to the underlying supporting tissues. On that basis, they may be chosen for use where the residual alveolar ridges show substantial atrophy.

The colour selected for posterior teeth should be the same as that chosen for the anterior teeth.

Selection of the material for posterior teeth involves deciding between the use of plastic or porcelain. As in the selection of material for the anterior teeth, the basis of choice should be a consideration of the relative advantages and disadvantages of the two materials as they apply to the patient in question. Porcelain posterior teeth have the particular merit of showing a very much reduced rate of occlusal wear relative to that which can occur in plastic teeth. Porcelain teeth can be difficult to set up when the available inter-ridge space is limited. It should also be remembered that patients who are being provided with replacement dentures, and who have plastic teeth on their existing denture, may not readily tolerate replacement dentures having porcelain teeth.

PREPARING A WRITTEN PRESCRIPTION

A written prescription should be provided which will assist the technician in the development of the trial dentures. The following points should be covered:

1. Details of the anterior and posterior teeth selected for use.

2. The type of articulator to be used. Required settings of the condylar guidance angle and/or of the incisal guidance angle should be provided where appropriate.

3. A request that the maxillary (or mandibular) cast should be positioned on the articulator via use of a face-bow record, where one has been obtained.

4. A request that the maxilla/mandible relationship registered by the occlusal rims be used to provide relative location of the two casts on the articulator.

5. A request that the condylar angulation of the articulator be set by use of the protrusive and/or lateral records of jaw relationship, where these have been obtained.

6. An indication of the baseplate materials to be used in the preparation of the trial dentures.

7. Details of any special aesthetic requirements not provided by the occlusal rims. For example, the need to provide a central diastema of given dimension may be indicated.

8. Details of functional requirements should be given. For example, a requirement that the teeth be set up in occlusal balance and where the lower teeth, in particular, should be set in relation to the alveolar ridges.

Where copying of some aspects of the existing dentures is desired for aesthetic and/or functional reasons, the provision of impressions of the existing dentures obtained using alginate in stock trays of the box form will be of considerable help to the technician in achieving this aim.

9. Whether contouring and/or stippling of the labial and buccal waxwork of the polished surfaces of the dentures is required.

FURTHER READING

Brodbelt RMW Walker GF Nelson D et al 1984 Comparison of face shape in the tooth form. J Prosthet Dent 52: 588
Broekhhuijsen ML van Willigen JD, Wright SM 1984

Relationship of the preferred vertical dimension of occlusion to the height of the complete dentures in use. J Oral Rehab 11: 129

Fay EF, Eslami A 1988 Determination of occlusal vertical dimension: a literature review. J Prosthet Dent 59: 321

Frush JP, Fisher RD 1959 Dentogenics: its practical application. J Prosthet Dent 9: 914

Grasso JE, Sharry JJ 1968 The duplicability of arrow-point tracings in dentulous subjects. J Prosthet Dent 20: 106

Heath MR, Boutros MM 1984 The influence of prostheses on mandibular posture in edentulous patients. J Prosthet Dent 51: 602

Lundquist DO, Luther WW 1970 Occlusal plane determination. J Prosthet Dent 23: 489

Payne AGL 1971 Factors influencing the position of artificial upper anterior teeth. J Prosthet Dent 26: 26

Saleski CG 1972 Colour, light and shade matching. J Prosthet Dent 27: 263

Toolson LB, Smith DE 1982 Clinical measurement and evaluation of vertical dimension. J Prosthet Dent 47: 236

Villa AH 1959 Gothic arch tracing. J Prosthet Dent 9: 624

Yurkstas AA, Kapur KK 1964 Factors influencing centric relations records in edentulous mouths. J Prosthet Dent 14: 1054

25. The principles of tooth arrangement

INTRODUCTION

The correct alignment of the teeth is essential to the production of a functionally effective and aesthetically pleasing denture. Failure to achieve occlusal balance, i.e. balanced occlusion and balanced articulation, may result in masticatory inefficiency and possible pathological change in the supporting and associated tissues, because of uneven distribution of masticatory forces and instability of the appliances. Incorrect alignment of the teeth may also give rise to speech difficulties.

ARRANGING THE ANTERIOR TEETH

The contribution of the anterior teeth to appearance will possibly be regarded as their prime function by the patient and his or her close acquaintances. There are, however, other functions of the anterior teeth which are equally important to the success of the denture. These include the incision of food and their contribution to occlusal balance and to the development of articulate speech. Aspects important to the attainment of occlusal balance are considered below, and the role of the teeth in speech has been referred to in Chapter 1.

Because of the individual nature of aesthetic requirements for each patient, only a general guide to arranging the anterior teeth can be given. The basis for restoration of the facial profile and lip contours has already been laid down by the contouring of the occlusal rims and the selection of the teeth, as described in Chapter 24.

The labial surfaces of the upper anterior teeth will be made coincident with the labial contour of the upper occlusal rim, and the incisal edges will be related to the occlusal plane developed during the jaw registration stage. These, together with the midline scribed on the upper rim and about which the upper central incisors will be orientated, provide a clear guide to the setting of the upper anterior teeth.

The lower anterior teeth contribute to lower lip support, to the development of occlusal balance, the incision of food and also assist in forming some speech sounds. They are generally arranged just anterior to the crest of the residual alveolar ridge, but must not be set further forward than the available width of the sulcus, or displacement of the lower denture may result when contraction of the circumoral musculature occurs.

The inclination of the anterior teeth

The inclination of the long axis of each tooth in both the anteroposterior and mesiodistal planes, and also their relationship to the occlusal plane, is of basic importance in establishing a natural appearance and functional effectiveness in the denture. This is not to imply that all artificial teeth should be set in the same way, but rather that, as artificial teeth should simulate natural teeth in appearance, it is essential that the normal or 'classical' orientation is appreciated as a basis for positional variations to be introduced. The classical inclinations of the teeth are also the basis for descriptions of required arrangements when writing prescriptions to the dental technician for the setting of the teeth.

The classical inclinations of the upper and lower anterior teeth and their relationships to the occlusal plane are as follows (Figs 25.1 and 25.2).

Upper central incisor. The long axis of this tooth is parallel to the vertical axis when viewed from the anterior, and slopes slightly labially when viewed

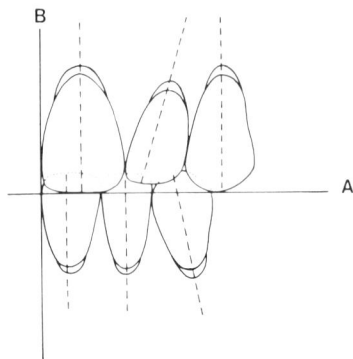

Fig. 25.1 The relationship of the anterior teeth to the occlusal plane (A), and the vertical axis (B), when viewed from the anterior aspect. The broken lines represent the inclination of the long axes of the teeth.

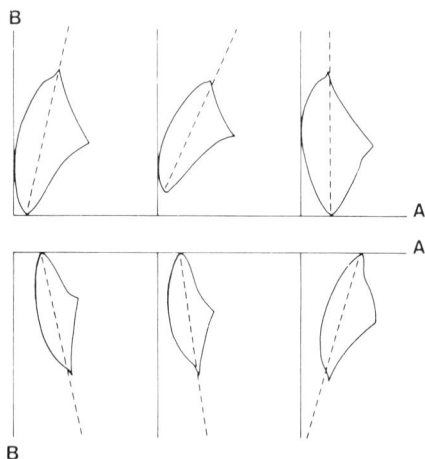

Fig. 25.2 The relationship of the anterior teeth to the horizontal plane (A), and vertical axis (B), in lateral view. The broken lines represent the inclination of the long axes of the teeth.

from the lateral aspect. The incisal edge contacts the occlusal plane.

Upper lateral incisor. The long axis inclines mesially when viewed from the anterior, and the tooth has a greater degree of labial inclination than that of the central incisor. The incisal edge is approximately 1–2 mm above the level of the occlusal plane.

Upper canine. The long axes are parallel to the vertical axis in both anterior and lateral views. The cusp contacts the occlusal plane.

Lower central incisor. Viewed from the anterior, the long axis is parallel to the vertical axis, and the

crown slopes labially when viewed from the lateral aspect. The incisal edge is some 2 mm above the level of the occlusal plane.

Lower lateral incisor. The long axis is parallel to the vertical axis when viewed from the anterior, and the crown has a labial inclination of lesser degree than that of the central incisor when observed from the lateral aspect. The incisal edge is some 2 mm above the level of the occlusal plane.

Lower canine. The long axis is inclined slightly mesially in anterior view, and is inclined slightly lingually when viewed from the lateral aspect. The tip of the cusp is slightly more than 2 mm above the level of the occlusal plane.

In providing variation from the above inclinations for an individual patient, a clear guide to the tooth positions which existed when the natural teeth were present may be available in the form of a photograph, or some other type of pre-extraction record. Where this assistance is not available, the patient may volunteer particular wishes in respect of such variations as spaces between the teeth, a crowding effect or rotation of some teeth. Generally, where variation from the normal is introduced, a reasonable degree of symmetry about the midline should be incorporated, since such variation tends to be symmetrical with natural teeth. For example, the mesial incisal angles of both lateral incisors might overlap the distal surfaces of the contiguous central incisors; or both central incisors might be rotated about the long axis, with the mesial incisal angles being rotated lingually. Subtle rather than marked irregularities may be more acceptable. Strongly rotated and tilted teeth should be avoided, because of the possibility of irritation to the lips and tongue by the incisal angles.

The relationship between the anterior teeth

Where an edge-to-edge relationship is developed between the upper and lower incisors, as may be used, for example, where a class III jaw relationship exists, there is, of course, no overbite or overjet present in the anterior part of the mouth. In the case of a skeletal class I or class II jaw relationship, the lower incisors are overlapped by the uppers. Wherever overbite is present, sufficient overjet must be provided to prevent interference of the teeth in speech and mastication. Further consideration of this important aspect of setting the anterior teeth is given below. Generally, however, with the class II relationship, in the interests of achieving occlusal balance, the overbite is reduced over that which would occur with natural teeth.

In setting the canine teeth, the lowers are set in relation to the upper canines such that during lateral excursions of the mandible an axial line passing through the tip of the cusp of the upper canine will contact the distal aspect of the lower canine (Fig. 25.3). This relationship is essential to the development of the correct intercuspation of the posterior teeth during lateral movements, as an aspect of balanced articulation. When the lower canine teeth have been set to provide for this canine relationship in lateral movements, the mesiodistal space available for the lower incisors is defined.

Slight irregularities of the lower incisors can be helpful in providing a non-artificial appearance to the lower denture, when it takes the form of slight rotation with a mildly crowded effect. Spacing of the lower incisors is only rarely necessary, and when present can sometimes be a source of tongue irritation. Where a class III jaw relationship is present, the space available for the lower incisors between the canines is often generous and, to avoid the use of excessively broad lower incisors, the addition of a fifth lower incisor may be considered.

Where a large overjet is present in the anterior region, difficulty may be experienced in that the space between the lower canines may be insufficient to place four incisor teeth of the correct proportional size to that of the upper teeth. Among methods by which this problem may be overcome is included crowding lower incisors of the correct size

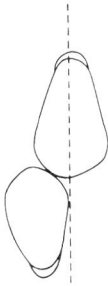

Fig. 25.3 Canine relationship during a left lateral excursion of the mandible.

into the available space, where the discrepancy is small. Where less space is available, the use of slightly narrower lower incisors might be aesthetically acceptable, and in an even more narrow situation the use of only three lower incisors may be resorted to.

ARRANGING THE POSTERIOR TEETH

The posterior teeth have primarily a functional purpose in aiding mastication and contributing to the development of some speech sounds, although the first premolars, being placed near the angles of the mouth, also contribute to denture aesthetics.

In order to develop functional efficiency in setting the posterior teeth, it is essential to aim for occlusal balance. While setting the posterior teeth is the province of the dental technician it is essential that the clinician has a clear understanding of the fundamentals of developing balanced occlusion and balanced articulation in complete dentures.

Occlusal balance

The contact movements which occur between opposing complete dentures may be considered in terms of protrusive and lateral movements. Hanau identified the factors involved in obtaining balance in protrusive movements of the mandible. The factors concerned are:

1. The condylar guidance angles
2. The incisal guidance angle
3. The cusp angles of the posterior teeth
4. The orientation of the occlusal plane
5. The prominence of the compensating curve.

These five factors are interdependent and, when one factor is changed, alteration is required in some, or all, of the others to maintain a state of balance. The 'laws of articulation' as expressed by Hanau define the relationship between the factors. Some of the relationships are referred to below and reference to the literature should be made for a fuller consideration of the laws.

Of the five factors listed above, the only one which is fixed by the edentulous patient is the condylar guidance angle. Where this is steeply inclined, a compensating curve of small radius, or high cusp angles on the posterior teeth, or a steeply

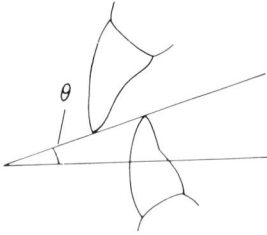

Fig. 25.4 Lateral view of upper and lower incisor teeth to illustrate the incisal angle (θ).

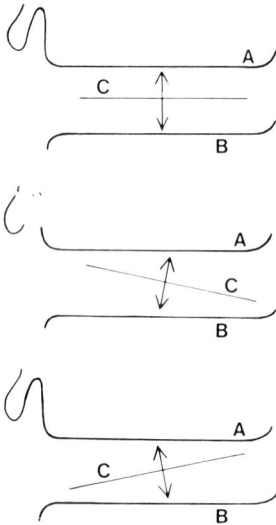

Fig. 25.5 Illustration of the effects of wide variation of the orientation of the occlusal plane on denture stability. The outlines represent the crest of the upper residual ridge (A), the crest of the lower residual ridge (B), and the occlusal plane (C). Tilting the plane down posteriorly (middle diagram) produces a tendency for the lower denture to be displaced anteriorly and the upper denture posteriorly. Tilting the plane up posteriorly (lower diagram) tends to produce the opposite effect in terms of the displacing forces developed.

angled occlusal plane are required to effect occlusal balance. All these factors tend to produce difficult conditions for denture management. An average value for the condylar guidance angle is some 30° and this is not regarded as a high value.

The function of the incisal guidance mechanism is to maintain the planned spacing between the casts on the articulator, and to impart an opening movement to the articulator as the casts move in imitation of the effect produced by the sliding of the lower incisors on the lingual aspects of the upper incisors, in protrusive and lateral movements.

The incisal angle is usually expressed as the angle made to the horizontal by a line drawn in the sagittal plane between the incisal edges of the upper and lower incisors, when the casts are mounted in the retruded jaw relationship (Fig. 25.4).

When the incisal guidance angle is steep, either high cusped teeth, or a steeply inclined occlusal plane, or a compensating curve of short radius are required to effect occlusal balance in protrusive movements. These factors should, if possible, be avoided in complete denture construction and a shallow incisal guidance angle should be chosen.

The orientation of the occlusal plane is developed during the jaw registration stage of denture production. In practical terms, its angulation may be varied slightly to assist in obtaining denture stability. Wide variation from being formed parallel to the ala–tragal line should be avoided, as this may result in resolved forces between the opposing dentures in occlusion, tending to displace the dentures (Fig. 25.5).

Protrusive movements

To help understand the effects of a protrusive movement of the articulator on the paths of movement of the inclined planes (i.e. the cusp angles) of the teeth, an example will be considered. Assuming that the condylar guidance angles on both sides are equal at 30°, and that the incisal guidance angle is 10°, a two-dimensional diagram can be produced as shown in Figure 25.6. Lines projected at right angles to the condylar guidance path and the incisal guidance path, as shown in the diagram, intersect at a point which may be termed the 'rotation centre'. Using a compass, and with the rotation centre as the central point, a series of arcs has been drawn which cut the line representing the occlusal plane. The angles at which these arcs cut the occlusal plane increase in value as the condylar mechanism is approached. With the upper teeth set as shown in the diagram, and the cuspal slope of the lower teeth set coincident with the paths of movement indicated by the series of arcs, balanced contact between the upper and lower teeth will be maintained when a protrusive movement is made along the paths of movement indicated. It will be noted that this

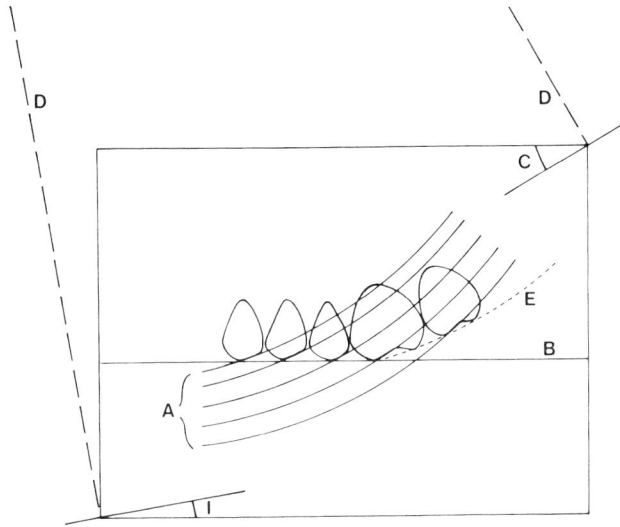

Fig. 25.6 Diagram to illustrate the way in which a compensating curve increases the effective cusp angles progressively towards the posterior. Condylar guidance angle C is 30°. Incisal guidance angle I is 10°. The two dashed lines D meet at the centre of rotation from which the series of arcs (A), which represent the paths of movement taken by the teeth in protrusion, have been produced. B, occlusal plane; E, compensating curve.

arrangement has the effect of increasing the effective cusp angle of the teeth progressively towards the posterior aspect, as the effective cusp angle is made up of the cusp angle of the tooth plus the angle of tilt provided. It will also be apparent that, to achieve these circumstances, the posterior teeth are set in a curved arrangement called a compensating curve, which may be considered as analogous to the curve of Spee of the natural dentition.

Lateral movements

During lateral movements, the right and left condyles are performing different actions. The side towards which the mandible moves is called the working side, and the condylar movement on that side may be considered to be largely rotational about a vertical axis. The side from which the mandible moves is called the balancing side and the condyle translates downwards and forwards and, in the example given above for protrusive movement, it would travel down at an angle of 30°. Consider the working side and balancing side separately.

The working side. Since only rotation has occurred, the condylar angle is effectively zero and the angles of movement are shallow, varying between 0° at the condylar guidance mechanism to 10° near the incisal guidance mechanism. The upper posterior teeth will need to be inclined outwards (buccally) to give the required shallow working angles (Fig. 25.7).

The balancing side. Translation down a 30° slope occurs. Assuming the incisal guidance angle to be less than the condylar guidance angle, the angles of movement increase as the condylar mechanism is approached. In order to provide the necessary balancing angle to maintain contact with the opposing lower teeth, the upper teeth will need to be inclined buccally (Fig. 25.7).

In this way, the buccal inclination of the teeth, as described, develops a lateral compensating curve (Fig. 25.8) which may be considered to be analogous to the curve of Monson of the natural dentition.

The factors involved in obtaining balance in lateral movements may be enumerated as follows:

1. The inclination of the condylar guidance angle on the balancing side.
2. The inclination of the incisal guidance angle.
3. The inclination of the plane of occlusion.

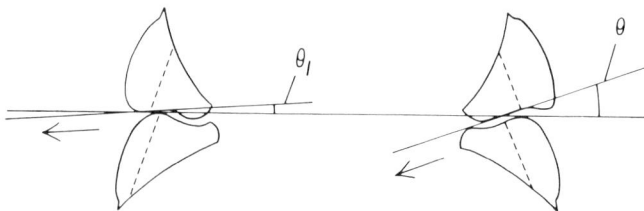

Fig. 25.7 Example of the buccal inclinations of the first molars in the coronal plane required to maintain balance in a right lateral movement when the condylar guidance angle is 30° and the incisal guidance angle is 10°. The direction of movement of the mandible is indicated by arrows. The working side angle (θ_1) is approximately 3°, while the balancing angle (θ) is some 19°.

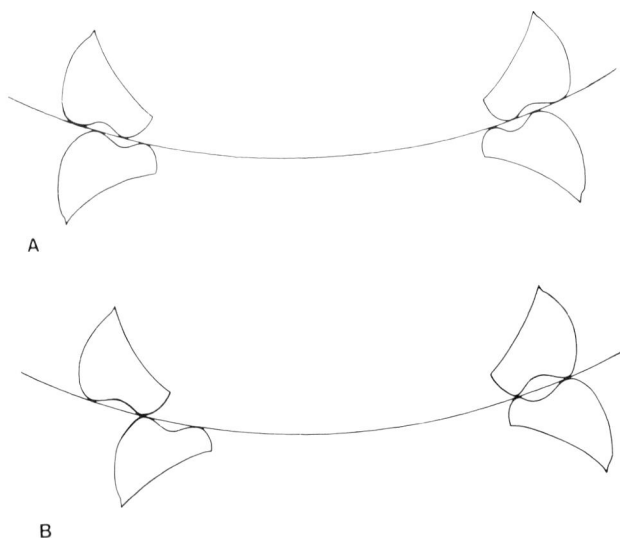

Fig. 25.8 Lateral compensating curve. **A** Tooth relationship in maximal intercuspal position, **B** Tooth relationship following a left lateral movement of the mandible.

4. The compensating curves.
5. The buccal cusp height of the lower teeth and the lingual cusp height of the upper teeth on the balancing side.
6. The cusp height of the teeth on the working side.
7. Bennett movement on the working side.

Arranging the posterior teeth

Just as the starting point for the setting of the anterior teeth for optimum function and aesthetics was a consideration of the axial inclination of the teeth, so the relatively complex factors involved in the setting of the posterior teeth can also be considered in terms of the axial inclinations of the teeth and their relationship to the occlusal plane. The correct location of the teeth in relation to the residual alveolar ridge in the buccolingual aspect is a clinical decision, and will be indicated by the position of the occlusal rim. Generally, for the lower denture, the teeth will be placed with the central fossae over or slightly buccal to the ridge crest, so that maximum stability to occlusal forces will result without encroachment on the tongue space. Placement of the teeth buccal to the ridge may result in displacement of the denture by interference with the action of the buccinator muscle. It is important in the case of each patient to visualise the space available between the buccal and lingual tissues, where minimal encroachment on the tissues will occur.

The axial inclinations and relationship to the occlusal plane for the posterior teeth are as follows.

Upper first premolar. The long axes of the tooth are parallel to the vertical axis. The buccal cusp contacts the occlusal plane, while the lingual cusp is some 2 mm above it.

Upper second premolar. The long axes are parallel to the vertical axis and both cusps contact the occlusal plane.

Upper first molar. The long axis slopes buccally when viewed from the anterior, and distally when viewed in lateral aspect. The mesiopalatal cusp contacts the occlusal plane, with the distopalatal cusp slightly above the occlusal plane. The buccal cusps are 1–2 mm above the occlusal plane.

Upper second molar. The long axis slopes buccally more steeply than the first molar when viewed from the anterior, and distally more steeply than the first molar in lateral view. All cusps are above the occlusal plane to a greater extent than those of the first molar, the buccal cusps more than the lingual, and the distal cusps to a greater extent than those of the mesial.

The inclinations and relationships are illustrated in Figure 25.9, where it can be seen that these arrangements form compensating curves both anteroposteriorly and laterally.

Lower first premolar. The long axes of this tooth are parallel to the vertical axis. The lingual cusp is below the occlusal plane, while the buccal cusp is some 2 mm above the plane.

Lower second premolar. The long axes are parallel to the vertical axis and both cusps are 2 mm above the occlusal plane.

Lower first molar. The long axis is inclined lingually in anterior view, and mesially when seen from the lateral aspect. All cusps are above the occlusal plane to a greater degree than those of the second premolar. The buccal and distal cusps are higher than the mesial and lingual cusps.

Lower second molar. The lingual and mesial inclinations of this tooth are more pronounced than those of the first molar. All the cusps are higher in relation to the occlusal plane than those of the first molar, and the buccal and distal cusps are higher than the mesial and lingual cusps.

Using the above inclinations in setting teeth having cusp angles of approximately 20° will provide a good basis for the development of occlusal balance where an average condylar angle (30°) and an incisal guidance angle of 10° are present.

Where the lower residual ridge has a broader arch form than the upper, such that in the retruded jaw relationship the lower ridge lies abnormally buccal to the upper, a special arrangement of the posterior teeth may be required to provide adequate space for the tongue and stability for the dentures. This relationship may be seen where a class III jaw relationship exists, and also where resorption of the residual ridges of a patient having a class I jaw relationship has reached an advanced stage. The arrangement of the posterior teeth which may be required is called a cross-bite arrangement. The cross-bite arrangement is such that the lingual cusp(s) of the lower teeth occlude in the central fossa of the upper teeth. In the normal arrangement, the buccal cusps of the lower posterior teeth occlude in the central fossa of the uppers. Using such an arrangement may remove the need to set the upper posterior teeth in a marked buccal relationship to the upper ridge, which would increase the risk of instability of the upper denture, while at the same time permitting the alignment of

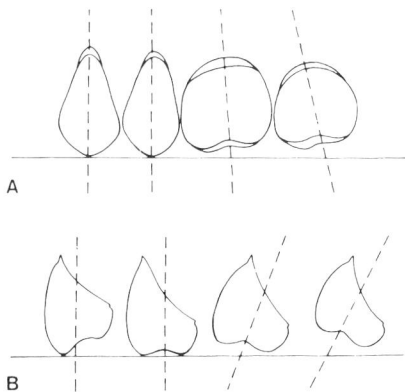

Fig. 25.9 Axial relationship of the posterior teeth to the vertical and horizontal axes: **A** lateral view; **B** anterior aspect.

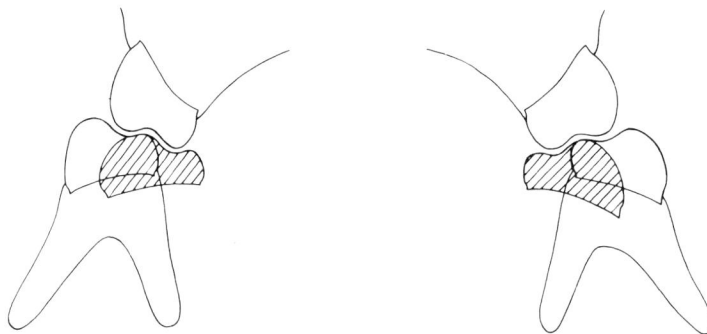

Fig. 25.10 Cross-bite relationship in the first molar region. The hatched areas indicate the normal tooth relationship.

the posterior teeth in a zone of minimum conflict with the environmental tissues (Fig. 25.10).

In practice, when setting the posterior teeth, the uppers are set in relation to the occlusal plane as described above. The lower posterior teeth are then set to occlude and articulate with the uppers, balance being obtained for each tooth, in turn, during setting.

The above description applies to posterior teeth having a definite cuspal form based on the anatomy of the human teeth. Where flat cusps or other non-anatomical forms of posterior teeth are chosen, there are two commonly employed approaches to setting the teeth. Where the biting surface has a flat form of greater mesiodistal dimensions than that of a tooth, the teeth are set to a flat plane and a 'balancing ramp' is used to provide three-point balance in protrusive movements of the mandible (Fig. 25.11). Such an arrangement may be suitable for use with the Bader cutter bar or with Hardy's V.O. teeth.

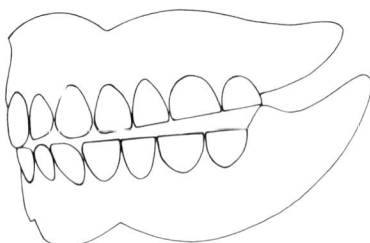

Fig. 25.11 Three-point balance using a balancing ramp posterior to the molar teeth, in conjunction with a flat arrangement of the posterior teeth.

With flat cusp or inverted cusp type teeth, the lower teeth are set to contact a template which has the form of a portion of the surface of a sphere with a radius of some 4 inches. This develops antero-posterior and lateral compensating curves. When the lower teeth are set, the uppers are set to occlude and articulate with them. This arrangement allows free sliding contact in anteroposterior and lateral movements (Fig. 25.12). As might be anticipated with this method of tooth arrangement, occlusal balance in the mouth may not be exactly the same as that developed on the articulator, and some occlusal correction may be necessary to satisfy the needs of the individual patient. Because of the absence of cusps, flat cusp and inverted cusp teeth present no difficulty where the ridge relationship is unfavourable and a cross-bite arrangement is required.

In setting posterior teeth of either the anatomical or non-anatomical type, it is important that the relationship between the upper and lower teeth in the buccolingual plane is such that the maximal value for buccal and lingual overjet, as provided for in the tooth design, is developed. Lack of adequate buccal overjet may result in cheek and tongue biting. Buccal overjet must be positively developed regardless of the cuspal form of the teeth used, and whether the tooth relationship is a normal one or of a cross-bite nature.

A further important point relating to the setting of the posterior teeth is that the teeth must not be placed over the retromolar pad region, as this will result in instability of the denture. Where there is a

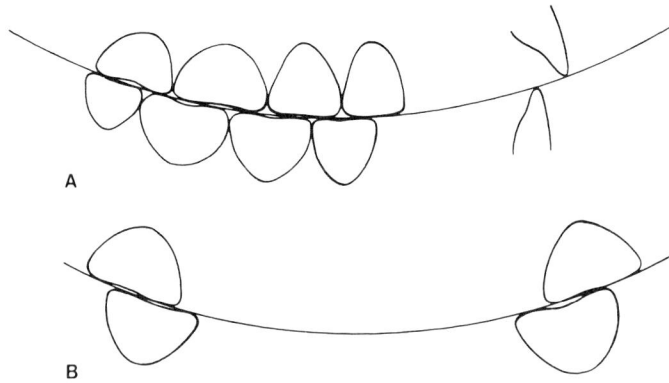

Fig. 25.12 Flat cusped teeth set in conformity with a template to develop lateral and anteroposterior compensating curves: **A** lateral view; **B** anterior view in the molar region.

lack of space for all the posterior teeth, a premolar tooth or, where the space disproportion is greater, one of the molar teeth should be deleted from the set-up.

FURTHER READING

Beck HO 1972 Occlusion as related to complete removable prosthodontics. J Prosthet Dent 27: 246

Frush JP, Fisher RD 1959 Dentogenics: its practical application. J Prosthet Dent 9: 914

Hanau RL 1926 Articulation defined, analysed and formulated. J Am Dent Assoc 13: 1694

Murrell GA 1970 Occlusal considerations in esthetic tooth positioning. J Prosthet Dent 23: 499

Nasr MF, George WA, Travalgini EA, Scott RH 1967 The relative efficiency of different types of posterior teeth. J Prosthet Dent 18: 3

Nimmo A, Kratochvil FJ 1985 Balancing ramps in non-anatomic complete denture occlusion. J Prosthet Dent 53: 431

Roraff AR 1977 Arranging artificial teeth according to anatomic landmarks. J Prosthet Dent 38: 120

Stephens AP 1970 Full dentures which occlude with natural teeth. Dent Pract Dent Rec 21: 37

Watt DM 1978 Tooth positions on complete dentures. J Dent 6: 147

Woelfel JB, Winter CM, Ishigari T 1976 Five-year cephalometric study of mandibular ridge resorption with different posterior occlusal forms. Part 1. Denture construction and initial comparison. J Prosthet Dent 36: 602

Zarb GA, Bolender CL, Hickey JC, Carlsson GE 1990 Boucher's prosthodontic treatment for edentulous patients, 10th edn. Mosby, St Louis

26. The trial denture stage of treatment

INTRODUCTION

The examination procedures which should be applied to check the satisfaction of trial dentures are considered in this chapter. Advice will also be given on the actions which are necessary where faults are identified in the course of the examination procedures.

Before proceeding to intra-oral examination, the trial dentures should be examined on the articulator. The arrangement of the teeth and the form of the polished surfaces should be checked for conformity with the prescription. Note should be made of the accuracy of adaptation of the baseplates to the casts. Where the dentures have been set up on an average value or adjustable articulator, lateral and protrusive movements should be made and the state of occlusal balance present in the dentition should be noted. Where unsatisfactory features are detected in the course of the above examination, they should be corrected before proceeding further.

The trial dentures should then be removed from the casts and the fitting surfaces checked to ensure that they are clean and free from any extraneous matter. All surfaces of the dentures should be checked to ensure the absence of any sharp areas which could traumatise the patient's tissues. To reduce the risk of cross-contamination arising, the dentures should then be placed in a suitable antiseptic solution. They should then be washed in running cold water before they are inserted in the mouth, at the commencement of the intra-oral check procedures.

If, in the course of intra-oral examination, the trial dentures are kept in the mouth for a period exceeding about 3 minutes, there is a risk that distortion will occur of any temporary base materials that have been used in their construction (e.g. wax or shellac). To avoid this risk, the denture should periodically be removed from the mouth and immersed in cold water for about 1 minute before reinsertion.

The number and order of application of the stages used in intra-oral examination of the trial dentures should duplicate those used in the checking and subsequent development of the occlusal rims at the jaw registration stage. Adopting a consistent approach to the examination procedures helps to ensure that no stage will be overlooked. The order in which the stages should be applied is as follows:

1. Checking extension, retention and stability
2. Checking aesthetics
3. Checking the vertical component of jaw relationship
4. Checking the horizontal component of jaw relationship.

CHECKING EXTENSION, RETENTION AND STABILITY

The upper trial denture should be inserted and the buccal and labial margins of the baseplate checked for conformity with the functional level of the sulcus, including the presence of adequate allowance for frenal attachments. The operator should make functional movements of the lips and cheeks of the patient and note whether any displacement of the denture occurs. Where displacement is seen to occur, the depth and/or thickness of the flange in the area concerned should be reduced until the problem has been overcome.

The posterior border of the upper baseplate should be seen to extend from one hamular notch to the other, along a line approximately 1 mm anterior to the vibrating line of the palate. Where necessary, the posterior extension of the baseplate should be adjusted until this requirement is satisfied.

Retention should be checked by applying a force at the premolar region on each side of the denture, in a direction away from the tissues and at right angles to the underlying alveolar surfaces. It should be noted that the retention of the trial denture is likely to be appreciably less than that of the completed denture, due to the absence of a post-dam seal, associated with poorer adaptation of the baseplate to the tissues. As a minimum requirement, the retention of the trial denture should be such that the denture will stay in position when the mouth of the patient is opened. Otherwise, difficulty will be encountered in the subsequent stages of the intra-oral examination procedure.

Stability of the upper trial denture should then be tested by applying force in a tissueward direction in the premolar and molar regions on each side of the arch in turn, and observing whether or not rotatory displacement of the denture occurs. Where displacement does occur, a likely cause is that the posterior teeth have been set in a position which lies excessively buccal to the underlying alveolar ridges. They will require to be reset into a position which provides an acceptable level of stability.

The upper trial denture should then be removed from the mouth and replaced by the lower denture. Testing of the extension of the lower denture should be carried out with the mouth in no more than the half-open position. This will ensure that the environmental musculature is in an acceptable state of relaxation. The operator should place two fingers of the left hand into light contact with the posterior teeth on each side of the denture. The thumb of that hand should simultaneously be placed under the chin of the patient, to provide mandibular support. The operator's right hand should then be used to apply functional movements to the lips and cheeks on the left side of the patient's face, note being made of the site and extent of any displacement of the denture which arises. The test should then be repeated on the opposite side, the role played by the operator's hands being reversed.

To test the lingual extension of the denture, the operator should use both hands to apply light finger pressure to the occlusal surface of the posterior teeth on each side, the thumbs being used to provide mandibular support. The patient should be asked to first fully protrude the tongue, then curl it upwards and backwards so that the tip lies on the posterior palatal tissues, and finally move the tongue laterally to the right and to the left to bring the tip of the tongue into contact with the cheek on each side. Note should again be made of the site and extent of any displacement of the denture which arises.

In all cases where displacement of the denture occurs, the denture flanges should be reduced in depth and/or in thickness in the areas concerned, until displacement no longer arises.

The retention and stability of the lower denture should then be tested by applying the same procedures as described for use with the upper denture. Additionally, testing the stability of the lower denture requires observations to be made of the functional relationship of the tongue to the lower denture. The position of the tongue relative to the denture should be observed with the mouth in the half-open position. The lateral margins of the tongue should be seen to be lying over at least part of the occlusal surfaces of the posterior teeth. When this position of the tongue is adopted, it can provide an aid to retention, helping it keep the denture in position as opening and closing of the mouth occurs. Note should be made of whether the lower denture remains in position on the denture-bearing tissues when the mouth is being opened and closed. Where either or both of these requirements are not met, there is an indication that the occlusal plane of the denture may have been set at too high a level, giving rise to 'walling-in' of the tongue. Alternatively, the position of the teeth or the form of the lingual polished surfaces may be causing 'cramping' of the tongue. Where either applies, consideration should be given to the need to redevelop the denture into a form which will provide improved stability.

CHECKING AESTHETICS

The upper and lower trial dentures should be inserted and the appearance of the patient noted in front face and lateral views, when the mouth is closed and also in a half-open position. The following features should be observed:

1. Whether the dentures provide adequate support for the lips and cheeks of the patient.

2. Whether the centre line of the dentition has been set in coincidence with the median line of the face.

3. Whether the occlusal plane is correctly aligned to the interpupillary and ala–tragal lines and to the level of the upper lip at rest.

4. Whether an acceptable display of the upper and lower anterior dentitions occurs when the mouth is in the half-open position.

5. Whether the size, form, texture, colour and arrangement of the teeth harmonize with the patient's facial features.

The patient should then be given a hand mirror and invited to comment on the appearance of the dentures. It should be pointed out to the patient that any modifications they require must be indicated at this stage. If requests for modification in tooth position are deferred to the subsequent insertion stage, they will be far more difficult to meet.

When either the patient or the operator consider that there is a need for relatively minor modifications to be made to the dentures, they should be carried out at the chairside. As examples of such changes, the alignment of some of the anterior teeth may be altered to provide a more personalised arrangement of the dentition, or the thickness of the flanges may be altered to provide an increase or decrease, as necessary, in the support provided for the facial tissues.

Where major modifications are required in the dentures, e.g. a change in the position of the centre line or the occlusal plane, it is advisable that the dentures be returned to the laboratory for resetting. In that case, the technician should be provided with clear guidance on the modifications which are required, both by provision of a written prescription and by indicating on one of the dentures the new position of the centre line or occlusal plane. The aesthetics of the modified dentures should then be checked at a subsequent visit of the patient, before finishing of the dentures is authorised.

CHECKING THE VERTICAL COMPONENT OF JAW RELATIONSHIP

Markers should be placed on the nose and chin of the patient, as used at the stage of registration of the vertical component of jaw relationship (see Ch. 24, p. 201). With the lower trial denture only inserted, the patient should be persuaded to adopt the position of rest jaw relationship. The distance between the markers should be determined and the measurement repeated until a consistent value has been obtained.

The upper trial denture should then be inserted and the patient persuaded to close the mouth to bring the posterior teeth into contact with the mandible in retruded jaw relationship. The distance between the markers should again be measured. The difference between this measurement and that obtained at rest jaw relationship indicates the freeway space, and its value should equal that selected for use at the jaw registration stage.

Other observations may also be made to confirm the presence of a freeway space in the trial dentition. The patient can be persuaded to adopt the position of rest jaw relationship and then asked to close the mouth to bring the teeth into contact. A distinct movement of the mandible should be observable as this action is performed.

Phonetic tests may also be used. These usually involve pronunciation of the letter 's', since this sound is made with the mandible positioned relative to the maxilla at the closest speaking distance. The patient may be asked to pronounce words containing the letter 's', e.g. 'Mississippi'. The teeth should be seen to come into close approximation as the 's' sound is made, but neither visibly nor audibly should actual tooth contact be noted, where an adequate freeway space is present. Alternatively, the patient may be asked to count slowly from one to ten and the relative positioning of the upper and lower anterior dentition observed as 'six' and 'seven' are pronounced.

Where an error is found to be present, it will be necessary to take a new registration of the vertical component of jaw relationship. The procedure for obtaining the new registration is considered below, in association with that for obtaining a new registration of the horizontal component of jaw relationship.

CHECKING THE HORIZONTAL COMPONENT OF JAW RELATIONSHIP

The upper and lower trial dentures should be inserted and the patient persuaded to close the mouth to bring the posterior teeth into contact, with the mandible in retruded jaw relationship. The relationship of the posterior teeth in this position should be observed. The teeth should be in a state of maximum intercuspation, coincident with that seen when the trial dentures were examined on the articulator.

When this condition is not satisfied, a new registration of the horizontal component of jaw relationship must be obtained. Where a new registration of the vertical component of jaw relationship is also required, this should be obtained initially.

The posterior teeth should be removed from the lower trial denture and the areas previously occupied by the teeth replaced by occlusal rims, constructed in modelling wax. Where a change in the vertical dimension of the dentures is required, the height of the rims on the lower trial denture should be adjusted until, when the patient closes the mouth to bring the upper posterior teeth into contact with the occlusal rims on the lower denture in retruded jaw relationship, an acceptable value of freeway space is found to be present. Where this involves a reduction in vertical height to provide an increase in freeway space, note should be taken of the relationship of the anterior dentition as reduction in height proceeds. If a point is reached in which contact of the anterior dentition arises, the anterior teeth should be removed as necessary from the lower denture and replaced by wax. To ensure the development of a correct record, it is important that the only contact between the dentures which arises when the patient closes to bring the dentures together in retruded jaw relationship is that between the upper posterior teeth and the wax rims on the lower trial denture.

In all cases, a new registration of the horizontal component of jaw relationship should now be obtained. A layer of softened modelling wax, approximately 2 mm deep, should be added to the occlusal surfaces of the wax rims on the lower trial denture. The dentures should be inserted and the patient persuaded to close the mouth with the mandible in retruded jaw relationship. Closure should cease as soon as it is judged that the cusps of the upper posterior teeth have penetrated the depth of the softened modelling wax added to the lower occlusal rims. Repeated mandibular closure should be applied to ensure that the position of retruded jaw relationship has been recorded. The freeway space which is present in the newly recorded position of horizontal jaw relationship should again be checked to ensure that it is still within acceptable limits.

The casts should then be remounted on the articulator in the relationship provided by the new registration and new trial dentures prepared by resetting of the lower teeth. The checks given for application at the trial denture stage should then be repeated at a subsequent visit of the patient. If necessary, the procedures for reregistration of the vertical and/or horizontal components of jaw relationship should be repeated until satisfaction is achieved.

PREPARATION OF THE CASTS FOR DENTURE FINISHING

When the trial dentures have been shown to be satisfactory, and before the patient is dismissed, observations must be made which will allow the casts to be prepared prior to the application of the finishing procedures. The observations which need to be made and the subsequent actions which are necessary can be considered under three headings:

1. The post-dam preparation
2. Relief areas
3. Undercuts and denture insertion.

The post-dam preparation

All complete upper dentures must be provided with a post-dam to ensure the development of a peripheral seal along the posterior palatal border. The border should extend from one hamular notch to the other, along a line approximately 1 mm anterior to the vibrating line. This will ensure that the maximum possible area of the posterior palatal tissues is covered, without encroaching on the movable tissues of the soft palate.

The extension of the posterior border of the upper trial denture has been developed to the required position at an earlier stage (see p. 222). The denture should now be seated on the upper cast and a line drawn on the cast at the level of the posterior border of the baseplate. A groove, approximately 1 mm deep, should then be cut along the full length of the line between the hamular notches. This provides a basic preparation for the post-dam and also serves to indicate the posterior finishing line of the denture. Further preparation of the post-dam should then be based on observations of the tissue displaceability present in the post-dam region.

An instrument such as a ball-ended burnisher should be used to determine the displaceability of the tissues in this region. Often, it will be found that displaceability will be at a maximum in the mid-lateral sections of the post-dam line. This finding relates to the presence of a relatively thick subepithelial layer of fibrous and glandular tissue, overlying the greater palatine nerves and vessels which emerge through the greater palatine foramina. In these sections, the basic post-dam groove may be deepened by an amount proportional to the observed level of tissue displacement, commonly by 1–2 mm.

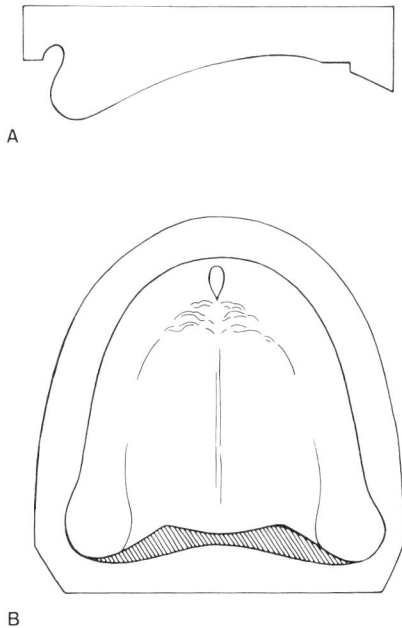

A

B

Fig. 26.1 Preparation of the maxillary cast to provide a post-dam on the upper denture. **A** Prepared cast shown in sagittal section, **B** Prepared cast shown in plan view.

Where tissue displacement permits, the post-dam preparation may also be increased anteriorly with the development of an area dam of Cupid's bow form. This can be beneficial in providing a degree of maintenance of post-dam action if, for any reason, it subsequently proves to be necessary to reduce the posterior extension of the denture. This form of post-dam preparation is shown in sagittal section and in plan view in Figure 26.1. In the development of the area portion of the post-dam preparation, the cast is trimmed to provide a chamfered form, tapering from zero depth at the anterior aspect of the Cupid's bow to a maximum depth at the previously developed posterior groove line.

Relief areas

Relief involves the provision of areas within the denture-fitting surfaces in which the dentures, in the absence of occlusal load, are spaced from contact with the underlying tissues.

The upper and lower denture-bearing tissues should be palpated, both digitally and by use of an instrument such as a ball-end burnisher, and note made of any anatomical features present which indicate a need for the provision of relief areas. These are as follows:

1. The presence of areas of varying tissue displaceability in the upper denture-bearing zone, in cases where the secondary impressions have been taken using a minimum-pressure procedure. The areas of minimum tissue displaceability should be noted as those which require relief. Unless relief is applied to these areas, when the denture is subjected to occlusal loading, tissue displacement will occur in some areas and the load will be concentrated on the remaining areas where the bone is thinly covered by mucosa, possibly giving rise to discomfort. The denture may also pivot about the area of high loading in function, giving an increased risk that denture fracture will occur. An area of minimum tissue displaceability often occurs along the mid-palatal raphe, especially where a torus palatinus is present.

2. The presence of a torus mandibularis in the lower denture-bearing zone.

3. The presence of bony spicules which show

sensitivity to pressure, in either the upper or lower denture-bearing zones.

4. The presence of the mental foramina within the lower denture-bearing zone, where they show sensitivity to pressure.

5. The presence of sharp mylohyoid ridges which are sensitive to pressure, where the lingual flanges of the lower denture are to extend over the ridges.

All areas which are found to require relief should be mapped out on the casts. Relief will normally be obtained by cementing metal foil of an appropriate thickness to the casts in the indicated areas.

It should be noted that relief will reduce the area in which dentures are separated from the under-lying tissues by a thin film of saliva. It will correspondingly reduce the retention developed by the physical forces (see Chapter 2). The provision of relief areas should thus be kept to the minimum compatible with denture comfort and stability.

Undercuts and denture insertion

The upper and lower casts should be examined for the presence of any undercuts which could prevent insertion of the denture. Where undercuts are present, the oral tissues should be examined in the areas concerned to determine if the undercuts are in soft tissues or hard (bony) tissues.

Where the undercuts are present in relation to soft tissues, a decision may often be made to extend the denture flanges into the undercut areas, as displaceability of the tissues may allow engagement of the undercuts during the insertion of the den-tures. Some reduction of the undercuts may prove to be necessary when insertion of the dentures is attempted, which will necessitate reduction of the undercut engaged by trimming of the fitting surface of the dentures in the areas concerned. This possible need should be anticipated by instructing the technician to thicken the flange in the undercut areas, so that, after trimming, a reasonable flange thickness will still be present.

Where unilateral hard tissue undercuts are present, it may be possible for them to be engaged by choosing an appropriate path of insertion for the denture. However, where bilateral or multiple un-dercuts are present of a depth greater than approx-

imately 1 mm, appropriate steps must be taken in relation to the forming of the denture flanges if insertion of the denture is to be possible. Three options are available for use:

1. Undercut of 1 mm should be retained to aid denture retention, any additional undercut being blocked out in plaster on the cast and the denture flange then being extended to the full depth of the sulcus (Fig. 26.2A).

2. The denture flange should extend only to the level providing 1 mm engagement of undercut on one or both sides (Fig. 26.2B).

3. The flange extensions into one or both of the undercut areas may be developed in a resilient lining material. The use of a modified acrylic type

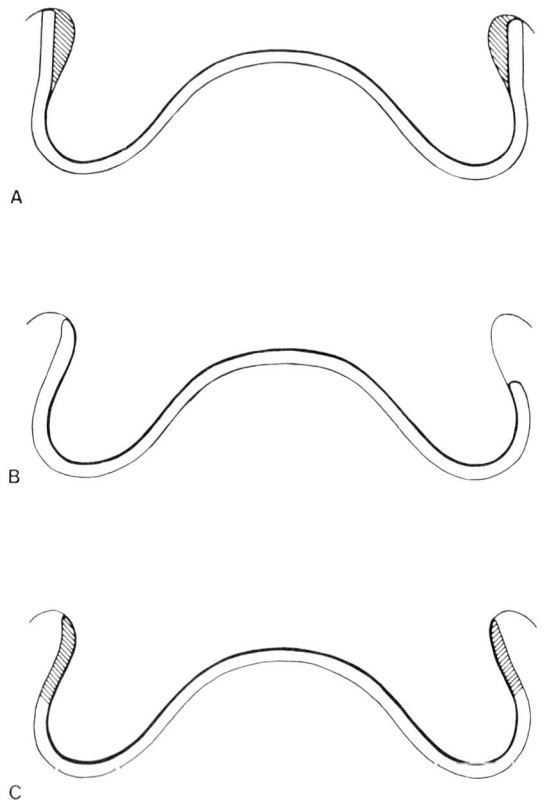

Fig. 26.2 Flange development in areas of hard tissue undercuts. **A** Undercuts in excess of 1 mm have been blocked out and the flanges extended to the base of the sulci, **B** Flange extended only to the level where 1 mm of undercut has been engaged on one side, **C** Flange extensions developed in a resilient lining material beyond the level where 1 mm of undercut has been engaged.

of material is preferable for this application, because of its superior bond strength to an acrylic resin base, relative to that achieved by a silicone type of liner (Fig. 26.2C).

None of these options provides an ideal result. Option 1 may provide excessive support for the facial tissues in the undercut area, and option 2 can provide deficient support for the facial tissues. With option 3, separation of the resilient lining from the main base may occur in a disappointingly short period. The general preference is for use of option 1, although option 3 may be chosen when the extra retention conferred by the resilient flanges is of special need.

PRESCRIPTION WRITING

When the trial dentures are returned to the laboratory for finishing, they should be accompanied by a written prescription providing the following information:

1. The colour and nature of the denture base material which is to be used.

2. Details of any modifications required in the polished surfaces of the dentures. For example, an indication for flange thickness to be increased in undercut regions, where reduction of the fitting surfaces may be required to permit denture insertion. Where contouring and/or stippling of the labial surfaces is required, this should also be stated.

3. Details of the site and depth of relief areas which are required, supplemented by the mapping out of the areas on the casts.

FURTHER READING

Brisman AS 1980 Aesthetics: a comparison of dentists and patients concepts. J Am dent Assoc 100: 345
Brodbelt RHW, Walker GF, Nelson D et al 1984 Comparison of face shape with tooth form. J Prosthet Dent 52: 588
Colon A, Kotwal K, Manglesdorf AD 1982 Analysis of the posterior palatal seal as related to the retention of complete dentures. J Prosthet Dent 47: 23
Ettinger RC, Scandrett FR 1980 The posterior palatal seal: a review. Aust Dent J 25: 197
Kemnitzer DF 1956 Esthetics and the denture base. J Prosthet Dent 6: 603
Lombardi RE 1973 The principles of visual perception and their clinical application to denture esthetics. J Prosthet Dent 29: 358
Silverman SE 1971 Dimensions and displacement problems of the posterior palatal seal. J Prosthet Dent 25: 476
Winkler S, Morris HF, Ortman HR, Staab RM, Baitz HC 1970 Characterization of denture bases for people of color. J Am Dent Assoc 18: 1349
Wright SM 1974 Prosthetic reproduction of gingival pigmentation. Brit Dent J 136: 367

27. The insertion stage of treatment

INTRODUCTION

The insertion of dentures represents an important event for the patient and, unless a careful approach is made to this stage of treatment, the success of the dentures may be prejudiced. While the preparation of the dentures following the trial stage will have been carried out by the dental technician, it must not be overlooked that the dentures are the responsibility of the dental surgeon, and the laboratory work must be carefully assessed to ensure that it is of an acceptable standard. Only then can a trial of the dentures in the mouth be contemplated. Even when this step appears satisfactory and the dentures meet the required clinical criteria, the manner in which information is presented relating to the use and care of the mouth and the appliances, and of any anticipated difficulties, will play an important part in the successful outcome of the treatment.

EXTRA-ORAL EXAMINATION OF THE DENTURES

This stage is carried out after delivery of the dentures from the laboratory, and before the patient arrives for the insertion appointment.

Each denture should be carefully checked for any faults which might be present. It is not uncommon for small nodules of acrylic resin to be present on the surface of the dentures. These result from the flow of acrylic resin into small surface or subsurface air spaces present on the master cast on which the denture was processed, or the investing gypsum. Any nodules must be removed using a scraper or similar instrument, or carefully ground off using a mounted stone. The surrounding denture base must not be damaged during this process. Common sites for such nodules are the fitting surfaces and between the teeth and, while they may be difficult to see, they are readily detected by lightly moving the tip of a finger over the denture surface. Other surface imperfections which might be present include those resulting from surface damage to the master cast. These may result from accidental knife marks or small chips of gypsum lost from the cast surface. The denture surface will require careful adjustment in the regions concerned, using a small mounted stone.

Where a relief area has been incorporated in the denture, the edges must be carefully examined to ensure that they are not sharp, as this could cause tissue damage when the denture is loaded in function.

The edges of any sharp relief area should be carefully smoothed, using a mounted stone to merge the margin into the surrounding denture base. The denture margins should be examined to ensure that their form is continuously curved and free of any sharp angles which may traumatise the tissues.

Finally, the dentures should be fitted together with the teeth in the maximal intercuspal position, as a means of detecting contact or interference between the posterior aspects of the denture bases, which will affect contact relations between the dentures when placed in the mouth. Any such contact will need to be removed by reducing the thickness of the upper and/or lower denture in the area(s) concerned.

Following the extra-oral examination of the dentures and completion of any required adjustments, the dentures should then be stored in a suitable antiseptic solution to await the arrival of the patient.

INTRA-ORAL EXAMINATION OF THE DENTURES

On the arrival of the patient, any existing dentures should be removed and the mouth carefully examined for evidence of any oral damage which might be present, as this may affect the patient's reaction to the new dentures. If any tissue damage is present, this should be pointed out to the patient and any necessary treatment instituted.

Extension, retention and stability of the dentures

Each denture should be assessed in turn, commencing with the upper denture. Where undercuts of an unyielding nature are present in the mouth, allowance will have been provided for these during the laboratory stages of denture production, in accordance with the instructions provided in the laboratory prescription. Because of the dimensional changes which accompany the processing of acrylic resin, resistance may be met on attempting to insert the denture. Should this occur, no attempt should be made to force the denture into place. Similarly, where undercuts associated with more yielding tissues are present, it may have been decided not to eliminate these in the denture, on the grounds that they may be useful as a means of providing additional retention. Such a denture may also meet resistance on attempted insertion. Where resistance is felt in the direction of the planned path of insertion, careful observation may enable the detection of tissue blanching in the region of resistance, where relief of the denture is required. A low viscosity pressure relief cream is a very useful aid for the detection of undercuts. The cream is applied to the denture base and an attempted insertion of the denture is made, the denture being removed when resistance occurs. Inspection of the denture base will show that the pressure relief cream has been removed from the area of contact with the tissues. The area from which the cream was removed should be carefully relieved and the whole process repeated until the denture is fully seated in position in the mouth.

Once seated against the basal tissues, the denture should be checked for accuracy of extension and effectiveness of retention and stability. These procedures, and the steps to be taken in the event of

any faults being detected, have been fully described in Chapter 26. Modified areas must be smoothed and polished on completion of the required adjustment.

The upper denture should then be removed and the lower denture placed in the mouth, following through a similar procedure to that outlined above for the upper denture.

Aesthetics

When any adjustments required to effect insertion of the dentures have been completed, both dentures are inserted into the mouth together and the appearance checked by the operator, as described in the previous section. This is to ensure that the form of the flanges and contours, as accepted at the trial stage and requested in the laboratory prescription, have been incorporated in the denture. Only errors in relation to excessive fullness of the flanges could be corrected at this stage by grinding and subsequent repolishing.

Poor aesthetics resulting from inadequate contouring, or displacement of a tooth or teeth from the position accepted at the trial stage, cannot be corrected at the chairside and will require reprocessing after correcting the deficiency, or possible remaking of the denture(s).

Occlusion

With both dentures in the mouth, the vertical and horizontal components of the jaw registration should now be verified. Because of the dimensional changes known to occur during processing between the trial denture stage and the production of the completed denture, an increase in the vertical height of the dentures is anticipated. This will result in a reduction in the freeway space of the order of 0.5–1 mm, when measured as described in Chapter 10. Correction of this error will take place during the process of selective grinding of the teeth (see below). It is, however, possible that an error in the jaw relationship has been incorporated in the dentures by virtue of the acceptance of an incorrect horizontal or vertical component or both, and this can generally be detected at this stage.

Occasionally, the tooth movement which occurs during processing results in gross interference between opposing teeth. This will be apparent when the patient is asked to close into the retruded jaw relationship. Where gross interference of this nature is observed, it is usually associated with a single premature contact and should be eliminated by grinding the offending contact(s), after first accurately locating the position using articulating paper. The vertical component of the jaw relationship can then be checked. Both the rest vertical dimension and the occlusal vertical dimension are measured to verify the presence of freeway space.

Where the freeway space is excessive or absent, one or both of the dentures may have to be remade. Only very rarely can sufficient tooth substance be removed by grinding to provide for freeway space without gross mutilation of the tooth surfaces.

The horizontal component of the jaw registration is then checked. While the occlusion will not be perfect at this stage because of processing changes, lack of coincidence between maximum intercuspation and the retruded jaw relationship can be readily detected. Where this exceeds a distance in excess of approximately one-quarter of the mesiodistal dimension of a cusp, it is unlikely to be correctable by occlusal grinding, and it will be necessary to reset the posterior teeth of one or both dentures, or to remake the dentures.

Where the occlusion is substantially correct, or has only a minor error which may be corrected by occlusal modification, the next step is that of perfecting the occlusion by selective grinding, following remounting on the articulator.

Remounting the processed dentures

The upper denture is mounted on an average value or adjustable articulator using a face-bow record, so that the denture is correctly related to the hinge axis of the articulator. The lower denture is then mounted on the articulator in the retruded jaw relationship by means of a wax interocclusal record. This is obtained by attaching a layer of modelling wax, approximately 2 mm thick, to the occlusal surfaces of the lower posterior teeth, while the upper denture is seated in position in the mouth. The wax on the lower denture is thoroughly softened, the denture placed in the mouth and the patient persuaded to close into the retruded jaw relationship. Closure is stopped just before com-

plete penetration to the opposing teeth occurs. If closure to contact of the opposing teeth is permitted, cuspal interferences may guide the mandible into an unacceptable position. Such a record may be referred to in the literature as a 'precentric registration'. The denture and the attached interocclusal record are removed from the mouth and placed in cold water to harden the wax thoroughly. The wax is then trimmed to remove any excess wax beyond the indentations of the cusps of the upper teeth, as the excess may form guiding planes which might influence the path of closure. The denture and the attached record is reinserted and checked for coincidence with the retruded jaw relationship. When satisfied with the accuracy of the wax record, it is used to assist attachment of the lower denture to the articulator with the dentures in the retruded jaw relationship. Selective grinding can then be carried out.

Selective grinding

The aims of selective grinding are to provide balanced contacts between the teeth in the retruded jaw relationship and in lateral and protrusive contact relations, and free sliding contact movements to eccentric positions without cuspal interferences. At the same time, the occlusal vertical dimension must be maintained.

Selective grinding to the retruded jaw relationship. After remounting the dentures on the articulator, the wax interocclusal record is removed and the occlusion observed. Typically, contact between the opposing teeth will occur towards the posterior aspect of the occlusal table. Using thin articulating paper interposed between the opposing teeth, the upper bow of the articulator is closed to record the points of first contact of the teeth. Those points will be marked by the articulating paper and a decision must be made as to whether the prominent cusp of the tooth, or the fossa or other region which it contacts, will need reduction. In general, where a premature contact is present only in the retruded position and does not cause interfering contacts when lateral excursions of the articulator are made, fossa reduction should be undertaken. Where a cusp produces premature contacts in the retruded relationship and also in lateral relationships, cusp reduction may be required. It should be

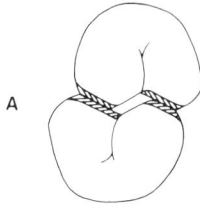

Fig. 27.1 Diagram to illustrate the effect of grinding cuspal inclines (shaded areas) to correct a minor mesiodistal error in occlusion. Note that the cuspal angles have been maintained. Buccal aspect. A, mesial.

appreciated that the vertical dimension of dentures having a normal occlusal relationship of the posterior teeth is maintained by the buccal cusps of the lower teeth and the palatal cusps of the upper teeth and their opposing fossae. Thus, once the originally planned occlusal vertical dimension of the dentures is restored, no further reduction of those parts of the teeth concerned with vertical dimension maintenance should be undertaken.

Where minor mesiodistal inaccuracy of the contact relations between the opposing teeth is present, grinding of the cuspal inclined planes may be required. This should be done in such a way that the cuspal angles are maintained. Grinding of the mesial inclined planes has the effect of producing a more distal position of the tip of the cusp and vice versa (Fig. 27.1).

Selective grinding for lateral excursions. Once balanced contact has been achieved in the retruded relationship, balance in lateral excursions may be sought. Thin articulating paper is placed between

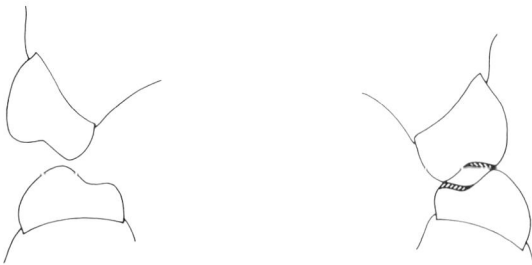

Fig. 27.2 Illustration of a coronal section through the molar region of a denture during a lateral movement with premature contact on the working side. To produce contact on the balancing side, the shaded areas will need to be reduced.

the opposing teeth and the condylar mechanism is operated to produce a lateral excursion to the right. If, when the buccal and lingual cusps are in contact on the working side, the balancing side of the denture teeth are out of contact (Fig. 27.2), the buccal cusps of the upper teeth and/or the lingual cusps of the lower teeth should be reduced. The lower buccal and upper palatal cusps must not be ground as these are required for the maintenance of vertical dimension. Similarly, if the lower lingual cusp and the upper palatal cusps occlude prematurely in a lateral excursion, the lower lingual cusp will need to be reduced.

Grinding the buccal upper and the lingual lower cusps to obtain balanced occlusion in lateral movements is often referred to as grinding to the B.U.L.L. rule.

Should the balancing side show premature occlusion between the lower buccal and the palatal upper cusps, the buccal cusp of the lower tooth may be reduced in preference to the palatal cusp of the upper tooth.

When balance has been achieved for the right lateral excursion, a similar procedure is followed to produce balance for the left lateral excursion.

Selective grinding for protrusive excursions. Following selective grinding to produce balance in the retruded jaw relationship and lateral excursions, the main premature contacts for protrusive excursions may be associated with the anterior teeth. This may require limited grinding of the incisal edges of the lower teeth, which should be carried out in such a manner as to simulate attrition of the teeth.

Final milling and polishing the teeth. In order to ensure that the movements of balanced articulation in excursions of the mandible can be achieved smoothly, selective grinding may be followed by the use of a paste of fine grit carborundum and glycerine. This paste is spread on the occlusal surfaces of the teeth and up to six contact sliding movements incorporating lateral and protrusive excursions can be made, without possible severe reduction of the cusps.

When selective grinding is complete, the tooth surfaces must be carefully polished, as rough tooth surfaces can be a source of severe irritation to the patient. Grinding will have been accomplished using fine grit mounted stones in a handpiece.

Where porcelain teeth have been used, repolishing with rubber-bonded abrasive wheels and polishing cups will be required, followed by a pumice slurry applied using a large-diameter buff revolving at high speed. Where acrylic teeth are concerned, a pumice slurry applied by means of a long filament heatless bristle brush will suffice.

The dentures are now ready for reinsertion into the mouth, when the vertical and horizontal components of the jaw registration are checked. If any lack of coincidence between maximum intercuspation and the retruded jaw relationship is present, the above procedure must be repeated. The vertical component of the registration should now coincide with that planned at the trial denture stage of treatment.

Following selective grinding with the dentures in the mouth, the patient should be questioned regarding evenness of posterior tooth contact, as most patients are able to detect slight pressure differences from one side to the other on closure. There should now be no pressure differences appreciated. As the patient brings the teeth into contact, there should be no movement of either denture, relative to the jaws, visible. No sliding contacts should be observable following the initial contact between the dentures, when the patient closes into the retruded jaw relationship.

Once satisfied that the occlusion is fully balanced, the patient is then given a hand mirror so that the new dentures can be inspected.

INSTRUCTIONS TO THE PATIENT

Prior to dismissing the patient after insertion of the dentures, instructions in the use and care of the dentures and the oral tissues must be given. Any anticipated difficulties which might arise should be discussed at this stage, and a further appointment must be given so that the progress of the patient can be reviewed.

Experienced denture wearers having oral tissues in good condition will already have views on denture management, whereas those receiving dentures for the first time will look to the dentist for advice in this new experience. It is advisable to give full information to both groups of patients and verbal instructions in the use and care of the dentures should be reinforced by the provision of written instructions. The advice given should be designed to enable the patient to adjust to the dentures as quickly as possible, and to understand the limitations of complete dentures.

The patient should be instructed in the insertion and removal of the dentures and should be asked to demonstrate this so that the dentist is certain that the patient has mastered the procedure. The points covered in verbal and written form should include.

1. Eating may be difficult at first. Food should be cut into small pieces and chewed slowly and carefully. Tough and sticky foods should be avoided in the initial learning period.

2. The dentures should be removed and cleaned after each meal. Cleansing of the dentures can be carried out using a soft brush with soap and cold water. A proprietary denture cleaner may be used, following the manufacturer's instructions.

3. The dentures should be removed at night and stored in water, to prevent drying of the appliances and possible consequential warping.

4. A warning that pain and soreness may occur with new dentures should be given, and that adjustment to the denture(s) may be required. The patient should be advised that, in the event of severe pain, the dentures should be removed from the mouth and placed in water. An appointment with the dentist to review the situation should be sought as soon as possible. It is helpful from the diagnostic point of view if the patient will return the dentures to the mouth on the day of the appointment, as otherwise painful areas are not always easily detectable.

5. The patient must be warned against attempting to adjust the dentures, as such a procedure can cause permanent damage to them.

Finally, an appointment is given to return in 7 days for review of the mouth and dentures. The patient should be urged to keep the review appointment even if it is felt by him or her to be unnecessary, as incipient tissue damage might be evident to the dentist and corrective measures could then be taken which will prevent possible discomfort.

FURTHER READING

Atkinson HF, Grant AA 1962 An investigation into tooth movement during the packing and polymerizing of acrylic denture base materials. Aust Dent J 7: 101

Budtz–Jorgensen E 1979 Materials and methods for cleaning dentures. J Prosthet. Dent 42: 619

Collett HA 1967 Motivation: a factor in dental treatment. J Prosthet Dent 17: 5

Guckes AD, Smith DE, Swoope CC 1978 Counselling and related factors influencing satisfaction with dentures. J Prosthet Dent 39: 259

Heath JR, Zoitopoulos L, Griffiths C 1988 Simple methods for denture identification: a clinical trial. J Oral Rehab 15: 587

Hickey JC, Boucher CO, Woelfel JB 1962 Responsibility of the dentist in complete dentures. J Prosthet Dent 12: 637

Hoad–Reddick G 1986 Gagging — a chairside approach to control. Brit Dent J 161: 174

Jankelson B 1962 Adjustment of dentures at time of insertion and alterations to compensate for tissue change. J Am Dent Assoc 64: 521

Lawson WA 1965 Information and advice for patients wearing dentures. Dent Pract Dent Rec 15: 402

MacCallum M, Stafford GD, MacCulloch WT, Combe EC 1968 Which cleanser? Dent Pract Dent Rec 19: 83

Rodegerdts CR 1964 The relationship of pressure spots in complete denture impressions with mucosal irritations. J Prosthet Dent 14: 1040

28. The review stage of treatment

INTRODUCTION

Following the insertion of complete dentures, an appointment to attend for review in approximately 7 days should be made for the patient.

At the review visit, the patient should be questioned concerning any difficulties which have arisen during the wearing of the dentures. A thorough examination should then be carried out of the oral tissues and the dentures. In the course of this examination, signs of tissue damage may be noted which link to the difficulties reported by the patient. In addition, signs of symptomless tissue damage may be noted.

A diagnosis should then be made of the cause of all problems revealed by the history and examination procedures. Appropriate treatment should be carried out to resolve these problems.

HISTORY OF THE PATIENT'S EXPERIENCES

Initially, the patient should be asked to give an account of any difficulties encountered when wearing the dentures, or which have occurred during insertion and removal of the dentures. Where specific complaints arise, secondary questioning should then be directed at obtaining information which will assist in diagnosis of the cause of the complaints. The complaints which commonly arise, and the appropriate questioning which should be applied, are as follows.

Pain

This is the commonest complaint made by patients, following the insertion of complete dentures. The patient should be asked to describe as fully as possible the nature of the pain. To assist categorisation, the patient may be asked, for example, if the pain is of a sharp and stabbing nature which is brought on by the application of biting pressure to the dentures. Alternatively, is the pain of a neuralgic type which may be likened to toothache, or is it better described as a burning sensation in one or both of the denture-bearing areas?

Subsequent questions asked should include the following:

1. How long has the pain been present, and is it relieved by leaving out the dentures?

2. Is the pain present continually when the denture is being worn, or does it arise only at certain times, e.g. at mealtimes, or when the denture is being inserted or removed?

3. Is the pain localised to a small area of the oral tissues, or is it widespread? The exact area affected by the pain should be established as far as is possible.

4. Have any analgesics or other medication been taken to try and relieve the pain?

Looseness of the dentures

The questions asked should include:

1. Do both dentures or only one seem to be loose, and, where the latter applies, which one is affected?

2. Does the looseness arise indiscriminately throughout the period when the denture is worn, or does it only arise when specific functions are being undertaken, e.g. eating or speaking?

3. Does displacement of the denture(s) seem to initiate in a particular area, e.g. does the back part of the lower denture rise when the tongue is moved?

Unsatisfactory aesthetics

Many patients are reticent about complaining of the appearance of dentures, fearing that they may be considered to be unduly vain. Careful and sympathetic questioning is necessary if the exact nature of the problem is to be established.

Initial questioning should be directed at finding out whether the patient's complaint relates to the display of the teeth, or to the support which the dentures provide for the cheeks and lips.

Where the complaint concerns the display of the teeth, secondary questioning should aim at determining the feature or features which concern the patient. For example: Do the anterior teeth seem to be too large or too small? Has the occlusal plane been set at too high a level, providing deficient display of the upper anterior teeth? Has the centre line been misplaced, or is the arrangement of the teeth unsatisfactory?

Where the problem relates to the support of the lips and cheeks provided by the dentures, the patient should be asked to indicate whether it is considered to be excessive or deficient, and whether it applies to a specific area or to the whole denture.

Speech problems

Questioning should be directed at determining the exact nature of the patient's complaint, e.g. does whistling or lisping arise during the pronunciation of the 's' sound?

Intolerance to denture wearing

Where the patient complains of an inability to wear the dentures continuously because of the development of nausea, the following questions should be asked:

1. For how long can the dentures be worn before they have to be removed?
2. Does taking out only one of the dentures remove the problem and, if so, which denture is concerned?
3. Has a similar problem occurred with any previous dentures worn by the patient?

Inefficient mastication

Where this complaint arises, the patient should be asked to indicate:

1. Does the problem arise when attempting to chew all types of food, or is it restricted to the chewing of certain types only, e.g. fibrous foods such as meat?
2. Are the masticatory problems accompanied by other difficulties, such as pain or looseness of the dentures?
3. Does adequate room seem to be present for the placement of food in the mouth, as chewing proceeds?

EXAMINATION OF THE ORAL CAVITY AND THE DENTURES

The dentures should be removed from the mouth and a detailed examination should be made of the oral tissues, with the help of a mouth mirror. Although particular attention should be paid to any areas where the patient has experienced pain, all the oral tissues should be examined, since symptomless tissue changes may be noted which require treatment. The site of all the observed tissue changes should be recorded, along with an indication of their intensity, which may vary from mild hyperaemia up to frank ulceration. In all cases where it is thought that a tissue change may be associated with underlying pathology, a radiographic examination should be carried out of the area concerned.

The dentures should then be examined, first extra-orally and then intra-orally. In the extra-oral examination, the state of cleanliness of the dentures should be noted. The denture surfaces should then be examined for the presence of any irregularities which may have caused tissue irritation. For example, nodules may be found on the fitting surfaces, or sharp margins may be noted on one or more of the teeth.

Intra-oral examination of the dentures should be carried out by the application of the procedures used to check the satisfaction of the trial dentures, which are described in detail in Chapter 26. Each denture should first be checked for extension, retention and stability. The aesthetic effect of the dentures should then be observed, with particular reference to any complaints relating to appearance raised by the patient. The occlusal vertical dimension of the dentures should be checked to ensure that an acceptable value of freeway space is present.

The intercuspal relationship of the posterior teeth should be noted when the teeth are brought into occlusion with the mandible in retruded jaw relationship. Finally, the patient should be requested to make protrusive and lateral movement of the mandible with the teeth in contact, and note made of the state of occlusal balance which is present.

Throughout the period of examination of the dentures, an attempt should be made to relate the observation of any faults which are found to be present with the complaints raised by the patient. For example, a finding of overextension in a denture may relate to complaints by the patient of pain and/or of looseness of the denture.

THE CAUSE AND MANAGEMENT OF PATIENTS' COMPLAINTS

Normally, diagnosis of the cause of a patient's complaints will be possible when the history of the experiences of the patient during denture wearing is considered in association with the findings of the examination of the oral tissues and the dentures. Occasionally, atypical conditions may be present which will require the patient being referred to an appropriate specialist before diagnosis is possible. A consideration of these conditions is considered to be beyond the scope of this text.

Once a diagnosis has been made, a decision must be made on the appropriate treatment which is necessary, e.g. modification of the dentures where this is indicated.

In this section, the common causes of patients' complaints will be considered and advice given on the treatment which should be provided. The subject will be discussed under the headings previously used in the presentation of the patient's complaints.

Pain

For convenience, the complaint of pain may be considered under three subheadings which correspond to the area of the oral tissues in which the complaint arises:

1. Cases in which the complaint of pain arises in a localised area of the oral tissues.
2. Cases in which the complaint of pain arises over a diffuse area, but one which is restricted to part only of the denture-bearing tissues underlying one or both of the dentures.
3. Cases in which the complaint of pain arises in a diffuse area extending over most, if not all, of the denture-bearing tissues underlying one or both of the dentures.

However, it should be noted that no clear division exists between the areas involved in the first two of the following sections. Cases will be encountered in which the presenting signs and symptoms overlap the boundaries of the areas of pain concerned in these two sections. Where this arises, the treatment provided must take account of the possible causes of pain and the appropriate treatment prescribed in the consideration of each of these sections.

Cases in which the complaint of pain arises in a localised area of the oral tissues

Where the complaint arises in the denture-bearing tissues, the likely causes are one or more of the following:

1. Overextension of the periphery of the dentures.
2. The presence of too deep or too sharp a postdam on the upper denture.
3. Irregularities present on the fitting surfaces of the dentures, not paralleled by the form of the corresponding areas of the underlying soft tissues.
4. Localised irregularities in the intercuspal relationship of the dentition, either in the position of maximum intercuspation, or during lateral or protrusive excursions of the mandible.
5. Excessive engagement of undercuts by the denture in a localised area.
6. Localised irregularities in the residual alveolar ridges, thinly covered with soft tissues, which have either not been relieved, or inadequately relieved, in the course of denture construction.
7. The presence of pathology, e.g. superficially placed buried roots, in the tissues supporting the dentures.
8. The presence of the mental foramina within the lower denture-bearing area, for which either no relief, or inadequate relief, has been provided in the course of denture construction.

Causes 1–5 inclusive will usually have produced clearly visible signs of inflammatory changes in the soft tissues in the areas concerned. Visual examination of the inserted dentures will usually indicate the area of the denture responsible for the tissue damage. Where necessary, pressure relief cream may be used to indicate the causative area(s) of the denture. Where causes 1–4 apply, the patient will usually complain of some discomfort being present whenever the dentures are worn, and that a more acute pain arises whenever biting pressure is applied. Where cause 5 applies, the patient may only experience severe pain when the dentures are being inserted or removed.

Visible signs of tissue damage will be seen in a proportion of cases where causes 6 and 7 apply, but only rarely where cause 8 applies. Where these causes are responsible for pain, the tissue areas concerned will be found to show increased sensitivity to pressure. Cause 7 will be identified by radiographic examination of the area. For cause 8, the mental foramina will be palpable within the lower denture-bearing zone. Again, pressure relief cream may be used to aid location of the portion of the denture associated with the area of the tissues where pain is arising.

Treatment of all the above causes except 4 and 7 will require modification of the dentures by trimming of the area(s) concerned, until the painful symptoms have been relieved. Treatment of cause 4 will require adjustment of the occlusion by selective grinding, until full occlusal harmony of the dentition has been established. Treatment of cause 7 will usually require surgery to effect resolution of the condition.

Where the complaint of pain arises in the mucosal surfaces of the lips, cheeks or tongue, the likely causes are as follows:

1. Irritation of the tissues arising from the presence of a sharp margin on one or more of the teeth.
2. Cheek biting, due to an inadequate buccal overjet having been developed in the posterior dentition.
3. Tongue biting, due to an inadequate lingual overjet having been developed in the posterior dentition, and/or the presence of too narrow an arch form, causing 'cramping' of the tongue.

Where cause 1 applies, treatment will involve smoothing and polishing of the sharp area of the tooth or teeth responsible for the condition.

For cause 2, where the cheek biting which has occurred is of a relatively mild nature, usually associated with development of only hyperaemia in the tissues concerned, resolution may be achieved by the grinding of appropriate areas of the teeth to develop an improved buccal overjet. Where the posterior teeth have been set in a normal relationship, this will involve reduction of the buccal surfaces of the lower posterior teeth. Where a cross-bite arrangement of the posterior dentition has been adopted, the buccal surfaces of the upper posterior teeth should be reduced instead. In both cases, the bucco-occlusal margins of the ground teeth should be rounded over and polished, to reduce the risk of further tissue trauma arising.

For cause 3, where tongue biting has occurred as a consequence of the presence of an inadequate lingual overjet being present in the posterior dentition, and the condition is of a relatively mild nature, treatment may be applied as described above for the condition of cheek biting. Where the posterior teeth have been set in a normal relationship, the palatal surfaces of the upper posterior teeth should be reduced and, for a cross-bite relationship, the lingual surfaces of the lower posterior teeth should be reduced, until an adequate lingual overjet has been achieved. Rounding over and polishing of the palato-occlusal or linguo-occlusal margins of the ground teeth should follow the above treatment.

Where tongue biting has occurred as a consequence of the arch form 'cramping' the tongue, and the condition is again of a relatively mild nature, grinding the lingual surfaces of the lower posterior teeth to increase the available tongue space may serve to resolve the condition. Where this treatment is applied, the linguo-occlusal margins of the posterior teeth should be rounded over and polished to reduce the risk of further tissue trauma arising.

Where cause 2 or 3 has resulted in severe tissue damage arising, especially where frank ulceration of the tissues has developed, treatment of the condition will usually require the posterior teeth being reset, or one at least of the dentures being remade, to provide adequate buccal or lingual overjet and/or adequate tongue space, as required.

Cases in which the complaint of pain arises over a diffuse area restricted to part only of the denture-bearing tissues underlying one or both of the dentures.

The cause of this condition is most commonly found to be the presence of anatomical abnormality in the tissue area concerned. A region where this condition is often encountered is the lower anterior alveolar region.

Here, digital and radiographic examination may reveal the presence of a sharp or irregular margin in the residual alveolar ridge, which may be associated with atrophy in the overlying mucosa. Pressure from a denture on such a tissue base may well stimulate a painful response. Other bony abnormalities in the lower denture-bearing tissues which may cause pain when pressure is applied by a denture include sharp mylohyoid ridges, and the development of the genial tubercles to form a bony shelf.

In the upper denture-bearing area, pressure from the denture may give rise to pain in the area of a torus palatinus, where the area has been either unrelieved, or inadequately relieved, in the course of denture construction. Also, in some cases, pain may arise where pressure from the denture is applied to the bone at the root of the zygomatic arch.

For all these conditions, relief of pain may be obtained by reduction of the fitting surface of the denture in the areas concerned, to reduce the pressure applied by the denture in the corresponding area. Where this is unsuccessful, treatment may necessitate surgical intervention. Alternatively, especially where surgery is contraindicated, the placement of a resilient lining in the denture may be considered.

Cases in which the complaint of pain arises in a diffuse area extending over most, if not all, of the denture-bearing tissues underlying one or both of the dentures

Two main causes may be responsible for this condition:

1. The presence of an excessive occlusal vertical dimension in the dentition.
2. Allergy or sensitivity to the denture base material which has been used.

Where cause 1 applies, the patient may complain of widespread pain arising in both the upper and lower denture-bearing areas. In the course of the examination of the oral tissues, inflammation of the denture-bearing tissues may be observed.

When an excessive vertical dimension is present in the dentures, the force applied by the masticatory muscles may be greater than that arising at the correct occlusal vertical dimension. Where an increase in force arises, the denture-bearing tissues may show an inflammatory response, with associated pain production in the tissues. The lower denture-bearing area is particularly liable to be affected, because the applied pressure is concentrated on a smaller area than that of the upper denture-bearing area. The space present between the teeth in speech will also be reduced, so that the patient may complain that a clicking sound occurs in the pronunciation of some sounds, as a consequence of tooth contact occurring. Difficulty may also be experienced in the production of sounds which involve contact being developed between the upper and lower lips, such as 'p', 'b' and 'm'. Where examination of the dentures shows the absence of an acceptable value for freeway space, treatment will require the remaking of one denture at least, at a reduced value of occlusal vertical dimension.

Where cause 2 applies, the patient usually complains of a burning sensation in the denture-bearing tissues, especially in the upper jaw. On examination of the oral tissues, those in contact with the dentures may show oedema and hyperaemia.

Acrylic resin is the denture base material which most commonly gives rise to this condition. Where allergy or sensitivity is suspected as being the responsible agent for a patient's complaint of pain, a patch test should be carried out. Details of the procedure involved in carrying out patch testing may be found in the literature relating to this topic, and are considered to be outside the scope of the present text.

Where a positive diagnosis of allergy or sensitivity to a denture-base material has been made, treatment will require the dentures being remade using an alternative material (e.g. vulcanite, where the allergy or sensitivity is to acrylic resin).

Looseness of the dentures

Where the patient complains that one or both of the

dentures is loose throughout the period they are being worn, the cause is likely to be one or more of the following:

1. Overextension of the periphery of the dentures relative to the level of the functional sulcus. Where intra-oral examination of the dentures shows one or more areas of overextension to be present, the areas concerned should be reduced to the correct level by marginal trimming. A complaint of looseness of the dentures due to this cause will often be accompanied by a complaint of pain arising in the tissues, in the area where overextension is present.

2. Incorrect shaping of the denture relative to the environmental musculature. This cause is particularly liable to produce a complaint of looseness of the lower denture. The teeth may not have been set in the neutral zone (zone of minimum conflict) causing, perhaps, cramping of the tongue. Alternatively, the polished surfaces of the dentures may have been incorrectly shaped, so that conflict arises between the dentures and the environmental musculature in the performance of functions such as speech. Where this cause applies, treatment will usually necessitate remaking of the dentures in a more acceptable form.

3. Inadequate retention may arise where the dentures are underextended relative to the level of the functional sulcus. Where the upper denture is affected, a deficient post-dam may have been provided. Alternatively, the condition may arise where faults have occurred in impression-taking or in the subsequent stage of preparing the master casts. Where features of the dentures other than inadequate retention are found to be satisfactory, relining or rebasing of the dentures may resolve the condition (see Ch. 23, p. 196, for details of the necessary impression procedures). In all other cases, treatment will involve remaking of the dentures.

Where the patient complains that the dentures are only loose when masticating food, the likely causes are one or more of the following:

1. Newness of the dentures, particularly where the patient has no previous experience of denture wearing. Where this cause is suspected, the patient should be encouraged to persevere. It may be helpful to reiterate previous advice that the den-

tures are 'foreign bodies' in their mouth and that it takes time for the tissues to adjust to their presence. It may take several weeks or even months for a patient who is new to denture wearing to learn the art of denture control. The patient should be reassured that with perseverance the position will improve and that food and dentures will no longer seem to be inexorably mixed at mealtimes!

2. Unilateral instability of the dentures arising in the course of mastication, as a consequence of the teeth having been set excessively buccal to the crest of the alveolar ridges. The lower denture is particularly liable to be affected, tilting from side to side as masticatory pressure is applied. Treatment will require resetting of the teeth into a more acceptable position relative to the alveolar ridges, or remaking of the dentures.

3. Bilateral instability occurring as a consequence of a lack of occlusal balance being present in the dentition. Where this cause applies, a face-bow record and wax precentric record should be obtained. The dentures should then be remounted on an average value or adjustable articulator and selectively ground to develop occlusal balance. The procedures for obtaining the necessary records and carrying out selective grinding are considered in Chapter 27 (pp. 231–233).

Unsatisfactory aesthetics

This complaint should arise only rarely if adequate care was taken in checking aesthetics at the trial denture stage. Where the patient does raise objections to the aesthetics of the dentures at the review stage, questioning will often indicate that the objections arise from comments made by the patient's relatives or friends.

Whenever possible, an attempt should be made to overcome the complaints by modification of the dentures. For example, where the complaint is that the dentures provide excessive support for the lips and/or cheeks, the denture flanges may be reduced in thickness until the required reduced level of support for the facial tissues has been obtained. Where the complaint is that the dentures provide inadequate support for the facial tissues, wax may be added to increase the thickness of the flanges until the required level of support has been achieved. Increasing flange thickness to provide greater support for the facial tissues is often referred to as 'plumping' of the dentures. The added wax is converted into the appropriate denture base material in the laboratory, before the dentures are returned to the patient.

Where the complaint of unsatisfactory aesthetics relates to the teeth, it may concern features such as the size or colour of the teeth, the position of the centre line and the degree to which the upper and/or lower anterior teeth show when the patient is smiling or talking.

Where modification of tooth arrangements is necessary to meet such complaints, remaking of the dentures will usually be necessary.

Speech problems

Where a patient is provided with complete dentures for the first time, a period of adaptation of a month or so may be necessary before the quality of speech approaches that which occurred when the natural dentition was present. In this period, the lips, cheeks and tongue will be adapting to the presence of the dentures, with gradual improvement in the quality of the sounds which are produced. The patient may be warned that this period of adaptation may be necessary when the dentures are inserted.

Some minor disruption of speech may also occur where replacement complete dentures are provided. The patient should be reassured that such a problem is likely to disappear in a month or so, as the tissues adapt to the presence of the new dentures.

Where speech problems persist beyond this time, modification of the dentures may be necessary. The sounds most likely to be affected are those associated with the pronunciation of the letters 's', 'p' and 'b'. This subject is considered in some detail in the parallel section relating to the review stage of partial denture treatment (Ch. 21, p. 176). The chapter should be consulted for details of the speech defects and of the denture modifications which are necessary to overcome them.

Intolerance to denture wearing

Where the patient complains of the development of nausea on or shortly after the insertion of complete dentures and indicates that the upper denture seems to initiate nausea, the likely causes are one or more of the following:

1. Overextension of the posterior aspect of the upper denture. Where the denture extends on to the movable tissues of the soft palate, the retching reflex may be stimulated.

2. The posterior extension of the upper denture is correct by 'normal' standards, but the denture covers areas of the posterior region of the hard palate which show abnormal sensitivity. This condition may relate to the presence of an enhanced amount or abnormal distribution of nerves in the tissues overlying the hard palate.

3. Incorrect development of denture form at the posterior palatal termination. Where a ledge is present at the junction of the posterior border of the denture with the palatal tissues posterior to the denture, irritation of the dorsum of the tongue may occur during deglutition and speech, giving rise to nausea. Enhanced sensitivity of the posterior region of the dorsum of the tongue has been said to occur in some patients as a consequence of the presence of an abnormal distribution of the glossopharyngeal nerves.

4. Inadequate retention being present in the upper denture. Nausea may arise when displacement of the denture occurs in function, bringing it into contact with the dorsum of the tongue, particularly where the latter shows enhanced sensitivity.

Where the patient indicates that the lower denture seems to initiate nausea, the likely causes are:

5. 'Cramping' of the tongue as a consequence of the provision of inadequate tongue space.

6. Overextension of the denture posterolingually, so that contact occurs in function between the denture and the tissues of the palatoglossal arch.

Where cause 1 applies, the treatment required will be reduction of the posterior extension of the upper denture to a level where it lies just anterior to the vibrating line. Where necessary, a new post-dam should be provided.

For cause 2, treatment will depend upon the severity of the condition. Where only mild nausea arises, not extending to actual retching, the patient may be asked to persevere with the wearing of the denture for a further trial period. With time, the tissues may adapt to the presence of the denture and the nausea will disappear without further treatment being necessary. Where this is tried but resolution of the nausea does not occur, or where the condition is found to be of a more severe nature at the initial review visit, it will usually be necessary to reduce the posterior palatal extension of the upper denture. Examination of the posterior palatal tissues should be carried out with an instrument such as a ball-ended burnisher and the area of enhanced sensitivity noted. The extension of the denture should then be reduced to avoid coverage of the corresponding tissue area. Minimum reduction of palatal coverage compatible with overcoming the complaint of nausea should be aimed at, so that optimal denture retention will be achieved. A posterior palatal seal, approximately 1 mm deep, should be developed around the new posterior palatal border of the denture.

It should be noted that a complaint of severe nausea due to enhanced sensitivity in the posterior palatal tissues is unlikely to be noted at the review stage without prior warning of the condition having arisen during earlier treatment stages. Often, it will have been necessary to reduce the palatal extension of the upper special tray, upper occlusal rim and upper trial denture baseplate to overcome nausea experienced in these stages. Where this applies, the palatal extension of the finished denture should be developed to a similar level. A denture of the so-called 'horseshoe' form may be necessary where an extensive area of the palatal tissues show enhanced sensitivity.

Treatment of cause 3 will require trimming of the polished surface of the upper denture in the region of the posterior palatal border, until the ledge has been removed.

Treatment of cause 4 will require action to improve the retention of the upper denture. This may be achieved by relining of the denture in appropriate cases, otherwise remaking of the denture may be necessary, as noted on page 240.

The treatment necessary to overcome cause 5 will depend upon the severity of the condition. Where the condition is of a mild nature, trimming of the lingual surfaces of the lower posterior teeth, and/or thinning of the lingual flanges of the lower denture, may provide sufficient increase in tongue space to overcome the complaint. Where the condition is more severe, treatment will usually necessitate remaking of the dentures to provide adequate tongue space.

Treatment of cause 6 involves reduction of the posterolingual extension of the lower denture until contact of the denture with the palatoglossal arch no longer occurs in function.

Where the patient complains of nausea, but this only develops several hours after the insertion of the dentures, the probable cause will be a reaction of the tissues to the bulk of the dentures. Where this problem arises, the patient may again be asked to persevere with the wearing of the dentures in the hope that adaptation will develop in time, and nausea will no longer be a problem. Where this is unsuccessful, the bulk of the dentures should be reduced by trimming of the polished surfaces. The palate of the upper denture should receive particular attention. Care should be taken that the reduction which is applied does not exceed the level at which the strength of the denture will be impaired.

In some instances, it may prove to be necessary to provide a denture with a metal palate (e.g. in cast cobalt–chromium alloy) to achieve a tolerable thickness in the palate. Singers in particular may present this special need.

Inefficient mastication

Where a patient complains of a difficulty in chewing all types of food, the cause is likely to be one or more of the following:

1. Inexperience in the wearing of complete dentures. When a patient wears complete dentures for the first time, an induction period is usually necessary in which the patient learns the art of muscular control of the dentures. This period may extend from 1 week to 6 months or even more, being dependent upon the ability of the patient's tissues to adapt to the presence of the dentures. In general, the older the patient at the time complete dentures are first fitted, the longer is the induction period likely to be. During the induction period, the patient is likely to experience difficulty in the mastication of food.

2. The presence of an excessive vertical dimension in the dentition. This may result in the patient experiencing difficulty in placing food on the occlusal table, and will require a conscious effort to increase mouth opening beyond the normal level each time food has to be placed in the mouth.

3. The occlusal plane of the dentures having been set at too high a level. Where this applies, the tongue and cheeks may experience difficulty in repositioning food on the occlusal table as mastication proceeds.

4. The presence of an inadequate vertical dimension in the dentition. One of the possible consequences of an excessive freeway space is that the power applied by the masticatory muscles may be reduced. This can give rise to inefficient mastication.

5. Lack of occlusal balance in the dentition. Where cuspal interferences arise in the course of mandibular movements, a reduction in masticatory efficiency is also likely to occur. This problem is particularly liable to occur where the patient has a ruminatory type of masticatory mechanism.

6. As an accompaniment of a complaint of looseness of the denture. Where the dentures are loose in the course of mastication of food, the efficiency of chewing is likely to be reduced.

7. As an accompaniment of a complaint of pain in the denture-bearing area. Where the patient is experiencing pain in the denture-bearing areas, the pain protection reflex may limit the force applied by the masticatory muscles in the course of the mastication of food. Decrease in applied pressure may result in decreased masticatory efficiency.

Where the patient complains of masticatory inefficiency, restricted mainly to the chewing of fibrous foods such as meat, the likely causes are one or more of the following:

8. The presence of anatomical-type posterior teeth whose cuspal form has been excessively reduced, usually in the course of selective grinding.

9. The use of flat-cusped or non-anatomical form of posterior teeth. Teeth of this type may provide poorer masticatory efficiency than that provided by teeth of an anatomical form.

10. The use of acrylic posterior teeth. This problem is particularly liable to be encountered where the patient has previously worn dentures provided with porcelain posterior teeth.

Treatment of cause 1 will require the patient being reassured that as muscular control of the dentures is developed, masticatory efficiency should improve. Where causes 2 or 4 applies, treatment will require remaking of the dentures to provide an adequate and yet not excessive value of freeway space. Treatment of cause 3 will require the dentures being remade to provide a more appropriate level of the occlusal plane. This need will have to be considered in association with the need to set the occlusal plane at a level at which acceptable aesthetics will be achieved, and some compromise in the level selected for use may be necessary. Guidance on the optimal position of the occlusal plane for achieving masticatory efficiency may be obtained by observing the level of the dorsum of the tongue when the tongue is at rest. The plane should be set at the observed level of the dorsum of the tongue. Treatment of cause 5 will require the dentures being remounted on an average value or adjustable articulator, via the use of a face-bow and wax precentric records, and selectively ground into a state of occlusal balance. The procedures for obtaining the necessary records and for carrying out selective grinding are considered in Chapter 27 (pp. 231–233).

Treatment of causes 6 and 7 will require resolution of the complaints of looseness of the dentures or pain in the denture-bearing areas, following the procedures considered on pages 240 and 237 respectively.

Treatment of cause 8 will require replacement of the posterior teeth by a new set, or remaking of the dentures.

Where cause 9 or 10 applies, the patient may be asked to persevere with use of the dentures for a further trial period. If no improvement in masticatory efficiency arises, it may be advisable to provide replacement posterior teeth, using anatomical-type posterior teeth where cause 9 applies and porcelain posterior teeth for cause 10.

Other complaints

The patient may raise one or more complaints at the review stage which have not been covered in the above list. For each of these, a diagnosis of the cause of the complaint should be made. This will be based on the history of the patient's experiences when wearing the dentures, considered in association with the findings of the examination of the oral tissues and the dentures. Appropriate treatment to overcome the cause of each complaint should then be provided.

One complaint that may be frequently encountered is that of excessive salivation, particularly where the patient has been provided with complete dentures for the first time. The only treatment normally required for this complaint is reassurance of the patient that the condition is likely to resolve in the fullness of time.

General note

In all instances where the peripheries, teeth or polished surfaces of the dentures have been modified at the review stage, the areas concerned must be carefully repolished before the dentures are returned to the patient.

Where severe tissue damage was noted at the review stage, an appointment for further review in approximately 7 days should be made for the patient, to see if the treatment provided has effected resolution of the condition. Where necessary, further treatment should be applied and the patient re-examined after the same interval. This procedure should be repeated until full resolution of the condition has occurred. Where extra-oral examination of the dentures showed a poor level of cleanliness to be present, the advice given to the patient at the insertion stage concerning care of the dentures should be repeated at the review stage.

At the conclusion of the review stage, the patient should be provided with information on the likely life of complete dentures and of the need to return for further reviews.

It may be pointed out to the patient that as a consequence of the changes which occur in the denture-bearing tissues and in the dentures, the average life of complete dentures is of the order of 5 years. However, considerable variation in this period may occur in individual cases. It is desirable that the patient should return for review at approximately yearly intervals. The oral tissues and the dentures can then be examined to determine if their condition is still satisfactory, or if further treatment is required. Of particular importance is the fact that symptomless changes can occur in the oral tissues which require treatment. For example, hyperplasia may develop in the tissues related to the peripheries of the dentures without the patient being aware of this occurrence.

The patient should also be encouraged to seek a further appointment for review whenever circumstances arise with the dentures which give cause for concern. For example, pain may develop in the oral tissues or the dentures may become loose or provide less efficient mastication of food than that present when the dentures were first fitted.

FURTHER READING

Kovats JJ 1971 Clinical evaluation of the gagging patient. J Prosthet Dent 25: 613
Kuebker WA 1984 Denture problems: causes, diagnostic procedures and clinical treatment. Quintess Int 15: 1035
Laine P 1982 Adaptation to denture wearing. An opinion survey and experimental investigation. Proc Finn Dent Soc 78(suppl 2): 159
McCabe JF, Basker RM 1976 Tissue sensitivity to acrylic resin. Br Dent J 140: 347
MacGregor AA 1983 Pressure-indicating pastes. J Dent 11: 264
Makila E 1974 Adjustment visits following provision of complete dentures. J Oral Rehab 1: 373
Miller EL 1973 Types of inflammation caused by oral prostheses. J Prosthet Dent 30: 380
Morstad AR, Peterson AD 1968 Post-insertion denture problems. J Prosthet Dent 19: 126
Murphy WM 1971 The effect of complete dentures on taste perception. Br Dent J 130: 210
Nagle RJ 1958 Post-insertion problems in complete denture prosthesis. J Am Dent Assoc 57: 183
Weiffenbach JM 1987 Taste perception mechanisms. In: Ferguson D B (ed) The aging mouth, Front Oral Physiol 6: 151
Yemm R 1972 Stress-induced muscle activity: a possible etiological factor in denture soreness. J Prosthet Dent 28: 133

PART IV

Special aspects relating to immediate denture treatment

29. Introductory considerations

DEFINITION

An immediate denture is a denture which is constructed before the extraction of at least some of the teeth which it replaces and which is inserted immediately after the extraction of those teeth.

This definition allows an immediate denture to be distinguished from a post-immediate denture, since the construction of the latter does not commence until all the teeth which it replaces have been extracted.

THE SCOPE OF IMMEDIATE DENTURE TREATMENT

An immediate denture can be either a complete denture or a partial denture. It may involve the immediate replacement of anterior teeth only, this probably being the commonest type of immediate denture. Alternatively, it may involve the immediate replacement of anterior and posterior teeth or, more rarely, may involve the immediate replacement of posterior teeth only.

THE SELECTION OF PATIENTS FOR IMMEDIATE DENTURE PROVISION

The decision as to whether or not an immediate denture is to be provided for a patient is based on weighing up the advantages and disadvantages of immediate denture treatment as they apply to the patient in question. The factors which need to be taken into consideration are as follows:

Advantages

1. The provision of an immediate denture can prevent a patient from being subjected to the possible embarrassment of having to appear in public in a partially dentate or edentulous state. Of particular importance from that regard is the aesthetic loss associated with the absence of some or all of the anterior teeth (Fig. 29.1).

Immediate dentures will thus be especially appreciated by persons whose daily life brings them into contact with the general public.

From the patient's point of view, this is probably the most important of the advantages offered by immediate denture provision.

2. By working from a baseline provided by the patient's standing natural dentition, it is possible to provide an artificial dentition which exactly duplicates, where indicated, the colour, size, form and arrangement of the natural teeth. This can be of particular significance where the replacement of anterior teeth is involved and can produce a result which should defy detection as being artificial.

3. Alternatively, where indicated, it is possible to introduce a known degree of modification to the appearance of the artificial dentition, relative to that of the patient's natural dentition. This can be achieved by introducing a different angulation of the teeth, or by a bodily repositioning of the teeth, which may be combined with a modification of the natural alveolar form by the carrying out of alveolar surgery in some cases.

Such procedures can play an important role in the cosmetic work of a dental surgeon.

4. The determination of the occlusal vertical dimension at the jaw registration stage of treatment is usually easier to carry out, and the result is more reliable, than applies when carrying out the same treatment stage for an edentulous patient. The

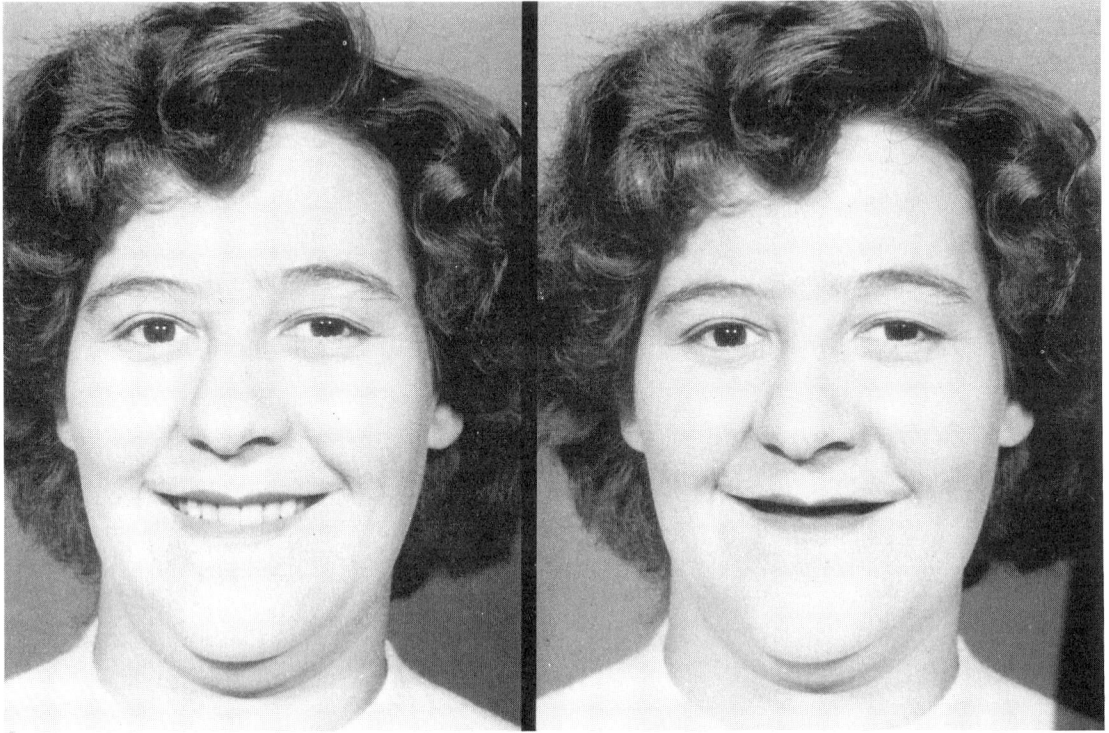

Fig. 29.1   Photographs of a patient (edentulous), with and without complete immediate dentures being worn.

reason for this difference relates to the presence of a partial or complete natural dentition in the patient undergoing immediate denture treatment, the height at which the upper and lower teeth contact usually providing a reliable guide to the required occlusal vertical dimension.

5. If a patient is rendered edentulous and left in that condition for several months prior to the provision of complete dentures, there is a risk that the lip and cheek muscles will tend to lose tonus and collapse inwards, thereby encroaching on the 'neutral zone'. Immediate replacement of teeth can help to reduce the risk of such changes occurring and so help to preserve the size of the neutral zone. As a consequence, patients who are provided with immediate dentures usually become accustomed to the presence of the dentures and learn to use them successfully in a much shorter period of time than applies where the patient has been left edentulous for a prolonged period prior to denture provision.

6. The provision of immediate dentures reduces the risk of interruption occurring in the patient's

normal speech pattern.

7. The provision of immediate dentures helps in preserving the patient's masticatory function. It is not necessary for the patient to have to adopt the 'soft' diet which is characteristic of the edentulous state and which, if unduly prolonged, may affect the general health of the patient.

8. When patients are subjected to a prolonged edentulous period, they tend to develop a more extreme range of mandibular movements than that normally present. This change arises through the patient trying to make the best possible use of the residual alveolar ridges as 'chewing blocks' for the mastication of food.

The increase in the range of mandibular movements can sometimes lead to the development of symptoms of the temporomandibular joint dysfunction syndrome. A more common finding, however, is that the operator will experience difficulty in persuading the patient to adopt the true retruded jaw relationship at the jaw registration stage of complete denture treatment.

These problems will be avoided where immediate dentures are provided.

9. An immediate denture has a splint action in covering over the blood clots which develop in the extraction sockets. This reduces the risk of post-operative haemorrhage occurring. It also prevents the risk of food entering the extraction sockets, so lessening the incidence of dry-socket formation.

10. The provision of a partial immediate denture prevents the risk that the teeth adjacent to the extraction site will tilt or drift into the space so created. Such a denture can thus serve a valuable role as a space maintainer, thereby facilitating the construction at a later date of either a removable partial denture or a fixed bridge.

Since tooth movement is particularly liable to occur in young persons, the provision of a partial immediate denture is of special value in persons of that age group.

Disadvantages

1. The major disadvantage arises from the fact that alveolar resorption will almost inevitably occur in the area or areas where teeth were extracted and immediately replaced. As a consequence, the denture is likely to show a progressive decrease in retention over a period of time. If a point is reached where the loss in retention of the denture becomes an embarrassment to the patient, it will be necessary to reline the denture in order to restore its retention to an acceptable level. It is not unusual to find that two relining procedures will prove to be necessary in the initial 6 month period following the insertion of the denture. The provision of a replacement denture is also often found to be indicated 6–9 months after the insertion of the immediate denture.

Before a patient is provided with an immediate denture, it is essential for them to be made aware of what will be involved and to ensure that they will be prepared to attend over the quite extensive treatment period.

2. Successful immediate denture treatment necessitates the full cooperation of the patient. As previously noted, treatment extends over quite a prolonged period of time. This can be expensive to the patient both in terms of the cost of the treatment itself and the indirect cost of having to take time off work. It is also essential that the patient should be prepared to spend the necessary time and effort in caring for both the denture and the oral tissues, especially in the early period following the insertion of the denture.

Thus, patients with a history of poor oral hygiene, or who have shown no obvious interest in maintaining their natural dentition, must be considered to be unsuitable for the provision of immediate dentures (Fig. 29.2). Careful selection of patients is, then, necessary if immediate denture treatment is to be successful.

3. The importance of both removable partial dentures and complete dentures being set up to achieve the best possible level of occlusal balance has been pointed out previously (Ch. 18 for removable partial dentures and Ch. 25 for complete dentures). This requirement is of special significance in immediate denture treatment since, if a traumatic conflict develops between the upper and lower dentitions, giving rise to a tendency for denture displacement, appreciable discomfort could arise, especially in the early period following the insertion of the denture.

The need for the development of occlusal balance applies equally to the anterior dentition as it does to the posterior dentition. Where immediate replacement of anterior teeth is involved, a problem can arise in relation to the development of occlusal balance, if the natural anterior dentition presents a condition of a deep overbite combined with a shallow overjet.

The traumatic conflict of such a dentition during the course of mandibular movements may well have

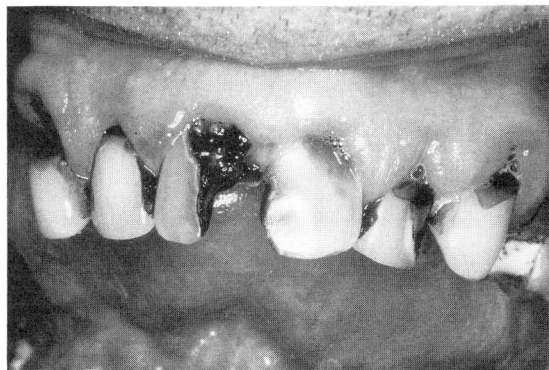

Fig. 29.2 A dentition severely damaged by dental caries.

led to a breakdown of the supporting tissues of the teeth and thus be the reason why extraction of the teeth is now required.

If such an arrangement of the anterior teeth was to be duplicated in the artificial dentition (especially in complete dentures), it is very likely that an unacceptable level of denture instability would arise. Overcoming the traumatic relationship found in a natural anterior dentition can, however, prove to be difficult. One possible solution is to set up the artificial anterior teeth with a reduced overbite relative to that present in the natural dentition. This is achieved by reducing the length of the teeth which are set up in the artificial dentition. If used alone, this solution is likely to produce an appearance which will prove to be unacceptable to the patient, especially where the reduction in length is applied to the upper anterior teeth.

A second possible solution is to set up the artificial anterior teeth with an increased overjet relative to that present in the natural dentition. This is achieved by setting up the upper anterior artificial teeth in a position which is anterior to the position occupied by their natural predecessors, and, thus, is only possible where upper anterior teeth are being immediately replaced. Care has to be taken to ensure that the upper anterior teeth are not set outside the 'neutral zone', otherwise denture instability will arise. It is inadvisable to attempt to achieve the same result by setting artificial lower anterior teeth in a position which is posterior to that occupied by their natural predecessors, as this would almost inevitably result in instability in the lower denture as a result of forces applied by the tongue.

By using a combination of the above solutions, it is possible to produce an acceptable level of occlusal balance in those cases where the degree of traumatic conflict present in the natural dentition is only minor or moderate in degree. Where, however, the traumatic conflict present in the natural dentition is of a severe nature, it may be advisable to explain the situation to the patient and advise against the provision of an immediate denture.

4. The medical/surgical history of the patient may contraindicate the multiple extractions which are commonly a feature of immediate denture treatment. Fortunately, the number of patients to whom this applies is relatively small, one example being patients who have had radiation therapy in the head and neck region for the treatment of a tumour.

The above are the factors which must be borne in mind during the examination of a patient, to determine the wisdom or otherwise of providing an immediate denture. In addition to a full clinical examination of the patient's oral tissues, details must be recorded of the patient's dental and medical/surgical history as well as such social factors as the patient's occupation. The nature and duration of immediate denture treatment must be explained fully to the patient, remembering that their full cooperation in the treatment plan is essential to success.

Except in the fairly infrequent instances where there are clear clinical contraindications to the provision of an immediate denture, it is usual to find that the advantages of providing an immediate denture far outweigh the disadvantages. There is undoubtedly a growing awareness in the general public of the existence of immediate denture treatment and many patients now ask about immediate dentures when the time comes for them to have to lose some or all of their remaining natural teeth. Under these circumstances, there would seem to be a good case for immediate dentures to be provided in all instances where it is feasible. Indeed, it does seem to be something of an anachronism that where the alternative procedure is used a patient can be left in an edentulous state for 6 months or so before dentures are provided. In distinction, the provision of an immediate denture can be said to be one of the most rewarding aspects of prosthodontic treatment in terms of the satisfaction which it can provide to both patient and operator alike.

TREATMENT PLANNING FOR COMPLETE IMMEDIATE DENTURES

When a decision has been made to provide a complete immediate denture in one or both jaws of a patient and there are both anterior and posterior teeth standing in the jaw or jaws involved in the treatment, a further decision has to be made as to which of two possible courses of action is to be followed:

1. The first possible course of action is to provide immediate replacement of all standing anterior and

posterior teeth in the jaw or jaws involved in the treatment, along with providing replacement of any already missing teeth. This course of action may thus involve the immediate replacement of 16 teeth in one jaw, or 32 teeth if both jaws are involved, or of any lesser number according to the number of natural teeth that are present. In treatments such as this, which involve the immediate replacement of a considerable number of teeth in one or both jaws, the disadvantage arises that alveolar resorption in the extensive extraction area or areas causes a gross change in the denture-bearing tissues. As a consequence, the denture or dentures will rapidly lose retention, giving rise to a need for early and repeated relining if retention is to be maintained at an adequate level.

Also, the amount of possible blood loss that can be associated with the extraction of, say, ten or more tooth roots in a single treatment session usually indicates a need for the extractions to be carried out with the patient hospitalised for 24 hours at least, so that facilities for a blood transfusion will be at hand, should that prove to be necessary.

This course of action does, however, have the advantage that the patient only has to face extractions on one occasion and, where the patient is of a particularly nervous disposition, or where there are other special indications for the extractions being carried out under general anaesthesia, this may prove to be a deciding factor.

2. The second possible course of action is to carry out the necessary extractions in two stages. Initially, all standing posterior teeth are extracted, with the possible exception of the first premolars where they are needed to maintain the vertical dimension. The patient is then left in this partially dentate condition for a period of at least 6 weeks but preferably for 3 months. Following this delay period, the construction of an immediate denture or immediate dentures is commenced and, when the denture or dentures are ready, the remaining teeth are extracted and the denture or dentures are inserted.

This course of action has the advantage of providing a reasonably stable tissue base posteriorly, so that the denture or dentures maintain adequate retention for a longer period of time than applies where the first course of action is used. It is also usual to find that the patient experiences less discomfort in the early days after denture insertion where the second course of action is used. Because of these advantages, the second course of action is the one most commonly chosen for use.

TREATMENT PLANNING FOR PARTIAL IMMEDIATE DENTURES

The need may arise for one or more teeth to be immediately replaced for a patient who is already wearing a removable partial denture. Where the latter denture has a connector which is constructed in a polymeric material such as acrylic resin, it is usually possible to add the teeth being immediately replaced to the denture, and this should be done wherever possible.

Where, however, the removable partial denture being worn by the patient has a metallic connector, it may be far more difficult or even impossible to add teeth to the denture. In that case, the construction of a new partial denture is indicated, carrying both the immediately replaced teeth along with the other teeth already missing from the dentition. The construction of an immediate partial denture will also be necessary for the patient who presents with a natural dentition within which one or more teeth need immediate replacement, but the patient does not have a partial denture available to which immediate additions could be made.

In all cases, the design of a partial immediate denture should follow the principles considered in Chapter 15 for designing a removable partial denture. Emphasis should, however, be placed on achieving a simple design form wherever possible, since the expected life of an immediate denture is limited to a period of about 6 months. For example, the use of an all-acrylic denture of the 'Every' type is to be preferred in the upper jaw, rather than the use of a more complex denture which includes a metallic base.

However, it should be noted that the use of a metal baseplate in an immediate denture can occasionally be necessary, such as where there is a close relationship present between the natural anterior dentition and the palate, and one or more of the upper anterior teeth needs to be immediately replaced.

FURTHER READING

Applebaum MC 1983 The practical dynamics of the interim denture concept: a comparison with the conventional immediate denture technique. J Am Dent Assoc 106: 826

Hondrum SO 1988 Interim dentures for the older patient who is medically compromised. Spec Care Dentist 8: 206

Johansen RE, Schwartz R, Harris WT 1988 The orthopaedic relator for fabricating immediate dentures. Gen Dent 36: 520

Johnson K 1986 The immediate maxillary full denture. I. Clinical observations. Aust Dent J 31: 44

Johnson K 1986 The immediate maxillary full denture. II. The dento-alveolar complex. Aust Dent J 31: 124

Johnson K 1986 The immediate maxillary full denture. III. The role of the immediate denture. Aust Dent J 31: 181

Ralph WJ 1979 The effects of dental treatment — biting force. J Prosthet Dent 41: 143

Sones AD, Wolinsky LE, Dratochuil FJ 1986 Osteoporosis and mandibular bone resorption: a prosthodontic perspective. J Prosthet Dent 56: 732

30. The classification of immediate dentures and class selection

CLASSIFICATION

Immediate dentures are normally classified in accordance with the form of replacement adopted for the anterior dentition. Two basic types can be distinguished:

Class I — Open face
Class II — Closed face or flanged.

Class II can be further subdivided, depending on whether or not extraction of the teeth being immediately replaced is combined with the carrying out of surgery on the associated alveolar bone, thus giving:

Class IIa — Closed face without alveolar surgery
Class IIb — Closed face with alveolar surgery.

In a Class I immediate denture no labial flange is present and the replacement teeth are designed so that a few millimetres of the neck of each of the anterior teeth enter the sockets vacated by their natural predecessors (Fig. 30.1). This open-face procedure is only used in the immediate replacement of anterior teeth. If posterior teeth are to be immediately replaced, either on their own or in association with the immediate replacement of anterior teeth, a flange is always used in the posterior region.

In the case of a Class IIa or IIb immediate denture, the appearance will normally be indistinguishable from that of a conventional partial or complete denture.

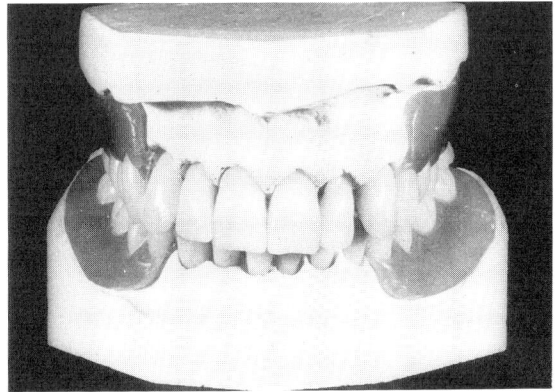

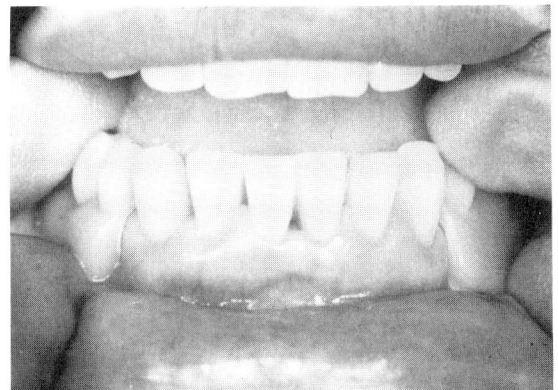

Fig. 30.1 **A** photograph of upper and lower complete open-face dentures following cast preparation and setting of the teeth. **B** photograph of a lower complete open-face denture after insertion.

CLASS SELECTION

When a decision has been made to provide an immediate denture (or dentures) for a patient, a further decision must then be made concerning the class (or classes) of immediate denture that should be provided. It should be noted that, where immediate dentures are to be fitted in both the upper and lower jaws of a patient, a decision as to the most appropriate class to use must be made separately for each jaw. For example, it may be decided to use a Class I denture in the upper jaw and a Class IIa denture in the lower jaw. Alternatively, it may be decided to use a Class IIb denture in both the upper and lower jaws. Other combinations are also possible, as any combination of the three classes may be selected for use in an individual patient.

In relation to the procedure to be adopted for class selection, this can sometimes be dictated by the personal preference of the operator. For instance, some operators always provide a Class I denture in the upper jaw and/or a Class IIa denture in the lower jaw. Although there are advantages to be gained in using familiar procedures, such an approach would not result in the most appropriate choice always being made. A wiser method of choice is one in which the special features of each class of immediate denture are considered in relation to the clinical findings of the jaw in question.

The special features associated with each class of immediate denture that need to be reviewed when making class selection can be listed as follows:

Class I — open face

1. This class is particularly indicated where it is desired to reproduce closely the existing natural anterior dentition of a patient, with no gross alteration in tooth position. When using a Class I type of immediate denture, the position of the neck of each tooth being immediately replaced is relatively fixed by the need for it to enter the socket vacated by its natural predecessor, so that only a minimal change in tooth angulation is feasible.

2. The absence of a labial flange, in combination with the use of a procedure in which the neck of each immediately replaced anterior tooth lies under the natural labial soft tissue flap, means that at the time the denture is inserted, and for some time afterwards, an excellent aesthetic result can be achieved. Indeed, the appearance of a Class I immediate denture is usually regarded as being superior to that achievable where a Class II immediate denture is used, at least in the early period following insertion.

3. The absence of a labial flange does, unfortunately, mean that a Class I immediate denture will have a relatively poor anterior peripheral seal. This seal will also be further decreased in the post-insertion period by alveolar resorption in the area or areas where anterior teeth were extracted. In this class of immediate denture, alveolar resorption is concentrated in areas around the necks of the immediately replaced anterior teeth, resulting in the possibility of the anterior peripheral seal of the denture being seriously disrupted after a relatively short period of time.

The implication of the anterior peripheral seal problem encountered where Class I immediate dentures are used is that it will only prove to be feasible to achieve an acceptable level of retention in such a denture where the anticipated retention factors in the rest of the denture-bearing area are favourable. For example, the presence of a relatively large denture-bearing area is desirable, preferably coupled with the presence of usable undercuts to aid retention. In the case of the upper jaw, the form of the palate is of importance, the presence of a relatively flat palatal vault being more favourable than the presence of a deep, 'V'-shaped form of palatal vault. Well-developed tuberosities would also favour good retention being achievable in the upper jaw. The absence of marked frenal attachments in either the upper or lower jaw would also be an asset.

Where examination shows that such compensatory retention factors are absent, then the use of a Class I immediate denture would generally be contra-indicated. Since good retention factors outside the region of the anterior alveolus are more commonly found in the upper jaw than in the lower jaw, the use of the Class I immediate denture is more common in the maxilla than it is in the mandible. However, in those instances where compensatory retention factors *are* found to be present in the lower jaw, a Class I denture can be beneficially applied and be just as successful as in the upper jaw.

4. A Class I immediate denture can be used to advantage where deep undercuts are present labially as well as elsewhere in the denture area, as engagement of labial undercuts would make it difficult to achieve insertion were a labial flange to be provided on the denture. Also, where a tight lip is encountered, the presence of a labial flange can be an embarrassment. Thus, in patients who present with a Class II or Class III skeletal jaw relationship, where a tight lip is often present in the upper or lower jaw respectively, use of a Class I immediate denture can be indicated.

Class IIa – closed face without alveolar surgery

1. Some of the special features that applied to the Class I type of immediate denture apply in a reverse sense to a Class IIa immediate denture. For example, the presence of a labial flange results in enhanced retention. Thus, for jaws where the anticipated retention factors are unfavourable, the additional retention arising from the presence of a labial flange is one of the main assets of the Class IIa immediate denture relative to use of the Class I type of immediate denture. Also, since the anterior peripheral seal is developed at the base of the sulcus in a Class IIa type of immediate denture, instead of being developed in the socket areas as occurs in a Class I type of immediate denture, adequate retention generally persists for a much longer period of time than applies where a Class I type of immediate denture is used.

2. In the use of a Class II type of immediate denture, the patient is accustomed to the presence of a labial flange from the time that the denture is first inserted. This situation can be contrasted with the position which can arise when a Class I immediate denture is used, where no labial flange is visible in the initial period following the insertion of the denture. However, after the denture has been worn for a period of several weeks a time arises when it usually proves to be desirable for a labial flange to be added to the denture. This helps to restore lip contour by replacing the area of the anterior alveolus lost by resorption. The addition of a labial flange also serves to strengthen the denture and helps to restore retention to an acceptable level. Patients often object, though, to the introduction of a labial flange when one was not present originally on the denture, claiming that it would detract from the natural appearance of the denture. As a consequence, when this happens, the operator may need to spend a considerable amount of time explaining to the patient why a labial flange is now indicated. This problem is avoided if a flange is present initially on the denture, as in a Class IIa immediate denture.

3. It is possible for the position of the artificial teeth to be modified, relative to that of their natural predecessors, where this is indicated on aesthetic or functional grounds.

4. When contemplating the use of a Class IIa immediate denture, it is necessary to ensure from the clinical examination of the patient that the tenseness and activity of the lip in the jaw concerned is such that the presence of a labial flange is going to be tolerated. Since this requirement is more commonly satisfied in the mandible than it is in the maxilla, then the Class IIa form of immediate denture is used more often in the lower jaw than it is in the upper jaw. There are, however, times when it will be found that the Class IIa immediate denture can be applied usefully in the upper jaw, and in such cases the labial flange is made as thin as is possible to avoid undue distortion of the lip occurring.

Class IIb – closed face with alveolar surgery

The first three of the special features listed for a Class IIa type of immediate denture are also applicable to the IIb type. In addition, there are further special features which apply only to the Class IIb type of immediate denture. Before these are listed, it may assist understanding of the subject if the rationale for carrying out alveolar surgery in association with immediate denture treatment is considered, along with the provision of an outline of the type of alveolar surgery commonly used in such work.

Basically, the aim of such surgery is to reduce the size of the anterior alveolus, care being taken, though, to leave sufficient alveolus present to provide adequate support and retention for the denture.

Perhaps the main indication for such alveolar surgery in immediate denture treatment arises in those cases where there is a need for the artificial anterior dentition to be set in a more retruded position than that occupied by their natural predecessors. This may arise in the case of a patient presenting with a gross Class II, division I skeletal jaw relationship, in which the upper anteriors are very protrusive and tend to occupy a position in which they rest on or anterior to the lower lip.

Although such an arrangement of the upper anterior teeth may be regarded as unsightly by some patients, there are others who are fully satisfied with their appearance. For those patients who are happy with such a tooth arrangement, it is generally inadvisable to try to persuade them to have the appearance of their teeth changed. Instead, it is wiser to restrict such work to those patients who ask if the appearance of their teeth could be improved. An approach which can then be adopted is to combine immediate replacement of the protrusive upper anterior teeth with alveolar surgery on the associated area of the upper anterior alveolus. Retrusion of the alveolar bone, along with a realignment of the replacement teeth in a more posterior setting, can produce a marked change in appearance. This can be illustrated in a sagittal section diagram of upper and lower central incisors before and after treatment (Fig. 30.2).

In relation to the procedure used in carrying out such alveolar surgery, one method commonly used in the past was reduction of the outer (labial) plate of compact bone. Here, the labial soft tissues were first elevated to expose the outer compact bony plate. Chisels, burs and bone files were then used to reduce the bulk of the bone, following which the soft tissue flaps were sutured back into place. The degree of bone removal thereby achieved is illustrated in Figure 30.3.

This method was capable of producing the required degree of bone reduction *but*, unfortunately, the bone form produced was not stable. This was because the sockets vacated by the extracted tooth roots were only marginally modified by the bone trimming process. As a consequence, a near normal degree of post-extraction alveolar resorption occurred, this being a process which is affected by the volume of blood clot in the sockets and the subsequent processes of tissue organisation, ossification

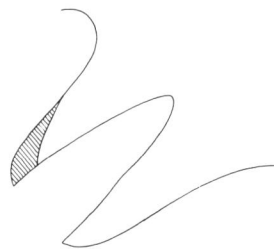

Fig. 30.3 Diagram to illustrate the bone removed in a radical alveolectomy operation (hatched area).

and bony remodelling. Thus, when a period of about 6 months had elapsed following the operation, and the degree of bone lost by alveolar resorption was now added to that lost by trimming of the outer bony plate, then inadequate bone could be left to provide effective support and retention for the denture. For this reason, the preference today is for the use of an alternative method of bone reduction which combines an interseptal alveolotomy with posterior displacement of the labial plate of compact bone. In this method, after the teeth to be immediately replaced have been extracted, fine forceps and bone rongeurs are used to remove the interdental bony septa lying between each pair of the extraction

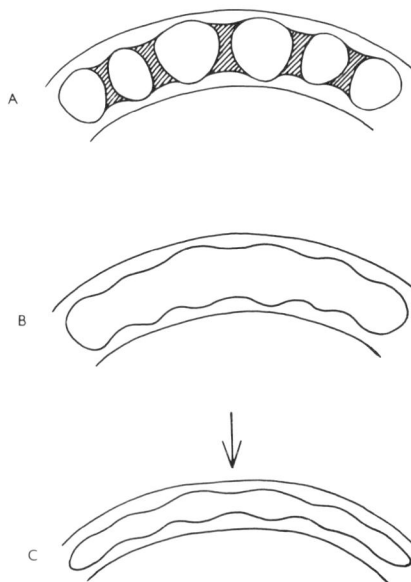

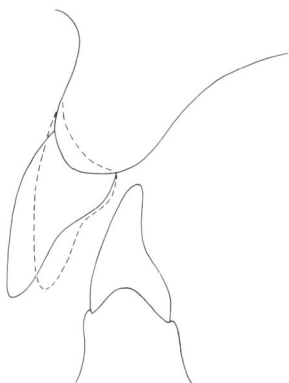

Fig. 30.2 Diagram of a sagittal section of the upper and lower central incisors before (solid line) and after (dashed line) treatment.

Fig. 30.4 Diagram to illustrate the sequence of events in interseptal alveolectomy. Plan views: **A** septa (shaded) removed; **B** continuous trough created; **C** labial plate depressed posteriorly.

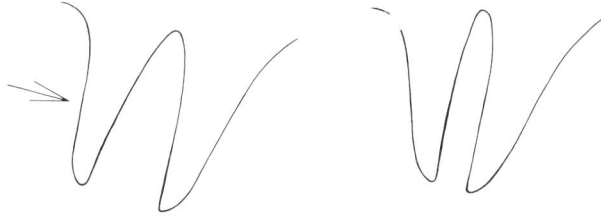

Fig. 30.5   Sagittal view of the effects of interseptal alveolectomy, prior to (left) and following (right) depression of the labial plate.

sockets, so creating a continuous trough between the inner and outer bony plates in the extraction zone. Vertical cuts are then made in the labial plate of bone at the distal ends of the extraction site. The cuts extend from the gingival margin level to about the level of the apices of the teeth on each side but must not be too deep, or the blood supply to the labial plate may be reduced excessively, leading to a risk of necrosis of the bony plate. The labial plate is

then elevated outwards to produce partial fracture at around the level of the root apices and is then manually pressed posteriorly to approximate it as closely as possible to the palatal (or lingual) bony plate. The changes which occur are illustrated diagrammatically in Figure 30.4 in plan view and in Figure 30.5 in a sagittal section view.

This method is capable of providing adequate

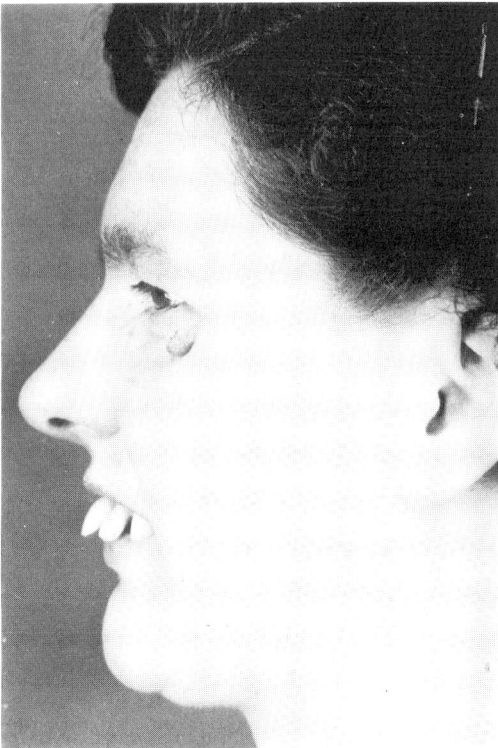

Fig. 30.6   Profile photograph of a patient showing the protrusive upper incisors often found in a Class II division I type of skeletal jaw relationship.

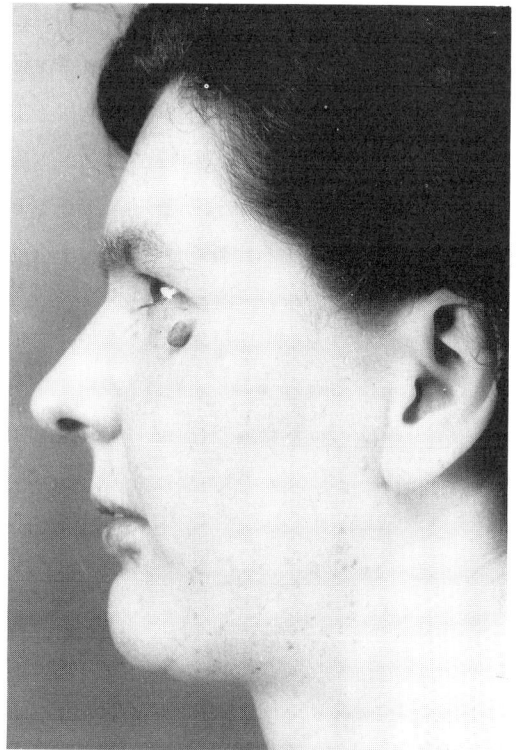

Fig. 30.7   Profile photograph of the same patient as in Figure 30.6 but after insertion of a Class IIb type of immediate denture following extraction of the upper anterior teeth and the carrying out of the interseptal alveolectomy form of alveolar surgery.

retrusion of the anterior alveolar bone to allow effective repositioning of protrusive incisors, as when trimming of the labial plate of alveolar bone is used. In distinction to the latter method of bone reduction, however, the septal alveolotomy method results in the extraction sockets being largely obliterated, so that only minimal blood clots are present. As a consequence, the degree of post-operative alveolar resorption that occurs appears to be reduced in comparison with that which normally occurs following tooth extraction. This results in immediate dentures of the Class IIb form maintaining adequate retention for a much longer period of time than normally applies when either a Class I or Class IIa denture is used. The need for a Class IIb immediate denture to be relined or rebased to counter the effects of alveolar resorption is correspondingly delayed and may, at times, even prove to be unnecessary over a period of about 6 to 9 months following the insertion of the denture.

The bone stability that occurs when the interseptal alveolotomy form of alveolar surgery is used is an important concept and can provide the rationale for a Class IIb type of immediate denture being selected for use, even where there is no indication for repositioning of the anterior teeth. Where this applies, the artificial anterior teeth can be set up anterior to the surgically reduced alveolus, to simulate the position of their natural predecessors.

To complete consideration of this chapter, the special features that are unique to the Class IIb type of immediate denture can now be considered, to add to the three features which, as previously indicated, it shares with the Class IIa type. These additional features are as follows:

1. It is a valuable procedure where it is desired to produce immediate retrusion of the anterior area of the alveolar bone to enable the artificial teeth to be set in a more retruded position. The sort of change in appearance that can thereby be provided is illustrated by comparing the profile appearance of a patient prior to treatment (Fig. 30.6) with that of the patient after a Class IIb immediate denture had been inserted, following extraction of the upper anterior teeth and the carrying out of the interseptal alveolotomy type of alveolar surgery (Fig. 30.7).

2. Where the alveolar surgery takes the form of an interseptal alveolotomy, accompanied by posterior displacement of the labial bony plate, subsequent alveolar changes will be minimal in extent. As a result, later and less frequent relining or rebasing will be required than applies when either of the other two types of immediate denture are used.

FURTHER READING

Kaldahl WB, Becher CM 1985 Prosthetic contingencies for future tooth loss. J Prosthet Dent 54: 1

31. The impression stage of treatment

INTRODUCTION

In common with the production of other types of removable prosthodontic appliances, the use of a two-stage impression procedure is strongly advocated in immediate denture treatment. This involves obtaining primary impressions using stock trays, followed by the taking of secondary impressions using special trays.

It is sometimes claimed that such a procedure is unnecessarily lengthy and hence expensive. However, the use of a stock tray will result in an uneven thickness of impression material with consequent potential inaccuracy of reproduction of the form of the oral tissues. In addition, it is very likely that there will be some portions of the denture-bearing area where the tray will be incorrectly extended relative to the sulci. Areas of overextension or of underextension will thereby arise in the impression and these will be transferred subsequently to the working cast and hence to the denture. If the denture is over-extended, it may well give rise to tissue irritation with attendant pain and discomfort for the patient, whilst underextension may give rise to retention problems. Extra visits to the dental surgeon may be necessary so that adjustments to the denture can be made to relieve the patient's discomfort and/or to develop the correct extension.

The risk of such problems arising can be greatly reduced by use of the advocated two-stage impression procedure, to the benefit of both the patient and the dental surgeon.

PRIMARY IMPRESSIONS

Choice of trays

Where both anterior and posterior teeth, or poste-

rior teeth only, are standing, stock trays of the 'box' form will normally be used to obtain primary impressions. Where, instead, only anterior teeth are standing, a 'combination' form of stock tray can be used. This has a 'box' form present anteriorly, but in the posterior regions it is shaped to match an edentulous ridge (Fig. 31.1).

Either metal trays or those made in a polymeric material may be selected for use. Metal trays have the advantage of possessing greater rigidity and they are reusable following cleaning and sterilisation. In distinction, trays made in a polymeric material are relatively inexpensive, allowing them to be disposed of after a single use. Lack of rigidity may, however, prove to be a potential source of error.

It is preferable to select trays which are perforated. The size of trays which are selected should be such as to adequately cover the required denture-bearing areas. Where doubt exists as to which of two trays to use, a better result will normally be

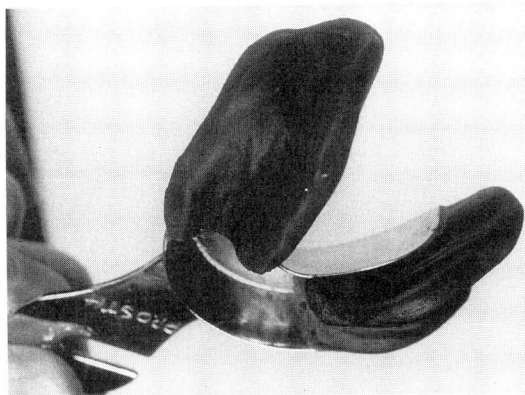

Fig. 31.1 Photograph of a stock tray which has been modified with impression compound to produce a 'combination' tray.

achieved by the choice of a tray which is a little oversize, rather than by choosing one which is undersize.

Preparation of trays

The quality of primary impressions can often be improved by making additions, using a suitable material, to the periphery or inner surface of a stock tray. Additions to the periphery should be made in all areas where the extension of a stock tray is short of the required denture-bearing area. Also, additions to the inner surface of a tray are indicated when there is found to be a gross discrepancy between the shape of the inner surface of the tray and that of the tissues in the area where the impression is to be taken. The palatal area of an upper tray often proves to be a region where such additions to the inner surface are needed. Impression compound is the material which is commonly used for making additions to trays where a hydrocolloidal or elastomeric impression material is to be used.

Finally, in the preparation of a stock tray, a layer of a suitable adhesive should be placed over the entire surface of the tray, including in the coverage any impression compound additions which are present. The adhesive which is used must be compatible with the chosen type of impression material, if adequate retention of the impression material within the tray is to be achieved.

Choice of impression material

Alginate is normally the impression material which is selected for primary impression taking in immediate denture treatment. This choice is based on the fact that alginate is relatively cheap to purchase, easy to manipulate and is usually sufficiently elastic in nature to be able to reproduce the many undercuts likely to be encountered in such work. However, where severe undercuts exist, alginate is liable to tear during withdrawal of the tray. If this problem is encountered, an alternative material with improved resistance to tearing may be selected. The preference usually falls on one of the elastomeric impression materials, a silicone type commonly being chosen for primary impression taking.

Impression-taking procedure

As alginate is the impression material which is commonly selected for use in immediate denture treatment, consideration of the impression-taking procedure will concentrate on this material.

It should be borne in mind that alginate is very liable to distort if abused, both during and subsequent to impression taking. Thus, for success, it is vital that correct procedures should be used in the manipulation of this material. The necessary procedures have been considered and explained in some detail in a previous chapter (Part II — Special Aspects Relating to Partial Denture Treatment, Ch. 16, p. 144 onwards). For convenience, they will be summarised briefly here:

1. Read carefully the manufacturer's instructions. Proportion powder and liquid correctly and mix for the recommended time in a clean bowl, using a clean spatula.

2. Place the mixed alginate in the chosen impression tray and on to tissue surfaces where trapping of air is liable to occur (e.g. on the buccal aspects of the maxillary tuberosities).

3. Rotate the loaded impression tray into the correct position, apply pressure to seat the impression to the required position and then apply border-moulding movements. Hold the tray in position without releasing or applying extra pressure until the alginate has set.

4. Release the impression from its seating position by the application of a rapid pull away from the tissues, then rotate it carefully out of the mouth.

5. Rinse the impression in cool running water. Check the impression for the presence of any imperfections. If any are found, repeat the impression until a satisfactory result has been obtained.

6. Treat the impression with a suitable antiseptic solution prior to casting-up (e.g. an aqueous solution containing 1000 p.p.m. of free chlorine).

Prescription writing

Preparation of study casts

The material to be used in the casting-up of the primary impressions should be specified. As the casts may need to be preserved for study purposes, in addition to being used for special tray production, it is usual for the impressions to be cast up using a mixture of equal parts of plaster of Paris and artificial stone.

Preparation of special trays

The information given should include:

1. The material of construction. It is preferable to use a polymeric material, such as self-curing acrylic resin, to ensure the tray possesses adequate rigidity and resistance to warpage.

2. The thickness of spacer to be used. This will be 3 mm where alginate is to be used as the secondary impression material, but can be a little thinner where an elastomeric impression material is to be used (see Table 9.1, p. 69).

3. The extension required. The posterior and peripheral extension should be indicated, preferably by the marking of lines on the study casts.

4. Perforations. An indication should be given as to whether or not perforations are required in the trays. Such perforations are essential where alginate is to be used and they are also required where an elastomeric material has been selected.

SECONDARY IMPRESSIONS

Choice of impression material

As at the primary impression stage, alginate is the impression material most frequently chosen for use. An exception will, however, apply in those instances where it was found to be necessary to use an alternative material to replace alginate at the primary impression stage, because of the presence of fairly severe undercuts, for example. The alternative material chosen for use when this eventuality arises is usually a silicone of the addition type.

Impression-taking procedure

The special trays to be used are first tried-in in the mouth of the patient and examined for satisfaction. They should fully cover the required tissue areas and have the required marginal extension. If any regions are found to be overextended, the trays should be trimmed to reduce the regions concerned to the correct level. Where, instead, there are found to be regions present where the extension is short of that required, then the deficiencies should be corrected by the application of greenstick impression compound.

A further necessary stage in the preparation for use of special trays is to apply a layer of an appropriate adhesive to the inner surface of the trays. The adhesive used must be a type specifically intended for use with the selected impression material.

The selected impression material is then prepared, the special tray is loaded and the impression is taken. Where alginate is the chosen final impression material, the impression taking procedure should be in accordance with that summarised in the section devoted to the primary impression taking procedure. Where, instead, an alternative impression material has been chosen such as silicone, the mixing and handling procedures should be in accordance with those given by the manufacturer concerned.

Prescription writing

1. Preparation of the working casts

The cast material to be used should be indicated. This will normally be a mixture of equal parts of plaster of Paris and artificial stone. This material is chosen because it provides a cast which is strong enough to withstand denture-processing procedures, but one which is capable of being trimmed without undue difficulty, such cast trimming being normally required in the course of immediate denture production.

2. Preparation of occlusal rims

Occlusal rims may need to be prepared for one or both of the patient's jaws, in order to be able to record the jaw relationship of the patient in the next clinical stage of treatment. Whether or not they are required is dependant on the number and distribution of teeth which are present, and this subject will be further considered in the next section.

Where it is found that occlusal rims will be necessary, the prescription for them should include:

1. The base material to be used, along with details of the required extension of the base.

2. The rim material to be used.

3. Details of any strengthening elements which are required.

4. Whether or not retaining elements are to be incorporated, to assist the retention of the occlusal rim.

FURTHER READING

Heartwell CM 1977 Conventional immediate complete dentures. Dent Clin North Am 21: 427
Lambrecht JR 1968 Immediate denture construction: the impression phase. J Prosthet Dent 19: 237
Lutes MR, Ellinger CW, Terry JM 1967 An impression procedure for construction of maxillary immediate dentures. J Prosthet Dent 18: 202
Ow R, Chia R 1983 The use of a sectional impression method for a complete maxillary immediate patient with a special indication. Singapore Dent J 8: 9.

32. The jaw registration stage of treatment

INTRODUCTION

The procedures which are adopted at this stage of treatment should be based on the principles considered in previous chapters of this book.

The presenting dentition may occasionally be a full natural dentition but, more commonly, it will be similar to that encountered in a patient who requires partial denture treatment. As a consequence, all of the procedures for establishing the correct vertical dimension and the correct horizontal jaw relationship which are utilized in partial denture treatment (see Part II, Ch. 17, pp. 153–156) can also be applied in immediate denture treatment. Of these procedures, the one which is found to be the most appropriate to use in both complete and partial immediate denture treatment will often be found to be that involving the use of occlusal rims, and so it will be considered in some detail.

REGISTRATION PROCEDURE UTILISING OCCLUSAL RIMS

Stage 1: Recording the occlusal plane and, where appropriate, the required degree of lip support. For cases where the natural upper anterior teeth are absent, the occlusal plane of the upper occlusal rim is adjusted to provide the required inclination (parallel to the interpupillary line) and the required level (normally, to extend 2 mm below the upper lip at rest).

For those cases where the natural upper anterior teeth are present, it is not necessary to develop an occlusal plane on the upper occlusal rim as in complete denture work. Instead, the satisfaction or otherwise of the plane present on the natural upper anterior dentition is noted. Where a change in the

anterior occlusal plane is felt to be indicated, the new inclination and/or level of the plane is indicated by drawing a line on the anterior teeth on the upper cast. An example of the sort of change that may be made is shown in Figure 32.1.

Stage 2: Adjusting the vertical height of the rim or rims until an acceptable value of freeway space has been achieved: In those cases where it is found that a stable contact occurs between the upper and lower natural dentitions at a height which provides an adequate and yet not excessive value for freeway space (normally 2–4 mm), the height of the occlusal rim (or rims) should be adjusted until the opposing rims, or rim and opposing natural dentition, just fail to contact when the upper and lower teeth are brought into the stable contact relationship. Such a situation is frequently found to exist in immediate denture treatment.

In the alternative cases in which it is found that either no natural tooth contact occurs *or* contact occurs at a vertical dimension providing an excessive freeway space, the height of the occlusal rims should be adjusted until contact of opposing rims and/or contact of rim and opposing natural dentition occurs at a height providing an acceptable value of freeway space.

Stage 3: Establishing the horizontal component of jaw relationship at the contact relationship of the standing natural teeth (where this provides

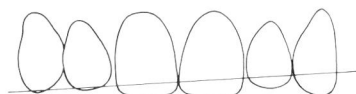

Fig. 32.1 Diagram to illustrate the marking of a new occlusal plane on the upper cast where the natural upper anterior teeth are standing.

adequate guidance); otherwise, in retruded jaw relationship.

The procedures which are used are similar to those previously described for establishing the correct horizontal relationship during the jaw registration stage of partial denture treatment, by the use of occlusal rims (see Ch. 17). For convenience, they are summarised below:

In the cases where a posterior rim segment in one jaw opposes a posterior rim segment in the other jaw, a notch is cut in the occlusal surface of one rim (usually the upper), a layer of wax about 2 mm deep is cut off the occlusal surface of the opposing rim segment and is replaced by a slightly higher mass of softened modelling wax. Alternatively, where a posterior rim segment in one jaw opposes a natural dentition in the other jaw, a layer of softened modelling wax about 2 mm deep is added to the occlusal surface of the posterior rim segment. In either case, the patient is then persuaded to close up until the teeth contact in a stable relationship at the required vertical dimension, or, where tooth contact does not occur at the required vertical dimension, to close up until the required height has been achieved in retruded jaw relationship.

An exception to the above method of registration using softened modelling wax applies where long free end saddles are present on the occlusal rims, especially in the lower jaw. If softened modelling wax was to be used to register on free end saddle regions, pressure development would be enough to cause the free end saddle (or saddles) to descend in a tissuewards direction in the course of the registration procedure. Such tissuewards movement of the free end saddle (or saddles) would not be paralleled when the rims and casts were assembled out of the mouth at the conclusion of the registration procedure, resulting in the casts now showing a different relationship from that seen in the mouth in the course of the registration procedure. To overcome this problem, a low-load method of registration needs to be adopted. The occlusal surfaces of opposing rim segments are trimmed until they just fail to meet at the required vertical dimension. Similarly, where a posterior rim segment is opposed by a natural dentition, the occlusal surface of the rim is reduced until it is just clear of meeting the opposing dentition at the required vertical dimension. Notches are cut in the occlusal

surface of the rim or rims, and a mix of plaster of Paris and water is placed onto the rims. The patient is then persuaded to close up until tooth contact in a stable relationship occurs, or to close into retruded jaw relationship at the required vertical dimension, in each case maintaining the closed relationship until the plaster has set.

In the case of *all* registrations, the casts and occlusal rims should be assembled via the wax or plaster registration and a check made that closure of the casts is not being interfered with by the presence of premature contacts on the heels of the casts. The relationship of the teeth on the casts should also be checked, to see that it is identical with that seen in the mouth at the time of registration.

AUXILIARY TASKS AT THE JAW REGISTRATION STAGE OF TREATMENT

1. Selection of the artificial teeth to be used

It is usual to select acrylic teeth for use in both the anterior and posterior regions of the mouth in immediate denture treatment. This choice is based on the fact that it is often necessary to trim the teeth in the course of immediate denture treatment and this task is very much easier to perform if acrylic teeth are used instead of porcelain teeth.

When selecting anterior teeth which are to be immediately replaced, guidance on the size, form, texture and colour of the replacement teeth is available by studying the corresponding features in the standing anterior teeth. Similarly, when selecting posterior teeth which are to be immediately replaced, guidance on the size, form and colour of the replacement teeth is available by studying the corresponding features in the standing posterior teeth. The same observations can also be used in the selection of anterior and/or posterior teeth which are to be used to replace missing teeth, in cases where there are some anterior and posterior teeth still standing. Where, however, all the anterior teeth *or* all the posterior teeth are missing, then selection of anterior teeth, or selection of posterior teeth where needed, will need to be made using the guiding principles considered in a previous chapter (Part I, Ch. 12 — Principles of Tooth Selection, pp. 87–96).

It should be noted that, when complete upper and lower immediate dentures are being provided for a patient, it is possible for teeth of a different colour to those of the natural dentition to be selected, where this meets the wishes of both the patient and the dental surgeon.

Once teeth of the required basic shade have been selected, a note should then be made of any alterations which are required to provide personalisation of the dentition. This can best be done by the provision of a suitably shaded (or coloured) diagram of the dentition, which will assist the dental technician to make the required alterations to the anterior and/or posterior teeth. Metallic restorations such as amalgam or gold inlays can be placed. Self-curing acrylic resins of the dentine type can be used to simulate composite or silicate restorations. Crack or fault lines on the labial surface of anterior teeth can be simulated using acrylic surface stains and appropriate colours of the latter material can also be used to simulate cervical staining.

When carefully done, such personalisation work can create a result which can defy detection as not being the natural dentition of the patient and result in a very satisfied patient.

An example of the application of personalisation to the anterior dentition of a Class II complete upper immediate denture is shown in Figure 32.2.

2. Determination of the depth of the periodontal pocket around each of the teeth which are to be immediately replaced

An estimation of the depth of a periodontal pocket can be made by examination of periapical radiographs of the teeth concerned. This method does, though, have the disadvantage of only providing information on the depth of pockets seen in a single plane. The results may also be distorted by a factor dependent on the magnification of the radiograph.

Because of the above problems, the preferred method is the use of periodontal measuring probes, which allow direct measurement to be made of pocket depth at several points around the circumference of a tooth.

The probes which are preferred have thin, narrow blades which are calibrated in millimetres. To determine the depth of a periodontal pocket, the blade is positioned in the gingival crevice and pressure is applied gently until the blunt end of the blade reaches the base of the periodontal pocket of

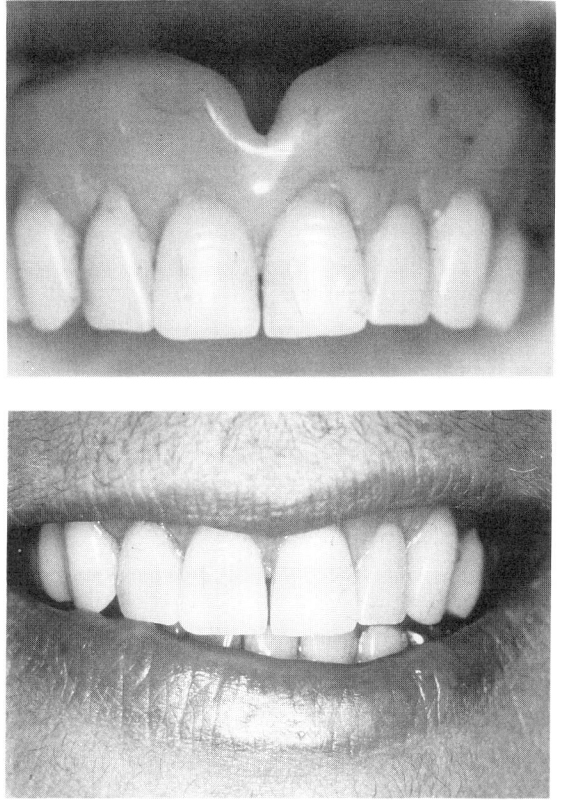

Fig. 32.2   **A** Personalisation of the anterior dentition in a Class II (closed-face) upper immediate denture and **B** the appearance when in the mouth.

the tooth under test. The depth of blade within the periodontal pocket is then read off on the scale and a note made of the value. The reading can then be repeated at a number of points around the tooth circumference and the average depth of the pocket for that tooth can be calculated. The same observations can then be made for each of the teeth in turn which are to be immediately replaced.

A diagram to illustrate the use of a pocket measuring probe appears in Figure 32.3.

3. Denture-finishing procedures

These are carried out at this stage of treatment *only* where immediate dentures are being provided which carry only the teeth being immediately replaced, since no trial denture stage of treatment is possible in such cases.

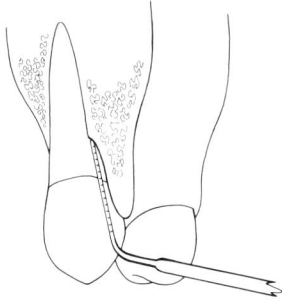

Fig. 32.3   The use of a periodontal measuring probe in the determination of pocket depths.

Where a complete upper immediate denture of this type is being provided, the correct position for the posterior border of the denture should be clinically determined and the displaceability of the tissues in that region should be noted by the use of an instrument such as a ball-ended burnisher. A post-dam preparation should then be made on the upper cast, utilising the method described for complete denture construction (Part III, Ch. 26 — The Trial Denture Stage of Treatment, p. 224). The same requirement applies to a partial upper immediate denture where a polymeric denture base material is to be used and a plate connector extends to the vibrating line.

In the case of upper or lower immediate dentures of both the complete or partial forms, the denture-bearing areas should be palpated and any areas which require relieving from direct contact with the tissues should be outlined on the cast. Such relief zones are usually achieved by the application of an appropriate gauge of metal foil to those areas of the casts which have been outlined.

4. Selection of the articulator which is to be used

A wide variety of articulators can be used in immediate denture treatment, but the type whose use is to be preferred is the simple adjustable type. The choice of this type of articulator, in preference to the use of a fully adjustable type, avoids undue complexity in the procedure and hence reduces cost, which may be considered to be an important consideration in the construction of an appliance which normally has an expected life span limited to

6–9 months. At the same time, the simple adjustable type does have an appreciable advantage relative to the use of a simple hinge type of articulator in that it allows teeth to be set up in a state of occlusal balance. The possession of occlusal balance is a very important requirement in immediate denture treatment, especially in the early period following the insertion of the denture. At that time the extraction sockets are not fully healed so that any tendency for denture displacement to occur in function, due to the presence of a traumatic contact in the dentition, could well prove to be very painful to the patient, in addition to possibly causing embarrassment.

PRESCRIPTION WRITING

The following information should be provided:

1. The type of articulator to be used.
2. The teeth to be used, along with information on any required personalisation of the dentition.
3. A request for the casts to be mounted on the chosen type of articulator, using the jaw registration provided. Where a face-bow record has been provided, this should be used in the mounting of the maxillary cast.
4. Requirements for the setting of the condylar inclinations and the angle of the incisal guidance table, where a simple adjustable type of articulator is to be used.
5. A request for the preparation of a trial denture or dentures, with the setting up of any anterior and/or posterior teeth missing from the dentition. An indication should be given of any special requirements for tooth arrangement.
6. Requirements should be given for the special cases where the teeth are to be set up and the denture then finished without proceeding to an intermediate trial denture stage. Such cases arise in those instances where an immediate denture carries only the teeth which are being immediately replaced and can apply to both partial and complete dentures.

The requirements are:

a. Any special arrangements which are required in the setting of the replacement teeth on the prepared master casts.

b. The colour and nature of the denture-base material to be used.

c. Where a partial upper immediate denture is to be provided which incorporates polymeric palatal connectors, details should be given of the position and depth of any peripheral seal lines which are required at the borders of the palatal connectors.

d. Details concerning any areas of the denture-bearing zone or zones which require relief.

FURTHER READING

Gilboe DB 1983 Centric relation as the treatment position. J Prosthet Dent 50: 685

Lundquist DO, Fiebiger CE 1976 Registration for relating the mandibular cast to the maxillary cast based on Kennedy's classification system. J Prosthet Dent 35: 371

McFee CE, Meier EA 1974 A technique for enhancing cosmetics in immediate dentures. J Prosthet Dent 31:385

Silverman SI 1985 Vertical dimension record: a three dimensional phenomenon. J Prosthet Dent 53: 420

Tallgren A, Tryde G, Mizutani H 1986 Changes in jaw relations and activity of the masticatory muscles in patients with immediate complete upper dentures. J Oral Rehab 13: 311

33. The trial denture stage of treatment

INTRODUCTION

This stage in treatment applies only to those immediate dentures which carry artificial teeth *in addition* to those providing immediate replacement of natural teeth, this being a condition which is satisfied by the majority of immediate denture cases.

The aims of this trial denture stage are two-fold:

1. To check the accuracy of the registration of the patient's jaw relationship recorded in the previous clinical stage of treatment, along with the accuracy of cast mounting achieved in the intervening laboratory stage in treatment.

2. To check the aesthetic satisfaction of artificial tooth selection and arrangement.

TRIAL DENTURE STAGE PROCEDURE

The trial denture (or dentures) should initially be checked on the articulator for conformity with the prescription which was provided. Where a simple adjustable articulator has been used, the state of occlusal balance which has been developed should be noted. If faults are found to be present such as with the state of occlusal balance or with the fit of the trial denture baseplates, then corrections should be made before proceeding further.

The trial denture(s) should then be removed from the cast(s) and checked for fitness for intra-oral trial. This involves checking the fitting surface(s) to ensure that they are clean and free from extraneous matter and the checking of all surfaces for freedom from any sharp areas which could traumatise the patient's tissues.

The trial denture(s) should then be immersed in a suitable antiseptic solution (e.g. an aqueous solution containing 1000 p.p.m. of free chlorine) to reduce the risk of cross-contamination arising. After being washed in running cold water, they are then ready for the intra-oral examination.

In order to ensure that nothing of importance is overlooked in the course of the intra-oral examination, it is desirable that the number and order of application of the stages which are used should be identical with those used at the trial denture stage in both complete and partial denture treatment. The order of these stages is as follows:

1. Checking extension, retention and stability.
2. Checking aesthetics.
3. Checking the vertical component of jaw relationship.
4. Checking the horizontal component of jaw relationship.

Each of these stages will be considered in turn:

1. Checking extension, retention and stability

Where an upper immediate denture is being provided, checks for extension, retention and stability should be applied initially to that denture. The denture should be inserted and the extension of any flanges which are present should be checked for compliance with the levels of the functional sulci. Where extension faults are found to be present, they should be corrected by making additions or subtractions to the baseplate as necessary.

As a preliminary to checking the retention of the denture, the fit of the baseplate in the mouth should be compared with the fit of the baseplate on the master cast. Where the fit of the baseplate in these two situations is found to differ, an indication exists that an error has occurred in the previous stages of

269

impression taking or cast preparation. Before proceeding further, it will be necessary to repeat these and other intermediate stages and to prepare a new denture for retrial.

Once the fit of the upper trial denture baseplate has been shown to be satisfactory, the retention of the denture should then be checked. This is achieved by applying a force to the denture along a path reversing the direction of the path of insertion and noting the resistance to displacement that arises. It should be remembered that the retention of the denture at this stage of treatment is likely to be appreciably less than that of the denture in the final (processed) form and due allowance must be made for this fact when assessing the adequacy or otherwise of the retention which is present. The presence of a reasonable level of retention is, however, a prerequisite for being able to carry out the subsequent procedures satisfactorily in the trial denture stage of treatment. Where necessary, consideration should be given to the incorporation of temporary wire clasps, positioned to engage undercuts on suitable abutment teeth, to help achieve the necessary level of retention.

The stability of the denture should then be tested by applying pressure in a tissuewards direction to the replacement teeth situated at or near the centre of each saddle. Where this gives rise to a rotatory displacement of the denture, the cause of the displacement must be sought and the appropriate remedy applied. Often, the cause of the displacement will be found to be that the replacement teeth have been positioned buccal or labial to the crest of the residual alveolar ridge to an excessive degree. Where this applies, the artificial teeth should be reset to bring them into a position where stability is achieved.

Once the extension, retention and stability of an upper trial denture have been found to be satisfactory, the same checks should then be applied to the lower trial denture, in those instances where both upper and lower immediate dentures are being provided. Where, instead, only a lower immediate denture is being provided, the checks will be made to that denture exclusively.

2. Checking aesthetics

The denture(s) should be inserted and the appearance of the patient noted when the mouth is closed and also with the patient providing a full smile. Where an upper immediate denture is being provided which carries replacement anterior teeth, the occlusal plane and (where appropriate) the centre line of the dentition should be checked for satisfaction. The level of the occlusal plane is best observed when the patient has the lips slightly apart. The patient should also be given a hand mirror and be invited to comment on the appearance provided by the denture(s) at this stage of the treatment.

If either the patient or the operator is unhappy with the aesthetic features of the dentures in any way, then chairside modification should be carried out until the required result has been achieved. It should be remembered that the observed appearance will depend not only upon the chosen artificial teeth and their arrangement but will also be influenced by the thickness of the flanges present on the dentures, via the lip and/or cheek support the flanges provide.

3. Checking the vertical component of the jaw relationship

Where, as is usual in immediate denture treatment, the occlusal vertical dimension is defined by the contact of opposing natural teeth, the denture should be inserted and a check made that both the natural teeth and the replacement teeth on the denture meet evenly at this vertical dimension.

Alternatively, in those cases where the natural standing teeth fail to meet at the occlusal vertical dimension, the denture(s) should be inserted and a check made that even contact of the natural teeth and the artificial teeth occurs at a vertical dimension which provides an adequate and yet not excessive value of freeway space.

Should the value of the freeway space which is present prove to be incorrect, it will be necessary for a new record to be taken of the vertical component of jaw relationship. The procedures used to obtain this required new record are considered in common with those used to deal with an error which is found to be present in the horizontal component of jaw relationship. The reregistration procedures which are adopted are based on those previously described for use in cases where such an eventuality proved to be necessary in the course of partial or complete denture construction (see Chs 19 and 26, respectively). For convenience, they are summarised in the following section.

4. Checking the horizontal component of jaw relationship

For those patients where the natural dentition provides a definitive intercuspal relationship in the horizontal plane, at the required occlusal vertical dimension, the denture(s) should be inserted and the patient persuaded to close into this relationship. For all other cases, the patient should be persuaded to close into the retruded jaw relationship.

In all cases, the intra-oral view of the intercuspal relationship of the natural and artificial dentition should be found to be identical with that developed on the articulator.

Where this requirement is not satisfied, or where an error was revealed in the course of the previous stage which involved checking the vertical component of jaw relationship, then a new registration must be taken.

In cases where an error was found to be present in the vertical component of jaw relationship, this should be corrected first. The artificial teeth should be removed from the denture(s) and the corresponding areas be replaced by wax occlusal rims. The height of these rims should then be adjusted until contact occurs between the rims and opposing natural teeth, and/or between opposing rim surfaces, at the required occlusal vertical dimension.

In all cases, a new registration must then be made of the horizontal component of jaw relationship. Where natural teeth oppose a rim surface, the registration is normally taken by adding softened modelling wax to the rim surface and then registering the indentations of the teeth into the wax as the patient closes in retruded jaw relationship. Where, instead, the registration is to be taken between opposing rim surfaces, a notch should be cut in the upper rim and about 2 mm should be removed from the surface of the lower rim in the area opposite to the notch. Softened modelling wax should then be built up on the cut-down surface of the lower rim to the extent judged to be just a little in excess of that needed to fill the notch in the upper rim. The patient should then be persuaded to close into retruded jaw relationship until the rim surfaces contact.

However, in cases where a decision had been made to use a low-pressure registration procedure when the original registration of jaw relationship was being taken (usually because of the presence of one or more free-end saddles) then such a low-pressure procedure should again be used in a reregistration.

When the new registration of the horizontal component of jaw relationship has been taken, a check should be made that the value of the freeway space which is present is still within acceptable limits. Such a check is always necessary because, unless the procedures used in the reregistration of the horizontal component of jaw relationship are applied with great care, there is a considerable risk that the previously developed vertical component of jaw relationship will be changed.

Following completion of the reregistration procedures, the casts should be remounted on the articulator to the given registration. New trial dentures should then be developed by resetting the replacement teeth. The checks listed for application at the trial denture stage of treatment should then be repeated at a subsequent visit of the patient. If necessary, the procedures for reregistration and trial should be repeated until satisfaction is achieved. Authority for finishing the denture(s) should only be given when both the patient and the operator are fully satisfied with the result at the trial denture stage.

When a satisfactory result has been achieved, two further observations should be made, where necessary, before the patient is dismissed:

1. Where a complete upper immediate denture is being provided, or a partial upper immediate denture is being provided which carries a palatal plate in a polymeric denture-base material which extends to the vibrating line of the palate, then the correct position for the posterior border of the denture should be clinically determined. Note should also be made of the displaceability of the tissues in this area via the use of an instrument such as a ball-ended burnisher. A post-dam preparation should then be made on the upper cast in the manner used in complete denture construction (see Ch. 26, pp. 224 and 225).

2. The denture-bearing area (or areas) should be examined and a decision made as to whether any

relief zones are required where the denture(s) will not come into contact with the underlying tissues. Where relief is required, the tissue areas concerned should be mapped out on the cast(s).

A very important final action before authorising the finishing of an immediate denture is that of taking steps to ensure that the denture will possess a free path of insertion. If, instead, modification to the denture should prove to be necessary before insertion can be achieved, the experience can be a very painful one for the patient, especially where the extractions were carried out under general anaesthesia.

Thus, during the construction of a partial immediate denture, all unwanted undercuts must be carefully blocked out on the master cast. In the construction of a complete immediate denture, the master cast must be surveyed and a decision made on how to deal with any undercuts which are found to be present (see the section on undercuts and denture insertion, in Ch. 26, pp. 226–227, for details of the available methods). In complete immediate denture treatment, the choice usually falls on option 2, in which the denture flanges in the undercut regions are only extended to engage 1 mm of undercut. Such an approach has been found to aid patient comfort, especially where the undercut flange(s) lie in the vicinity of the immediate extraction areas.

PRESCRIPTION WRITING

The following information should be provided to assist the technician:

1. Details of the required positioning and arrangement of the artificial teeth which are to be set up on the trimmed master cast(s) as successors to the teeth to be immediately replaced (see Ch. 34)

2. Information on any characterisation which requires to be applied to the artificial teeth, preferably aided by the provision of diagrams indicating the site and colour of the required additions.

3. Information on the sites where any colouring or stippling of flanges is required.

4. Where a partial upper immediate denture is being provided which is to carry a palatal plate in a polymeric denture base material, details of the depth and position of any peripheral seal lines which need to be placed at the borders of the palatal plate.

5. Information on the site and depth of relief areas which need to be placed within the denture-bearing area(s), accompanied by a mapping out of the areas on the casts.

6. Information on the procedures to be used to ensure that the immediate denture(s) will have a free path of insertion, when processed and finished.

7. Details of the nature and colour of the denture base which is to be used.

FURTHER READING

Fay EF, Eslami A 1988 Determination of occlusal vertical dimension: a literature review. J Prosthet Dent 59: 321
Hardy IR, Kapur KK 1958 Posterior border seal — its rationale and importance. J Prosthet Dent 8: 386
L'Estrange PR, Vig PS 1975 A comparative study of the occlusal plane in dentulous and edentulous subjects. J Prosthet Dent 33: 495
Tryde G, McMillan DR, Christensen J, Brill N 1976 The fallacy of facial measurements of occlusal height in edentulous subjects. J Oral Rehab 3: 353
Yemm, R, El-Sharkawy, M, Stephens CD 1978 Measurement of lip posture and interaction between lip posture and resting face height. J Oral Rehab 5: 391.

34. Cast preparation in immediate denture treatment

RESPONSIBILITY FOR CAST PREPARATION

From the historical point of view, cast preparation has sometimes been regarded as a laboratory task and, as such, has been delegated to a technician to perform. In the absence of a knowledge of the clinical factors which apply to the case in question, such a method of cast preparation will involve arbitrary estimation of the degree of reduction to be applied to a cast and may well result in it being either over- or under-trimmed. Over-trimming of the cast will result in the production of a denture with a cross-section less than that of the alveolar ridge. As a consequence, it may not be possible to insert the denture. Alternatively, if insertion is achieved, pressure between the denture and the underlying tissues may give rise to appreciable discomfort for the patient. Where, instead, the cast has been under-trimmed, a denture with an oversize cross-section will result, with corresponding loss of retention.

Because of these problems, a wiser approach, and one favoured by the authors of this textbook, is that of regarding cast preparation as a clinical responsibility, which should be carried out by the clinician who is treating the patient. Having recorded the medical, surgical and dental history of the patient and having carried out a full clinical examination of the patient's oral tissues (including the periodontal condition and the examination of radiographs), the operator will be able to base the amount of cast trimming on a reasoned assessment of the clinical findings. Accordingly, there will be a reduction in the risk of discrepancy arising between the cross-section of the denture and that of the alveolar ridge, to the mutual benefit of both the patient and the operator.

CAST TRIMMING PROCEDURES

1. In the following descriptions where the object under consideration is referred to in the singular, the plural is inferred where two dentures are to be produced. Prepare a duplicate of the master cast unless a second cast of an adequate standard is already available. Sometimes, the primary cast remains undamaged in the course of special tray construction, in which case it will serve as a record.

The duplicate cast will be used in the subsequent stage in which artificial teeth are set up in lieu of those natural teeth being immediately replaced. It enables the artificial teeth to be set up to exactly duplicate their natural predecessors where this is indicated. Alternatively, it allows the artificial teeth to be set in a new arrangement, modified to a known degree relative to the arrangement of their natural predecessors, in those cases where such a change in arrangement is thought to be indicated by both the patient and the operator.

It is also desirable that the record cast should be stored for a period of about 6 months after the immediate denture has been inserted. The record cast will then serve to provide evidence of the appearance of the natural dentition in case the patient, over that period of time, should complain about the appearance of the immediate denture.

2. Information is recorded on the master cast concerning certain features of each of the teeth to be immediately replaced. The features recorded are as follows:

a. A pencil line is scribed around the gingival margin of each tooth.

b. A line is drawn to indicate the long axis of each tooth.

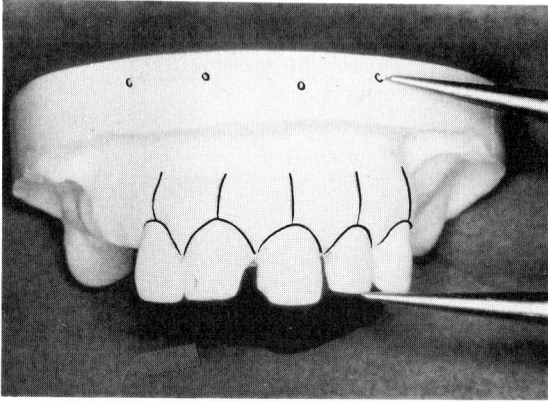

Fig. 34.1 Anterior view of an upper cast showing: lines scribed around the gingival margins of teeth to be immediately replaced; lines drawn along the long axis of each tooth being immediately replaced; use of dividers to transfer the position of the incisal edge of each anterior tooth being immediately replaced.

c. Dividers are used to record the position of the incisal edge of each anterior tooth.

An example of the records so obtained is shown in Figure 34.1.

The records help to facilitate arranging the artificial teeth in a subsequent stage in a manner duplicating that of the natural dentition. Alternatively, the artificial teeth can be set in a new arrangement, differing from that of the natural dentition by a known amount, in cases where such a change is indicated.

3. Trim the master cast by an amount judged to be appropriate for the class of immediate denture being provided, taking into account the clinical features which apply to the case in question.

Since the guiding principles which govern cast trimming procedures vary with the class of immediate denture being provided, they will be considered in turn on an individual basis:

1. Class I immediate denture (open face)

Here, the master cast is trimmed to allow for the changes which occur in the soft and hard tissues of the alveolar ridge in the immediate extraction area at the time the denture is inserted, along with those changes which occur to the soft and hard tissues of the alveolar ridge in the immediate extraction area in a period of about 2–3 months following the insertion of the denture.

It should be noted that this procedure is only applied in replacement of anterior teeth. The stages involved in the cast trimming procedure are as follows:

1. Trimming is applied initially to one tooth only. Where possible, choose as the starting point a tooth which has standing teeth adjacent to it on either side, as this facilitates the development of contact points in the subsequent stage in which the replacement tooth is waxed into position. The crown of the chosen tooth is then carefully removed from the cast down to the level of the pencil line previously scribed around the gingival margin of the tooth. All the other standing anterior teeth are left intact at this stage.

2. A socket form is then prepared for the cut-off tooth. The way in which the socket form is prepared is a matter of considerable importance, as it can have a marked influence on the prognosis for a successful outcome for the denture. To ensure a successful result, the socket form must be designed to satisfy two criteria:

a. Firstly, it must take into account the processes of healing and bony remodelling which will occur in the extraction area over a period of about 3 months following the extraction of a tooth. Studies have shown that this involves the loss of bone labially and on the crest of the ridge, with lesser changes occurring palatally (or lingually) (Fig. 34.2).

If the socket form is designed so that its form, internally, anticipates the form of the residual alveolar ridge as it is thought it will become in a

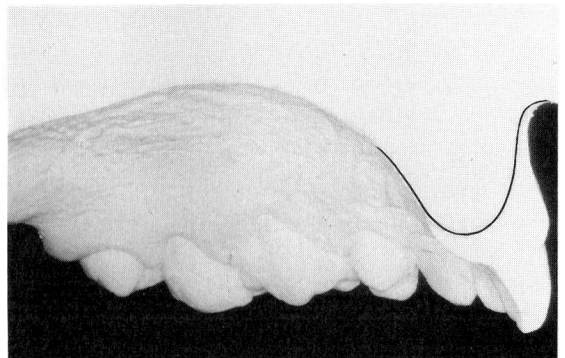

Fig. 34.2 Sagittal section of an upper cast. The line drawn on the cast indicates the anticipated effect of resorption in the 21 region of the alveolar ridge.

period of about 3 months following tooth extraction, and the neck of the replacement tooth is shaped to coincide with that of the resorbed alveolar ridge, then the replacement tooth will automatically come to lie in a ridge-fitting state, with little or no need for post-insertional trimming of the tooth (Fig. 34.3).

If, for any reason, the patient then fails to attend the usual follow-up appointments subsequent to the insertion of the denture, there will be minimum risk of the denture giving rise to ridge damage. Thus, the advocated procedure for socket preparation carries a built-in safety factor. This arrangement can be contrasted with the undesirable one which often arose in the past, when the socket preparation used involved cutting a hemispherical cavity in the cast within the confines of the scribed gingival margin around a tooth. This results in the production of a corresponding hemispherical mass of acrylic resin on the neck of the tooth. Unless such a mass is trimmed down in stages, as healing and bony remodelling occurs in the extraction area, there is a risk that it will take up a part of the region that otherwise would have become the new bony ridge, resulting in the formation of an irregular ridge with a scalloped shape. The simple hemispherical form of socket preparation, despite being quick and easy to prepare, is, then, best avoided because of the possibility that it could have a destructive influence on the alveolar form.

b. The second criterion which governs the design of a socket preparation is the need for it to be done in such a way that the labial soft tissue flap will be fully supported by the replacement tooth for as long a period as is possible, following the insertion of the denture. Otherwise, the excellent initial aesthetics of the open-face type of immediate

denture could be lost quite rapidly. As an example of such a risk, consider a case in which an anterior tooth having fairly advanced periodontal disease present (periodontal pocket depth 6 mm) is to be replaced by an open-face type of immediate denture. If the replacement tooth in such a case was carried to a depth of only 3 mm below the gingival margin labially, then there would be a gap of 3 mm between the end of the tooth and the crest of the bony alveolus. The 3 mm section of the labial soft tissue flap overlying the gap between the tooth and the bone would lack support from either the replacement tooth or the bone. As a result, it tends to be pulled inwards by the contracting blood clot in the socket and in doing so it drags upwards and inwards the tissue flap overlying the tooth, resulting in rapid loss of the socketed appearance of the replacement tooth (Fig. 34.4). Since much of the benefit of the open-face type of immediate denture stems from the natural appearance achieved by the socketing of the replacement teeth, then the rapid loss of the socketed appearance is clearly undesirable and steps must be taken to ensure that the labial soft tissue flap will be fully supported. At the same time, it is necessary to ensure that the replacement tooth stops short of actually entering the bony crypt. Otherwise, the patient could experience severe discomfort when contact occurs between the bony crypt and the replacement tooth, as minor movements of the denture occur during the mastication of food and at other times.

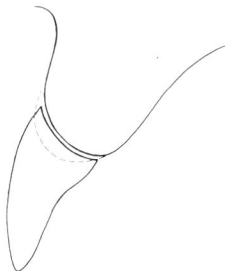

Fig. 34.3   The relationship of the artificial tooth to the resorbed alveolar ridge. The dashed line represents the form of the ridge prior to extraction of the natural tooth.

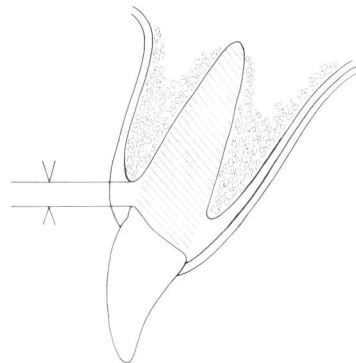

Fig. 34.4   Sagittal section to show a 3 mm section of unsupported labial soft tissue flap which tends to collapse into the blood clot (shaded) in the socket, resulting in the part of the soft tissue flap overlying the tooth being pulled upwards, with loss of the socketed appearance.

In order to ensure that socket preparation meets the above criteria it should be carried out as follows: Working just inside the scribed pencil line around the gingival margin of a tooth, cut a slot on the labial part of the circle to the depth of the periodontal pocket present on the labial part of the tooth, as measured in the jaw registration stage of treatment (Fig. 34.5A). Cut a second slot on the palatal (or lingual) part of the circle to a constant depth of 1 mm (Fig. 34.5B). In between the two slots, trim the cast to develop a convex form, in anticipation of the shape of the residual alveolar ridge as it will become in a period of about 3 months following the insertion of the denture (Fig. 34.5C).

A plan view of the prepared socket for one anterior tooth appears in Figure 34.6a, whilst a photograph of the socket prepared on 21 appears as Figure 34.6b.

By using a cast preparation procedure in which the neck of a replacement tooth is carried labially to the base of the measured periodontal pocket, it is possible for open-face immediate dentures to be provided successfully for patients even though quite a marked degree of periodontal disease is present at the time of treatment. There is certainly no need for the provision of open-face immediate dentures to be restricted to patients with anterior teeth free from

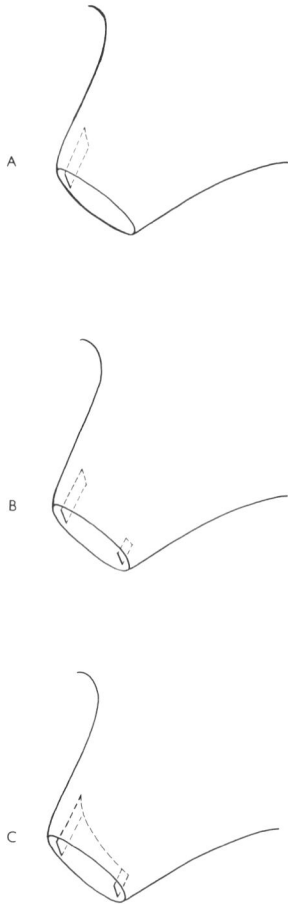

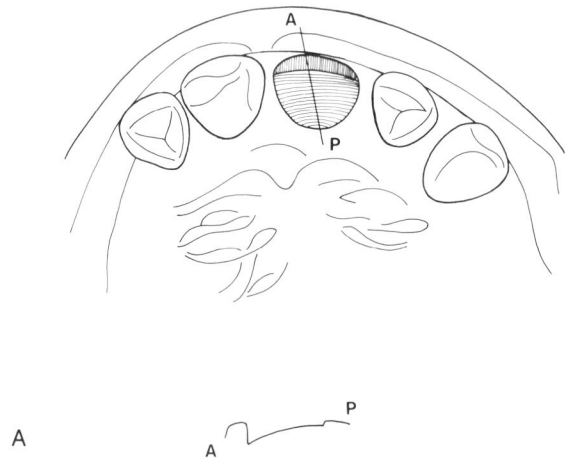

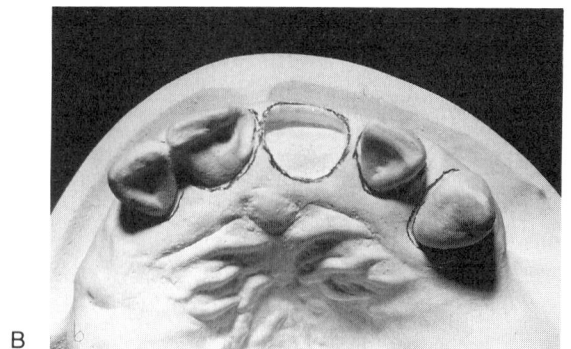

Fig. 34.5 Sagittal section of a cast of the upper anterior alveolus in the 11 area. A Slot cut in the labial part of the tooth root to the depth of the periodontal pocket on the labial aspect of the tooth. B Second slot cut on the palatal aspect to a depth of 1 mm. C Development of a convex form in between the two slots anticipating the shape of the residual alveolar ridge as it is considered that it will become in a period of about 3 months after the insertion of the denture.

Fig. 34.6 A Plan view of the prepared socket for one anterior tooth. B Photograph of the prepared socket in 21.

periodontal disease, as has sometimes been suggested in the literature.

3. When preparation of the first socket has been completed, the corresponding replacement tooth is set up. The neck of the tooth is trimmed to allow it to fit right to the base of the prepared socket labially and so that elsewhere it fits as closely as possible on the convex form of the socket. Developing a snug fit on the labial extremity of the neck of the tooth is important if optimal aesthetics are to be achieved. However, if a small gap is left between the convex form of the prepared socket and the corresponding concavity developed by the trimming of the remaining part of the neck of the replacement tooth, it will be filled in by the inflow of denture base material in the subsequent packing and processing stage.

During the setting up of the replacement tooth, the duplicate cast and the records taken of the incisal edge position and the angulation of the original natural tooth are used to ensure correct positioning is achieved (Fig. 34.7).

4. The procedures for socket preparation and the setting up of a replacement tooth are repeated on a one-at-a-time basis for each of the remaining anterior teeth which are to be immediately replaced. During cast trimming, it is important that great care should be taken not to damage the portions of the cast which lie between each of the socket preparations. These portions of the cast represent the interdental bony septa and they are not removed in the course of tooth extraction. Should such a portion of the cast be accidentally removed, a corresponding raised area will be developed on the processed denture. Unless this raised area is re-moved during the denture-finishing process it will become impacted on the interdental septa of bone when insertion of the denture is attempted, and will either prevent the denture from being seated into the correct fully inserted position and/or will give rise to considerable pain for the patient.

2. Class IIa immediate denture (closed face without alveolar surgery)

For this class of immediate denture, the master cast is trimmed to allow for the changes which occur in the soft and hard tissues of the alveolar ridge in the immediate extraction area at the time the denture is inserted.

It should be noted that in the case of Class II (closed-face) immediate dentures, the trimming that is applied to the master casts takes little account of the changes in shape of the residual alveolar ridges which occur by the process of alveolar resorption, subsequent to the insertion of the denture.

Since such dentures have to fit over the visible external form of the alveolar ridges, if the cross-section of dentures (via trimming of the master casts) was also reduced to allow for alveolar resorption, then they would clearly be too small to be capable of being fitted at the insertion stage of treatment.

The stages involved in this cast-trimming process, which can be applied in the immediate replacement of both anterior and posterior teeth, are as follows:

1. Carefully remove from the master cast the crowns of *all* the teeth which are to be immediately replaced, doing so down to the level of the pencil lines previously scribed around the gingival margin of each tooth.

2. Trim the master cast to allow for the reduction in the height of the ridge which occurs when a tooth is extracted and which results from the collapse into the socket area of the now unsupported soft tissue flaps (Fig. 34.8).

The dimension of the reduction in ridge height which so occurs is dependent on the degree of periodontal disease present when the tooth is extracted. If 'D' mm is the average of the depths of the periodontal pockets measured at a series of points around the circumference of a tooth (as

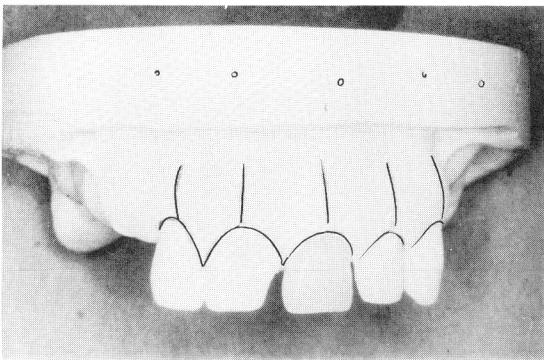

Fig. 34.7   The first replacement tooth set in position.

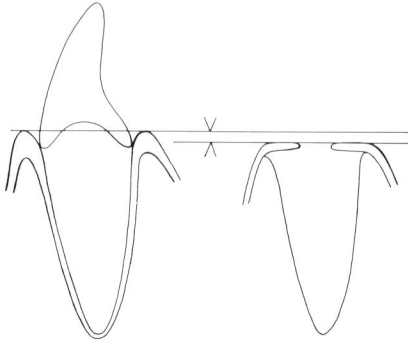

Fig. 34.8 Sagittal sections in the lower central incisor region to show the reduction in height of the alveolar ridge which occurs as a result of the collapse into the socket of the unsupported soft tissue flaps, following the extraction of a tooth.

determined in the jaw registration stage of treatment), then the reduction in height of the alveolar ridge arising when the tooth is extracted will be D mm minus an allowance for the thickness of the soft tissue flaps.

The latter thickness is normally estimated to average 1 mm. Thus, the reduction in ridge height which occurs will be $D - 1$ mm and, if the average depth of the periodontal pocket was found to be 5 mm, the ridge height should be reduced by a distance of 4 mm. Similarly, if the average depth of the periodontal pocket was found to be 3 mm then 2 mm should be trimmed off the height of the ridge, and so on. The easiest way of reducing the height of the alveolar ridge by a given amount is to first cut a central hole to the required depth, using a depth gauge to assess the hole dimension. The height of the ridge is then reduced until the hole has just been erased (Fig. 34.9). A very minimal degree of rounding-over is then applied to the sharp superior margins of the trimmed ridge, both labially and lingually (or palatally).

It should be noted that trimming as described above leads to the production of a rather strange and basically square-section form of ridge, especially in the lower jaw. A temptation may so arise to further trim the margins of the ridge labially and lingually (or palatally) to produce a ridge with more of a semicircular form, akin to the form of ridge commonly seen in patients who have been edentulous for a year or more (Fig. 34.10). Such a temptation must, however, be resisted as it could result in the production of a very unsatisfactory immediate denture. To explain that point, it is necessary to consider what may happen to the ridge when an anterior tooth is extracted.

In order to break the fibres of the periodontal membrane which hold the tooth in position in its bony crypt, it is usual for the operator to attempt rotatory movements of the tooth. Since very few anterior teeth have roots with a circular cross-section, rotation can only occur by some outward movements of the bony plates. This outward pressure on the bony plates which develops as an attempt is made to rotate a tooth usually results in a partial fracture at about the level of the apex of the tooth of the labial plate, which is weaker than the lingual or palatal plate. This, then, allows the plate to displace labially and the tooth to rotate. When extraction of the tooth has been completed, it is usual for the operator to apply digital pressure to the displaced bony plate in an attempt to reposition it. As a result of spring tension in the area of partial fracture it is, however, usual to find that the plate tends to move slightly outwards again when the applied pressure is released (Fig. 34.11). A situation is thus created in the alveolar ridge which is exactly opposite to that achieved by the excessive trimming of the master cast. When an attempt is made to insert the denture prepared using the over-trimmed

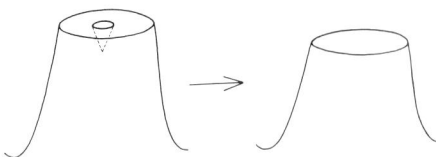

Fig. 34.9 The left diagram shows a central hole cut to the required depth ($D - 1$ mm). The right diagram shows the height of the ridge reduced until the central hole has been erased.

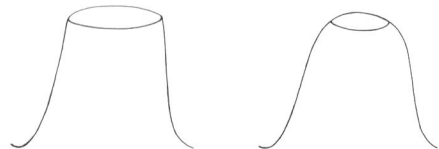

Fig. 34.10 The form of the ridge developed by correct trimming is shown on the left. The right shows an incorrect form caused by excessive trimming of the labial and lingual ridge margins.

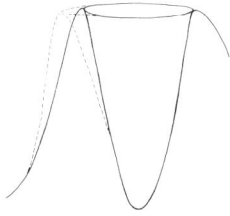

Fig. 34.11 The dashed line indicates the final position of the labial plate after tooth extraction.

cast, it may prove to be impossible to achieve full insertion. Alternatively, if the denture does seat in position correctly, considerable pressure will be developed on the labial plate. This may result in the soft tissues and the bone becoming denuded in the regions where pressure points exist, in as short a period of time as 24 hours, but in all cases it is likely to give rise to considerable discomfort for the patient.

3. When correct trimming of the master cast has been completed, the chosen artificial teeth are set up in lieu of those being immediately replaced.

As setting up proceeds, use is made of the duplicate casts and the records which were taken of the position of their natural predecessors, to ensure correct positioning. Care is also taken to ensure that the best possible level of occlusal balance is achieved in the setting of both the anterior and posterior teeth.

3. Class IIb immediate denture (closed face with alveolar surgery)

For this class of immediate denture, the master cast is trimmed to allow for the change in alveolar form in the immediate extraction area which it is planned to achieve surgically. The procedure can be applied in the immediate replacement of both anterior and posterior teeth, but it is normally reserved for use in the replacement of anterior teeth only.

The stages involved in the cast preparation procedure are as follows:

1. Carefully remove from the master cast the crowns of *all* the teeth which are to be immediately replaced, doing so down to the level of the pencil lines previously scribed around the gingival margins of each tooth.

2. Trim the master cast by an amount corresponding to the amount of bone which it is planned to remove surgically from the alveolar ridge. Where the alveolar surgery is to take the form of a thinning of the outer cortical plate of bone, the cast trimming has to be done on an arbitrary basis, assessing via radiographs and other clinical records the amount of bone removal that it is thought can be achieved. Hence the importance of cast trimming being carried out by the operator who will also be responsible for carrying out the bone surgery. Where, instead, the bone surgery is going to involve an interseptal alveolectomy in combination with a posterior displacement of the labial plate of compact bone, then guidelines have been suggested to assist cast trimming. Of the various methods which have been suggested, the following is the one which is preferred. Note that some variation may have to be made, though, by the operator to take account of the special clinical features of the case in hand:

a. Mark the trimming area:

(i) Looking down on the cast in plan view, draw a line in a mesiodistal direction which bisects each of the gingival margin circles on each tooth being immediately replaced, except for the last tooth at each end of the replacement arch, where the line deviates outwards by about 25° from the mesiodistal direction.

(ii) Draw a line on the labial surface of the cast, half-way between the most labially situated point on each of the gingival margin circles of each tooth being immediately replaced and the base of the sulcus (Fig. 34.12).

b. Trim off those portions of the cast which lie labial to the demarcated trimming area (Fig. 34.13).

c. Round over the sharp superior and inferior margins of the trimmed area of the cast (Fig. 34.14).

3. Once cast trimming has been completed, using a method appropriate for the selected type of alveolar surgery, the trimmed master cast is then duplicated. Either agar-agar, a laboratory type of alginate duplicating material, or a silicone material is used for this purpose, the duplicate cast being prepared in a mix of equal parts of plaster of Paris and artificial dental stone. Two sheets of modelling wax are then laid down to extend to the peripheral outline of the duplicate cast. The wax sheets on the duplicate cast are then flasked, packed and processed using clear acrylic resin. After smoothing,

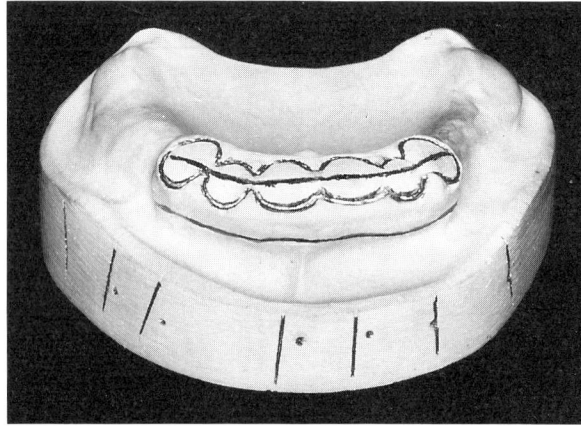

Fig. 34.12 The areas marked for trimming, showing the outlines of
the gingival margins, and, on the labial surface, a line midway
between each gingival margin and the base of the sulcus.

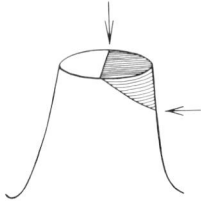

Fig. 34.13 Sagittal section of one anterior tooth on a lower
master cast. The portion of the cast which is removed from
between the two trimming lines is shown as the hatched area on
the labial side of the cast.

polishing and sterilisation, the clear acrylic sheet
serves as a template for use during the subsequent
alveolar surgery (Fig. 34.15). When a point is
reached in the surgical procedure where it is
thought that an adequate amount of bone has been
removed from the alveolar bone, the template is
tried-in in the mouth. If the template fits into
position satisfactorily, it provides an indication that
the immediate denture will, likewise, fit satisfacto-

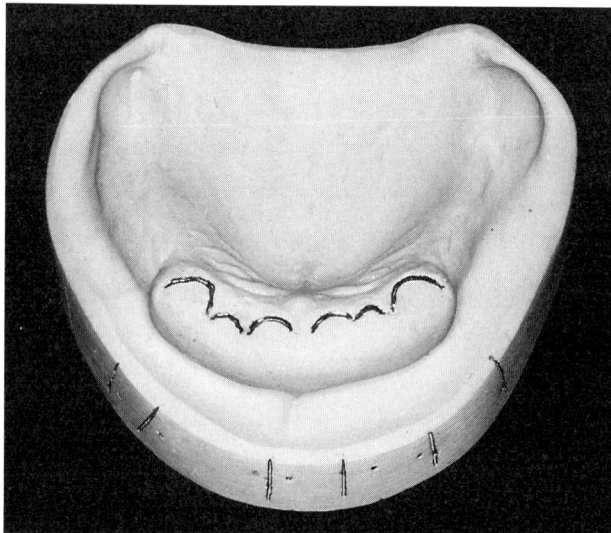

Fig. 34.14 The appearance of a cast after the superior and inferior
margins of the trimmed area have been rounded over.

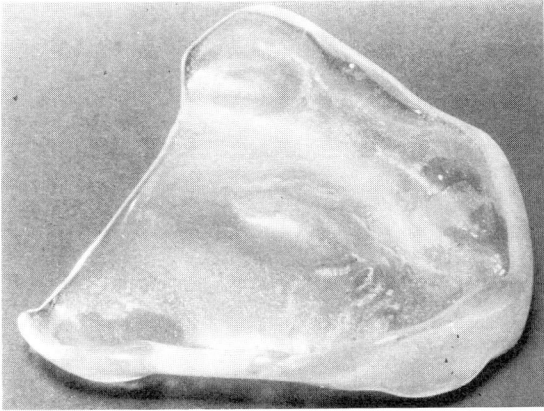

Fig. 34.15 Clear upper acrylic template for use during alveolar surgery.

rily, allowing the alveolar surgery to be terminated. If, however, it is found that the template cannot be inserted, then there is an indication that further removal of alveolar bone is still needed. The particular value of using a template made in clear acrylic resin is that in those instances where the template cannot be inserted it often proves to be possible, by observing any blanching of the underlying tissues, to observe where the bony areas are situated which are obstructing insertion of the template, so indicating the areas where further bone removal is still needed. The process of trial insertion of the template, followed by further bone removal, is repeated as necessary until full insertion has been successfully accomplished.

Following the preparation of a clear acrylic template on the duplicate of the master cast, the artificial teeth are then set up on the master cast in lieu of the natural teeth which are to be immediately replaced. As in the case of other classes of immediate dentures, use is made of the duplicate casts and the records which were taken of the position of the natural dentition, to help to ensure that the required positioning of the replacement teeth is achieved. In the case of the artificial anterior teeth, the position of the teeth depends upon the reason why the Class IIb procedure for immediate denture construction was selected. Where it was selected to meet a need for change in the arrangement of the anterior dentition, e.g. where the overbite/overjet relationship needs to be modified in the presence of a gross Class II, division I malocclusion, the replacement anterior teeth are set close to the new form of the surgically modified alveolar ridge. Where, instead, use of the Class IIb procedure was decided upon because of the stability of the alveolar form in the post-operative follow-up period which applies, the replacement anterior teeth can be set up anterior to the new ridge form to simulate the position of their natural predecessors. Alternatively, an intermediate setting of the anterior teeth may be adopted where both patient and operator agree that such a setting is indicated.

FURTHER READING

Bates JF, Stafford GD 1971 Immediate complete dentures. British Dental Association, London
Drummond JR, Duthie N, Yemm R 1983 An immediate denture technique for replacing the last natural teeth. Br Dent J 155: 297
Jerbi FC 1966 Trimming the cast in the construction of immediate dentures. J Prosthet Dent 16: 1047
Jones HS 1970 Immediate replacement of lower anterior teeth. Dent Survey 46: 28
Withrow G, Crandall EM, Clark IR 1990 An efficient method to make surgical templates for immediate dentures. J Prosthet Dent 63: 363
Young L Jr, Gatewood RR, Moore DJ, Sakumura JS 1985 Surgical templates for immediate denture insertion. J Prosthet Dent 54: 64

35. The insertion stage of treatment

DENTURE PREPARATION

Before attempting to insert an immediate denture, it must be carefully inspected extra-orally to ensure that it is in a satisfactory condition. The fitting surface should be examined to check for the presence of any non-anatomical irregularities which, if left in situ, could result in the patient experiencing considerable discomfort when wearing the denture. Such irregularities can include nodules of denture base material which arise due to the presence of air cavities on or just below the surface of the cast on which the denture was processed. Any irregularities which are found to be present should be trimmed away, using a small cutting instrument or stone, care being taken not to damage the surrounding area of the denture.

The occlusal and polished surfaces, along with the margins of the denture, should be checked for the presence of sharp areas or blemishes which could traumatise the patient's oral tissues. If any such problems are found to be present, the area concerned must be smoothed and repolished.

Where a denture of the Class I type is being provided, special attention should be paid to ensuring that no unwanted extensions of the denture base material are present interdentally, in the open-face region of the denture. As previously noted, such extensions can arise if the master cast is accidentally damaged in the interdental areas, during the preparation of the sockets. Unless they are removed, the extensions can prevent the denture fitting into the intended position and/or can give rise to appreciable discomfort for the patient.

When adjudged satisfactory, the denture should be thoroughly cleaned and then be immersed in a suitable antiseptic solution (e.g. an aqueous solution containing 1000 p.p.m. of free chlorine) for a period of 10 minutes. For dentures which are composed solely of non-metallic materials, the period of immersion in the antiseptic solution can be safely increased to longer periods of time. However, for dentures which include metallic elements in their composition, the period of immersion should be limited to 10 minutes, to avoid the risk of corrosion of the metalwork arising.

The use of a disinfection procedure is very important at the insertion stage of immediate denture treatment, as the denture will be introduced to an environment in which open wounds are present, in the form of the immediate extraction sockets.

SURGICAL TREATMENT

The use of local analgesia is generally considered to be preferable in immediate denture treatment, as it can provide adequate working time for any necessary surgical procedures, in relative safety. General anaesthesia can, however, be used as an alternative, where both the patient and the operator agree that it is desirable. Where local analgesia is to be used, the choice of block injections rather than localised infiltration injections can be advantageous where feasible since, when a series of localised infiltration injections is used, the accompanying tissue oedema can disrupt the initial fit of the immediate denture.

Once an adequate level of analgesia has been achieved, the teeth which are to be immediately replaced are extracted. Appropriate procedures must be adopted to ensure that the cortical plates of the alveolar bone are left intact in the course of tooth extraction. This is especially important where an immediate denture of the Class I (open-face)

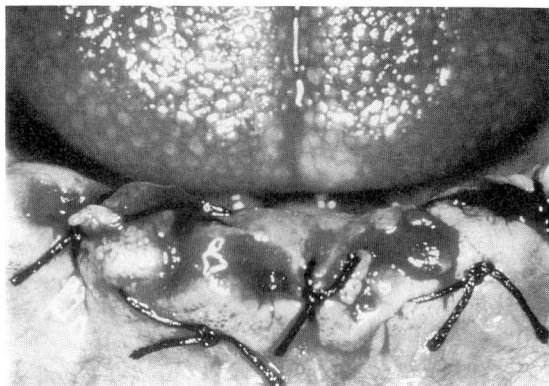

Fig. 35.1 The lower alveolar ridge following interseptal alveolectomy and suturing of the soft tissue flaps.

form is being provided, as the loss of the labial bony plate would seriously disrupt the appearance of such a denture.

Where an immediate denture of the Class IIb form is being provided, the planned form of alveolar surgery is then carried out. An outline of the methods that may be used to effect a reduction in the size of the alveolar ridge in the immediate extraction area has been provided previously (see Ch. 30). For further information on this subject, an appropriate text on oral and maxillofacial surgery should be consulted.

When it is considered that the planned reduction in the size of the alveolar ridge has been achieved, an attempt is made to insert the clear acrylic template which had been produced on a duplicate of the trimmed master cast. Where necessary, bone reduction is continued until full insertion of the template is possible.

Reduction in size of the alveolar ridge results in the soft tissue flaps overlapping when they are brought together. To aid healing of the flaps by first intention, they are trimmed until they just approximate, and then are sutured together using a series of interrupted sutures (Fig. 35.1).

DENTURE INSERTION

On completion of surgical treatment, the insertion of the immediate denture(s) should follow without delay. Where both upper and lower dentures are being provided, it is usual for insertion of the upper

denture to be carried out initially, followed by the insertion of the lower denture. Providing that appropriate action had been taken to deal with any undercuts which were found to be present in the course of the trial denture stage of treatment, then a partial or complete immediate denture should show a free path of insertion.

Some interference with the path of insertion may, however, arise as a result of the dimensional change in the denture base material which occurs during processing. Also, a limited amount of undercut may have been deliberately left in situ on one or more of the denture flanges, with the aim of increasing the retention of the denture. In cases where interference does arise when trying to insert the denture, no attempt should be made to force the denture into place. Instead, action should be taken to try and find the region(s) where the interference is arising, these often being highlighted by blanching of the underlying tissues. After detection, the region(s) of the denture responsible for the interference are relieved, after which insertion of the denture is again attempted. This procedure is repeated, if necessary, until full insertion of the denture has been achieved.

The inserted denture is then checked for satisfaction using the same procedures, applied in the same order, as were used at the trial denture stage of treatment (see Ch. 33, pp.269–271). Where both upper and lower dentures are being provided, the extension, retention and stability of the upper denture are checked first, followed by the application of the same checks to the lower denture. During the checking of denture retention, it should be borne in mind that where local analgesia was used in the surgical stage of treatment, oedema of the denture base tissues may result in a disruption of retention in the initial period following denture insertion. This problem usually resolves after the denture has been worn for 20 minutes or so.

The aesthetics of the denture(s) is then checked. The observed appearance of the denture(s) should coincide with that approved during the trial denture stage of treatment.

The occlusion of the dentition should be observed when the patient closes into a definitive position dictated by the interdigitation of the natural dentition, or into retruded jaw relationship, to accord with the method used when recording the horizontal component of jaw relationship in the jaw registration stage of treatment. In this position, the natural and/or artificial teeth should meet evenly in a horizontal relationship coinciding with that seen at the trial denture stage of treatment and an acceptable value should be present for the freeway space.

Where an occlusal error is found to be present, thin articulating paper coupled with observation should be used to denote where interference is arising. The area(s) concerned should then be reduced by careful stoning. This process of oral selective grinding is continued until even contact of the dentition has been established at an acceptable value for freeway space. Fortunately, errors in the occlusion are less common and are often reduced in severity in immediate denture treatment, relative to the position found in the treatment of edentulous patients. This difference is due to the fact that the presence of at least some natural teeth in immediate denture treatment usually allows a more reliable assessment to be made of both the vertical and horizontal components of jaw relationship than often applies in complete denture treatment. This is a fortuitous occurrence, as it is generally considered to be inadvisable to remount the denture(s) immediately after insertion on a simple adjustable articulator and then to selectively grind them, as in complete denture treatment (see Ch. 27). If used in immediate denture treatment, it would be necessary for the newly inserted dentures to be removed from the mouth of the patient for the period of time required to remount the dentures and carry out selective grinding, which will be at least 45 minutes. Over this time, changes associated with the initiation of the wound healing process will be occurring in the area where the teeth being immediately replaced have been extracted. Also, when local analgesia has been used, sensation will be returning to the same area. As a consequence, when an attempt is made to reinsert the denture(s) on completion of the selective grinding process, the action may prove to be a difficult if not impossible one to achieve and will almost certainly provide a very painful experience for the patient. This problem is particularly apparent where an immediate denture of the Class I type is being provided.

On successful completion of all the check stages, including any necessary correction of the occlusion, any areas of the denture(s) which needed to be modified are carefully smoothed and, except for the fitting surface, are repolished. The denture(s) are then reinserted as soon as possible.

INSTRUCTIONS TO THE PATIENT

On completion of the denture insertion procedures, the patient is then given instructions on the care of the denture (or dentures) and the oral cavity. As at the insertion stage of partial or complete denture treatment, this is accomplished by combining orally given instructions with the provision of a printed sheet of information, which can then be studied at leisure by the patient.

In the case of the instructions given orally to the patient, these are designed to cover only the initial period of 24 hours following denture insertion. The main points which are covered at this time are as follows:

1. The denture(s) should be worn continuously, both by day and by night, for the initial period of 24 hours following insertion. No attempt should be made by the patient to remove the denture(s) during this period, even for the short time required for denture cleansing. Especially in those instances where a Class I type of immediate denture has been provided, a warning is given that if the denture is removed by the patient then they may not be able to get it to go back into the same position. This could result in the appearance of the denture being irreparably damaged.

2. The patient is asked to avoid mouth washing for the initial period of 4 hours following denture insertion, in order to allow time for consolidation of the blood clots in the extraction sockets to occur without interruption. After this time, light rinsing out of the mouth using warm (not hot) water after each meal is advised to ensure that any food which has been left in the mouth will be removed as far as is possible.

3. The patient is advised to keep to a fairly soft diet over the initial 24 hour period.

4. A warning is given that some discomfort is likely to be experienced in the early hours following the extraction of teeth. The use of a suitable analgesic can be advised, such as two tablets of paracetamol taken at intervals of not less than 4 hours.

5. If bleeding from the sockets should persist for longer than the initial hour or so after the extractions were carried out, the patient should return to the surgery straight away. In case this problem should develop outside surgery hours, the patient is given a telephone number to call for an emergency service to be provided by the operator.

A final action at this stage in immediate denture treatment is for the patient to be given an appointment for the first review stage. This will normally be held about 24 hours after denture insertion.

FURTHER READING

Conny DT, Tedesco LA 1983 The gagging problem in prosthodontic treatment: I. Identification and causes. J Prosthet Dent 49: 601

Conny DT, Tedesco LA 1983 The gagging problem in prosthodontic treatment: II. Patient management. J Prosthet Dent 49: 757

Demmer WJ 1972 Minimizing problems in placement of immediate dentures. J Prosthet Dent 27: 275

Holt Jr RA 1986 Instructions for patients who receive immediate dentures. J Am Dent Assoc 112: 645

Holt RA, Stratton RJ, Donoghue T 1985 Prevention of cross contamination during immediate denture delivery. Quintess Int 11: 787

Wictorin L 1969 An evaluation of bone surgery in patients with immediate dentures. J Prosthet Dent 21: 6

36. The review stages and after-care in immediate denture treatment

THE FIRST REVIEW

Whenever possible, this is carried out about 24 hours after denture insertion. Initially, the patient's experiences over this period of denture wearing are recorded, including details of any problems which have been experienced.

The denture(s) are then very carefully removed from the mouth, after which they are thoroughly cleaned using a soft brush, soap and water. The patient is also given an antiseptic mouthwash and asked to gently rinse out their mouth, in order to remove any debris that is present. The condition of all of the oral tissues is then examined in detail, special attention being paid to the extraction sockets and the areas involved in any alveolar surgery.

It is not unusual for a patient to experience some degree of low-level discomfort during the initial 24 hour period following the insertion of an immediate denture. This is often due to pressure between a denture flange and the underlying soft and hard tissues. Where the history of the patient's experiences includes a complaint of pain being experienced in one or more localised areas of the denture, examination of the tissues may reveal signs of early inflammatory changes and thus give a clear indication of the problem site or sites. Where no change in the soft tissues can be seen, disclosing wax or pressure relief cream may be used to indicate the area(s) where pressure is arising. The pressure must then be relieved by trimming the fitting surface of the denture in the area or areas concerned. Trial reinsertion and denture trimming are continued until the pain problem has been resolved. If a point is reached during the trimming of the fitting surface of the denture where it is considered that any further reduction in flange thickness would result in the production of a dangerously sharp margin on the flange, then it is advisable for further relief of pressure to be provided by reducing flange depth rather than by further reducing flange thickness.

Another complaint that may be raised by the patient is that the denture(s) appear to be loose. Fortunately, this is not a commonly voiced complaint. The usual cause of looseness at this stage in immediate denture treatment is undertrimming of the master cast, relative to the reduction in size of the alveolar ridge that actually occurs after tooth extraction and, where relevant, the carrying out of alveolar surgery. The only effective solution to this problem will normally be found to be relining or rebasing of the denture, using one of the methods which are considered in a later section of this chapter which deals with denture after-care.

In addition to the two complaints considered above, it is also possible that the patient may raise any of the other complaints listed in the previous chapters devoted to the review stage in partial denture treatment, or in complete denture treatment, according to the type of immediate denture that has been provided (see Ch. 21, pp. 174–177, and Ch. 28, pp. 237–244). It should be noted, however, that such complaints are often not raised by the patient until the second or a subsequent review stage has been reached.

When any necessary modification to the denture(s) has been completed, all areas which have been trimmed are smoothed and, except for the fitting surface, are repolished.

The patient is then provided with further oral

instructions, and is told that these will apply until further notice:

1. The denture(s) should now be taken out of the mouth after each meal and be cleaned using a toothbrush, soap and water. Where any natural teeth are present, they should be cleaned using a toothbrush, toothpaste and water, and then the mouth should be thoroughly rinsed out. The denture(s) must then be returned to the mouth as soon as possible. Where a denture of the Class I type has been provided, the method of inserting the denture is demonstrated to the patient with the help of a hand mirror, with emphasis on the importance of ensuring that the neck of each immediately replaced anterior tooth is positioned behind the corresponding labial soft tissue flap. The patient is warned that unless this procedure is followed, the appearance of the denture may suffer.

2. Apart from the time required for cleansing, the denture(s) should continue to be worn both during the day and overnight, until notified otherwise.

A further appointment is then arranged for the second review, which will normally be about 1 week after the first review.

THE SECOND AND SUBSEQUENT REVIEW STAGES

On returning to the surgery for the second review, the patient is asked whether any problems have been experienced whilst wearing the denture(s). The oral cavity and the denture(s) are then examined in detail with the help of a mouth mirror where necessary. Joint consideration of the history and the examination procedures should then allow a diagnosis to be made of the cause of any problems which were reported by the patient. Appropriate action can then be taken to try and overcome these problems. Where the action which is taken involves denture modification using small mounted stones or similar cutting instruments, the area(s) which have been modified must be carefully smoothed and, except for the fitting surface, must be repolished before the denture(s) is returned to the patient. Another appointment is then arranged for a further review.

The procedure which was used at the second review is then repeated at the third and subsequent review stages, which are normally held at increasing intervals of time. For example, the following schedule of visits may be selected:

Third review appointment — 2 weeks after the second review.

Fourth review appointment — 3 weeks after the third review.

Fifth review appointment — 4 weeks after the fourth review.

Subsequent review appointments are then held at approximately monthly intervals for as long as proves to be necessary.

In addition to these set appointments, the patient is asked to arrange one or more additional appointments should they experience any special problems that, they feel, need urgent attention. It has been found that having the assurance of the availability of such extra appointments can aid the patient's psychological adaptation to denture wearing and so, indirectly, can help to achieve success in immediate denture treatment.

THE AFTER-CARE OF IMMEDIATE DENTURES

As a consequence of alveolar resorption in the area(s) where teeth were extracted, it is very likely that an immediate denture will gradually lose retention with the passage of time from the insertion stage. Eventually, a stage is likely to be reached when the looseness of the denture becomes such as to prove a source of embarrassment to the patient. When that happens, relining of the denture is indicated where this is possible, in order to restore retention to an acceptable level.

The time at which a need for relining first arises varies markedly from patient to patient, being dependent on a number of factors. One factor which has considerable influence on the time interval which elapses before relining is required is the class of immediate denture which has been provided. For a denture of the Class I (open-face) type, this time interval may be as short as 6 weeks, although more commonly it will be in the range of

2–3 months. In contrast, the time interval where a denture of the Class IIb type has been provided may be 6 months or, occasionally, even longer. For dentures of the Class IIa type, the time interval will be intermediate between these two extremes, a typical value being of the order of 4 months.

Another controlling factor is the number of teeth that were extracted and immediately replaced, the time before relining is required being approximately proportional to the number of teeth involved. Yet another controlling factor is what may be called the 'personal bone factor' of the patient. This relates to the fact that the rate at which alveolar resorption occurs, other factors being equal, varies from person to person, being influenced by features such as hormonal, age and sex differences.

In the case of immediate dentures of the Class I type, when the time arrives for relining to be required, it will often be found that the addition of a labial flange will also be indicated. Where this double requirement arises, it may be possible for the reline and flange addition to be carried out as a joint procedure.

For complete immediate dentures, probably the most satisfactory way of carrying out a reline is to use the denture as a tray to take an impression of the denture-bearing area. The impression material is then replaced by conventional denture base material in a subsequent laboratory procedure. This method is described and explained in detail in Chapter 23 (p. 196) in a presentation that deals with impressions for relining and rebasing complete dentures. For convenience, the essential steps in the procedure can be summarised as follows:

1. Examine the fitting surface of the denture for the presence of undercut areas. If any are found to be present, they must be removed by careful stoning of the area or areas concerned.

2. Check the extension of the denture. As a consequence of alveolar resorption, some areas of the denture may now be overextended, in which case they must be reduced by stoning to the level of the functional sulcus. Other areas may be found to be underextended, where, for example, flange extension was reduced to alleviate pain caused by the pressure of the flange on the underlying tissues. Any areas of underextension must be built up to the level of the functional sulcus using additions of green-stick impression compound. Where the addition of a labial flange is required on a Class I denture, the flange should be developed to the required form by moulding softened impression compound in the area concerned, making sure the compound is sealed to the labial margins of the denture and that adequate clearance is allowed for the labial and/or buccal frenae, where necessary.

3. A mix of zinc oxide–eugenol impression material is prepared in accordance with the manufacturer's instructions. The fitting surface of the denture is dried, along with the drying of the inside surface of any compound additions, and the dried areas are then coated with an even layer of the mixed impression material. The denture is then seated in position in the oral cavity, after which the patient is persuaded to bring the opposing dentitions into contact in the retruded jaw relationship. The occlusion should now show the same interdigitation as that present before the reline procedure was commenced. After the occlusion has been checked the patient is now asked to open the mouth, so enabling border moulding movements to be made around the margins of the denture. The denture is then supported in position until the impression material has set. The denture can then be removed from the oral cavity and the impression surface checked for satisfaction. If necessary, the impression is repeated. After approval, the denture is then immersed in a bath of antiseptic for 10 minutes before going to the laboratory for application of the procedures by which denture base material replaces the lining of impression material in the denture.

4. The relined denture is then again immersed in an antiseptic solution for 10 minutes, prior to the return visit of the patient for reinsertion of the denture. At the latter visit, the denture is checked for satisfaction once again, following through the same check stages as used at the original insertion stage.

After the first reline of an immediate denture, it is likely that a gradual decrease in retention will be found to occur as a consequence of continuing alveolar resorption in the area where the immediately replaced teeth were extracted. The rate at which alveolar resorption occurs is now, however, likely to be considerably reduced relative to the rate in the early post-extraction period. Even so, it will often be found that a second reline will become necessary within the normal life span of an immediate denture (of the order of 6–9 months), if an adequate level of retention is to be maintained. The need for a second reline is particularly likely to be found to be necessary where a Class I type of immediate denture has been provided.

The relining procedure as described above for application in complete denture treatment can also be used to reline the saddles of a metal base partial immediate denture, if the metalwork of the saddles has been designed to give a layer of non-metallic denture base material on the fitting surface of the saddles. The same procedure is not, however, normally used to reline a partial immediate denture having a connector structure in a polymeric denture base material. This is because when the reline impression is taken, the impression material would enter the undercut areas likely to be present around the standing natural teeth. When the impression material is converted to denture base material in the subsequent laboratory procedure, reproduction of the undercut regions would prevent the relined denture from having a free path of insertion. Because of this difficulty, it is often suggested that, when a partial immediate denture bearing a polymeric connector structure shows the need for relining, it is wiser to provide a new partial denture than to attempt to reline the existing denture by use of the method described above. Relining carries with it the major disadvantage that the patient has to lose the use of the denture for the period required to carry out the associated laboratory procedure, which often is in the range of 12–24 hours. Thus, one of the chief advantages arising from the provision of an immediate denture may be breached — that of preventing the patient from having to appear in public in either an edentulous or partially dentate condition.

For a proportion of patients, this disadvantage is of sufficient magnitude for them to refuse to have their immediate denture relined using a conventional type of denture base material. Where this problem arises, the use of alternative procedures must be considered.

One such alternative is the construction of a replacement denture, the patient being able to continue to wear the immediate denture until the replacement denture is ready for insertion. The clinical stages which are used in the provision of a replacement denture are considered in detail in Chapter 38.

Another alternative which may be considered is that of temporarily relining the immediate denture, using only clinically applied procedures which can be carried out whilst the patient is still in the surgery. This method utilises one of the available range of tissue conditioners as the relining material. Although tissue conditioners are intended to be used to help produce a healthy tissue base prior to other dental treatment, they can perform a valuable auxiliary role as relining materials in immediate denture treatment.

Their viscoelastic nature at, and for some time after, the insertion stage allows them to be used when relining any type of immediate denture, including partial immediate dentures which carry a polymeric type of connector structure. However, on the debit side, it is not feasible to use impression compound additions to build up any deficiencies in flange extensions which are found to be present, prior to placing the tissue conditioner lining.

Tissue conditioners are often supplied by manufacturers in the form of a powder and liquid. The procedure for using such materials for the relining of an immediate denture can be summarised as follows:

1. Check the extension of the denture flanges. Reduce any areas of over-extension found to be present and then repolish the margins where reduction was applied. Note that when this relining procedure is being used it is not necessary to remove any undercuts which are present on the fitting surface, but the fitting surface should be thoroughly dried.

2. Make a mix of the tissue conditioner in accordance with the manufacturer's directions. Apply the paste to the fitting surface of the denture.

3. Insert the denture and persuade the patient to close into the retruded contact relationship. Check that the occlusion is satisfactory. Ask the patient to open the mouth and then apply border-moulding movements around the denture. Support the denture in position until gelling is under way.

4. Carefully remove the denture and immerse it

in a bath of warm (not hot) water to accelerate further gelling. After removal from the water bath, cut off any excess tissue conditioner which has flowed on to the occlusal or polished surfaces of the denture.

5. Reinsert the denture. The patient is now able to leave the surgery wearing the denture, with the retention now restored to a satisfactory level.

Unfortunately, the tissue conditioner lining has only a short satisfactory life. It tends to harden and crack over a period of about 3–4 weeks as a consequence of the leaching out of some of the constituents. The lining may also tend to become rather unhygienic as a result of particles of food becoming embedded in the lining.

Thus, once a tissue conditioner lining has been placed in an immediate denture, the patient needs to attend review visits at intervals of 3–4 weeks. Often, it will be found necessary at these visits to clean the surface of the lining and then place a further tissue conditioner lining over the initial lining.

Both of the alternative procedures noted above carry financial implications for the patient, in that they are likely to prove to be more costly than, say, two relines using a conventional denture base material. However, for the patient who is not prepared to be without an immediate denture, even for the time required for the placement of a lining in a conventional denture base material, the cost of using one of the alternative procedures may well be felt to be justified.

Irrespective of the procedure selected for use in the after-care of an immediate denture, it is highly desirable that the status of the denture should be checked between about 6 and 9 months after the denture was inserted and a decision made as to the need for further treatment.

At this time it may well be found that the denture is again becoming rather unretentive, although the rate at which alveolar resorption is now occurring is likely to have fallen to a rate which is characteristic for the patient under treatment. It is generally considered to be undesirable to reline a denture more than twice, when a heat-curing type of denture base material is used, because of a cumulative tendency for warpage of the denture to occur. Thus, in those instances where two relines have already been carried out with use of a heat-cured denture base material as the lining, it may well be considered preferable that a new denture should now be provided to replace the immediate denture.

Where, instead, the patient was provided with a replacement denture to wear in lieu of the original immediate denture, if this denture has now also become loose, then the provision of a further replacement denture is indicated.

Finally, where a tissue conditioner has been used for relining the immediate denture, provision of a replacement denture may again now be thought to be indicated to save both patient and operator from the tedium of having to continue to reline the immediate denture at intervals of 3–4 weeks.

FURTHER READING

Atkinson HF 1960 Some aspects of immediate denture treatment. Aust Dent J 5: 221

Carlsson GE, Bergman B, Hedegård B 1967 Morphological changes of the mandible after extraction and wearing of dentures: a longitudinal clinical and x-ray cephalometric study covering 5 years. Odontol Rev 18: 27

Kelly KE 1967 Follow-up treatment for immediate denture patients. J Prosthet Dent 17: 16

Lassila V 1985 Adaptation in maxillary immediate denture treatment. Prac Finn Dent Soc 81: 210

McCarthy JA, Moser JB 1978 Mechanical properties of tissue conditioners. I. Theoretical considerations, behavioral characteristics and tensile properties. J Prosthet Dent 40: 89

McCarthy JA, Moser JB 1978 Mechanical properties of tissue conditioners. II Creep characteristics. J Prosthet Dent 40: 334

Nairn RI, Cutress TW 1967 Changes in mandibular position following removal of the remaining teeth and insertion of immediate complete dentures. Br Dent J 122: 303

Wical KE, Brusse P 1979 Effects of a calcium and vitamin D supplement on alveolar ridge resorption in immediate denture patients. J Prosthet Dent 41: 4

PART V

Special appliances and procedures

37. Treatment of the elderly

INTRODUCTION

Dental treatment for the elderly has taken on a new impetus over the past few years, as a substantial treatment need in this section of the community has been recognised. The number of ageing and elderly individuals in the community has increased and will continue to do so into the next century, especially in those aged over 75 years. Improved health and socio-economic status have contributed to increased longevity, while the number of births has remained essentially static.

While there is clear evidence of improved dental health within the population, the retention of teeth into later life brings with it many restorative challenges, since tooth wear, dental caries often in unusual sites on the teeth, periodontal disease and general health problems may arise. In addition, there is a very large number of people who are edentulous or partially edentulous at the present time. Also, there are those who may require removable prostheses to be provided in the future. All the treatment referred to will be required at a stage in their lives when adjustment to new circumstances can be difficult in the extreme. The conversion from dentate to denture-wearing status can be difficult for younger adults and is significantly more so for the older patient.

PHYSIOLOGICAL AGEING CHANGES

There are certain physiological changes that occur with increasing age. In the healthy subject these are not a cause of concern, as the only consequences are a diminution in the reserve capacity of organs. They do not of themselves cause illness (Table 37.1).

FUNCTIONAL DISORDERS

Changing physiology and increasing possibility of pathology occurring with age can produce a very different response to illness in the elderly, when compared to younger subjects. Surveys have shown that, on average, elderly persons may have three or four different pathological processes occurring at the same time.

Not only do the elderly suffer multiple medical pathologies but also multiple social problems. Further detailed discussion of these important considerations is beyond the scope of this book and reference to the gerontology literature should be made. However, some of the disorders of the organic systems which may exceed physiological changes have direct relevance to prosthodontic treatment and may be considered in the following functional groups.

1. Sensory system. Deficiencies in visual, auditory, taste and olfactory facilities.
2. Motor systems. Disorders affecting joint and muscle function or secondary to central nervous system defects.
3. Cardiovascular disorders.
4. Affective disorders.
5. Cognitive disorders.

1. Sensory systems

Visual

Often, patients are required to contribute to treatment in, for example, tooth selection and the acceptability of the appearance of prostheses. For the elderly patient, good lighting and ensuring that the patient has their spectacles available is essential.

Table 37.1   Some physiological ageing changes of dental significance

System	Physiological change	Implications
Skin	Loss of elasticity Capillary fragility Decrease in thickness Decrease in lipids	Wrinkles Easily damaged Change in colour Dryness
Muscle	Decrease in strength	Easily fatigued Reduced mobility
Bone	Progressive bone loss	Increased bone resorption
Cardiovascular	Diminished aortic elasticity	Increased pulse and systolic pressure
Respiratory	Reduction in elastic recoil	Decreased vital capacity Posture important
Nervous	Elevated threshold for touch, temperature and pain Kinaesthesia diminished Taste/smell diminished Vision and hearing disturbances	Potential for injury Position sense is decreased Reduced interest in food and nutrition may suffer Sight and communication difficulties
Liver	Hepatic blood flow altered Enzyme activity altered	Drug metabolism and clearance affected
Kidney	Reduced renal blood flow Diurnal excretory pattern altered	Reduced excretion of drugs and metabolites
Bladder	Increased dysinhibition	Incontinence

Where necessary, the patient should be accompanied by a companion. These are the minimum provisions to ensure sensible cooperation.

Hearing

Hearing loss is common in the elderly and can be a potent barrier to good communication and understanding. Distracting extraneous sounds in the clinic, speaking over other conversations in the same room and even background music can block all or parts of a direct conversation with a patient who is hard of hearing. This can mean that essential instruction to the patient may go unheeded and good rapport is impossible to develop.

Taste and smell

A patient whose gustatory and/or olfactory senses have been diminished, perhaps unnoticed, over a lengthy period, may become very conscious of this when a new denture is provided and as a result can lay the blame for the sensory loss on the denture treatment.

2. Motor systems

Discussion of damage to the central nervous system through strokes, Parkinsonism or neurological disease, while having clear implications in the delivery of a prosthodontic service, is beyond the immediate scope of this book. As a consequence of these disease processes, mobility problems may be such that domiciliary treatment may be required and mandibular dyskinesia may be present, posing problems of access and in the securing of jaw relations. Degenerative joint disease is a very common form of chronic arthritis in the elderly, producing pain and stiffness in a variety of joints. The patient's mobility is severely affected, and he or she may be unable to sit in a dental chair in the normal way, for example. Consideration should be given to the type of floor covering which is used, as slippery floors and any obstructions to a clear passageway such as looms of services to the dental chair must be avoided. Furniture should be robust and secure, since it may be used as a resting point for the elderly patient to lean on, and door handles should be of the lever type so that those with limited manual dexterity can operate them.

3. Cardiovascular system

Postural hypotension is common in older patients, where a form of venous pooling on rapid change in posture between a horizontal and vertical position occurs. The cause is related to alteration in the baroreceptor response in older subjects because of changes in the autonomic nervous system. Thus, an older patient who may have been in the dental chair in a recumbent or semi-recumbent position must be given adequate time to achieve adaptation to the change in posture when the dental chair is placed upright, or possibly when attempting to stand after treatment. The older patient should be carefully observed in these circumstances, in case collapse should occur.

4. Affective disorders

The need for major life adjustments as a person enters old age is common and may be related to loss, which may be of a physical, sensory or interpersonal nature. Loss of, or marked reduction in, physical capabilities and the need to curtail an active life style may occur. In addition, there may be loss in intellectual capabilities, hearing problems, and problems in acquiring new skills. At the interpersonal level there may be loss of friends or family through bereavement. Economic position and social status may also deteriorate. The consequence of these losses is often a depressive reaction of varying severity. Patients may associate the onset of their emotional disturbance to a particular illness or loss — perhaps even the loss of their natural teeth, or the provision of a new denture. Complaints are not commonly presented as emotional complaints but as somatic ones, perhaps related to aspects of prosthodontic treatment such as atypical facial pain or other forms of discomfort.

5. Cognitive disorders

These are disorders such as senile and presenile dementias and are the result of an early loss of higher judgemental and abstraction skills. In the extreme case the individual progressively loses all memory function and ultimately loses basic orientation to space, time and even themselves. The early stages are those in which forgetfulness, confusion and behavioural aberration may occur. They are included here to discriminate them from the affective disorders for which treatment is available as, to date, there is no known effective treatment apart from general supportive care for the cognitive disorders. Some 20% of those over 80 years of age are subject to cognitive disorders to some extent.

ORAL CHANGES IN THE ELDERLY

These include the following.

Oral mucosa. Reduction in thickness of the epithelial layers with decreased elastic properties of the connective tissue occurs. The tissues are consequently more susceptible to trauma and disease. The use of resilient lining materials may need to be considered for some denture patients.

Bone. Osteoporosis and resorption occur and may be particularly evident in the edentulous mandible.

Teeth. Loss of tooth substance mainly resulting from attrition is evident and may be marked where there has been loss of some natural teeth for several years, or abnormal habits (e.g. bruxism) have developed. The colour of the teeth becomes darker and the enamel and dentine become friable.

Periodontium. Decrease in the fibrous and cellular components, and irregularity in structure occurs.

Gingivae. The gingivae become smooth and shiny as stippling is lost. The epithelium is thinned and easily damaged.

Oral hygiene. Neglect of oral hygiene may occur because of the physical inability of the patient to undertake it, or because of lack of motivation.

Tongue. Reduction in the functions of the taste buds occurs. Atrophy of the circumvallate papillae may be evident. Fissuring is common. Varicosities may be present on the ventral surface.

Saliva. While there is little evidence of decrease in the volume of saliva produced as a result of the ageing process alone, xerostomia is a common side-effect of pharmacotherapy. Thus, frictional effects may be seen in the mouth with localised mucositis. For denture wearing subjects, retention may be reduced and pain and inflammation may result from the rubbing of a denture against the dry mucosa. The selection of an impression material which will not be adherent to the dry mucosa will be required. A saliva substitute may be helpful to the patient.

Lips. Reduction in the vermilion borders, skin wrinkling and possibly inversion of the commissure occurs, which may lead to angular cheilitis. Care with the provision of lip support for denture patients will be necessary.

Neuromuscular changes. Progressive strength and control diminution occurs, so that it may be difficult to sustain a resting posture and to consistently achieve the retruded jaw relation. Dyskinesia of the mandible may be evident.

TREATMENT OF THE ELDERLY

The mere fact of the advanced chronological age of a patient does not necessarily mean that the treatment regime to be followed will differ from that of a younger age group. However, as indicated above, there may be many additional matters of a medical and/or social nature to take into account. Treatment may be slow and tedious, requiring an understanding of the ageing process and all its ramifications and of the way that it has affected the particular patient being cared for.

The development of good communication and rapport is essential. Short appointments will suit some and these should be arranged at a time which does not significantly alter the patient's daily routine. A feeling of security is very important, so a careful explanation of what is being done, as well as safe surroundings, will assist the treatment process.

FURTHER READING

Abelson DC 1985 Denture plaque and denture cleansers: a review of the literature. Gerodontics 5: 202

Ambjornsen E, Rise J 1985 The effect of verbal information and demonstration on denture hygiene in elderly people. Acta Odontol Scand 43: 19

Cohen B, Thomson H 1986 Dental care for the elderly. Heinemann, London

Douglass CW, Gammon MD, Atwood DA 1988 Need and effective demand for prosthodontic treatment. J Prosthet Dent 59: 94

Duxbury AJ, Hayes NF, Thakkar NS, Wastell DG, Kelly A, Leach FN 1985 Clinical trial of a mucin-containing artificial saliva. IRCS Med Sci 13: 1197

Greebny LM, Schwartz SS 1986 A reference guide to drugs and dry mouth. Gerontology 5: 75

Hoad–Reddick G 1988 Changes in population, prosthetic need and dental disease in the elderly. J Br Inst Surg Tech 2: 3

Hoad–Reddick G, Grant AA, Griffiths CS 1987 Knowledge of dental services provided: investigations in an elderly population. Commun Dent Oral Epid 15: 137

Lappalainen R, Nyyssonen V 1987 Self-assessed chewing ability of Finnish adults with removable dentures. Gerodontics 3: 238

MacEntee MI, Weiss R, Morrison BJ, Waxler–Morrison NE 1987 Mandibular dysfunction in an institutionalised and predominantly elderly population. J Oral Rehab 14: 523

Weiffenbach JM 1987 Taste perception mechanisms. In: Ferguson D B (ed) The aging mouth, Front Oral Physiol. 6: 151

38. Replacement dentures

INTRODUCTION

All patients who have been provided with complete dentures will require their replacement, following a period which will vary between different patients.

The principal factors which will determine the interval between dentures for patients include:

1. The rate at which the form of the tissues has changed. For example, rapid changes will be expected in a patient who has been provided with an immediate denture. On the other hand, a patient provided with a denture after healing following extraction is complete, may not show significant tissue contour changes for 5 or more years. There may be considerable individual variation between patients in relation to the rate at which resorption of the residual alveolar ridge occurs following tooth loss. The factors which may play a part in ridge resorption are considered in Part I (Ch. 2).

2. Occlusal wear, which may affect the appearance, the occlusion and articulation, and the vertical dimension of occlusion.

3. Damage to the dentures. For example, that resulting from: local abrasion due to inappropriate cleaning methods; fracture of the teeth or base caused by dropping the denture; or colour change following the use of hot water during cleaning.

PROLONGED DENTURE USAGE

It is desirable that denture patients should have a dental examination at regular intervals, e.g. annually, so that the health of the oral tissues and the fit of the dentures may be assessed. However, many patients fail to do this and continue to wear their dentures for many years beyond the time at which the appliances would be considered unsatisfactory when examined by a dentist.

That such patients are able to continue to control dentures which, on examination, are ill-fitting, unstable, poorly retentive and have occlusal inaccuracies is a result of a process of adaptation related to developed muscular skills and motivation. Such a patient may stabilise the upper denture during mouth opening by placing the posterior aspect of the tongue against the palate of the denture. At the same time, the lower denture is held in place by the lateral borders of the tongue. On closure of the mouth, the mandible is protruded into an apparent class III jaw relation, in order to provide occlusal contact for the worn denture teeth.

Frequently, the soft tissues show the effects of denture-related trauma such as inflammation, hyperplasia and hyperkeratinisation

REPLACEMENT DENTURES

When replacement dentures are contemplated for such patients as described above, it is essential that the well-tolerated features of the existing dentures are retained. This is especially so for the older patient. The capacity for adaptation to the multiple oral stimuli that will be produced by a new denture, of different form to the existing denture, diminishes with increasing age.

In particular, for the older, successful denture wearer to achieve habituation to replacement dentures in the minimum of time and inconvenience, it is important to preserve:

1. The contours of the dental arch and polished surfaces.

2. The spatial relation of the teeth to the surrounding tissues.

3. The areas of contact of the denture base and the supporting tissues.

In order to accomplish this, a method known as the *copy denture method* may be used to produce replacement dentures. As will become apparent in describing this method, the term is somewhat misleading in that it aims to copy only the *desirable features* of the existing dentures.

Copy casts

Attempts are sometimes made to copy existing dentures by means of an impression of the polished surfaces and teeth. A cast produced from this is used as a guide for the technician to copy the existing denture. While this may be satisfactory as a guide to produce a similar arrangement of the anterior teeth, for example, significant changes will occur in the other features, which are critical from an adaptation point of view.

Preliminary treatment

The copy method is recommended for use where successful dentures are to be replaced. Where dentures have not been successful, a studied approach to denture production, as described in the earlier chapters of this text, must be used.

As with all prosthodontic treatment, the first stage to be achieved for the replacement of successful existing dentures is to bring the oral tissues to a healthy state. The recovery of damaged tissues is essential prior to the commencement of other stages in treatment.

If no surgical or other form of intervention is required, the adaptation of ill-fitting dentures to the supporting mucosal tissues should be improved. This can be accomplished using a temporary lining of a tissue conditioner material within the dentures.

The occlusion of the existing dentures may also be modified using self-curing acrylic resin, in order to correct existing occlusal errors. If it is judged that some change in the extensions of the denture are required, such adjustments should also be carried out at this stage. It is recommended that, where major changes are judged to be necessary, these

should be undertaken by first modifying the patient's existing dentures. This will provide an opportunity to test the response of the patient before producing the replacement dentures as, up to this stage, the required changes are all reversible. Should the patient be unable to cope with the modifications, the copy method should proceed without them.

The effect of these preliminary procedures will be to eliminate, or at least minimise, traumatic effects to the supporting mucosa.

The copy method

When satisfied that the condition of the patient's oral tissues is optimal, and that tolerance of proposed changes has been achieved, the copy method can be applied.

A suitable duplicating flask is selected. The object is to record the form of the occlusal, polished and fitting surfaces of the dentures using alginate impression material in a two-part flask. The flask may be of metal or plastic, and the two parts must fit together accurately and be large enough to contain a denture.

First visit

The patient's denture is cleaned, decontaminated and dried. Mixed alginate is placed on the polished and occlusal surfaces to minimise air entrapment and the denture is then invested, with the polished surface down in the lower part of the flask (Fig. 38.1).

When set, the alginate is trimmed so that the surface is smooth and level with the borders of the denture. Petroleum jelly is coated on the exposed alginate surface.

A fresh mix of alginate is then prepared, most of which is placed in the exposed fitting surface of the denture, being careful to avoid air entrapment. The upper part of the flask is then filled with the remainder of the alginate and both parts of the flask are brought together.

When the alginate has set, the excess is trimmed away and the flask opened. The dentures are removed from the investing alginate, cleaned and returned to the patient.

Two sprue holes are cut in the alginate in the

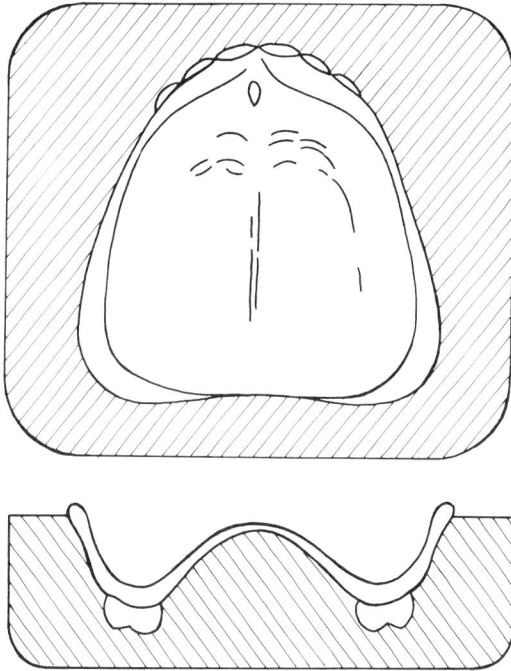

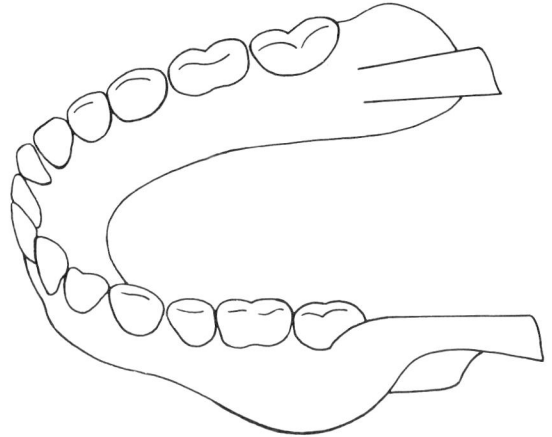

Fig. 38.3 Appearance of a lower denture with sprues still attached after removal from the mould.

Fig. 38.1 Upper denture positioned, with the polished surface down, in the lower part of the flask. The hatched area represents the alginate investment. **A** Plan view. **B** Cross-section through the flask.

by the mix emerging from the second sprue.

After the resin has cured, the all-pink replicas can be removed from the mould (Fig. 38.3). The sprues, flash and any pimples on the acrylic due to air blows in the alginate are cut away using a rotating stone. The replicas are then smoothed with sandpaper and lightly polished until they are suitable for insertion in the mouth.

Second visit

Any undercuts in the fitting surfaces of the replicas are removed and any overextension of the borders reduced.

An impression is obtained using a low-viscosity silicone or zinc oxide–eugenol paste. Where undercuts are present in the mouth, it is advantageous to use silicone impression material, to facilitate removal of the replica denture from the cast which will be produced from it. The impression may also then remain in the template denture during the subsequent trial stage. Care is taken to maintain the existing horizontal jaw relationship, if it has been decided that this should remain unaltered.

Wax is added to or subtracted from the occlusal surfaces of the replicas, until even contact is established in the retruded contact position at the desired occlusal vertical dimension.

The jaw relationship is preserved with the aid of a small quantity of impression paste spread on the occlusal surface of the lower denture, which is

lower part of the flask, from the extension to the rear part of the impression of the polished surface of the denture. The mould is reassembled and the sprue holes checked to ensure that they are large enough to permit a fluid mix of self-curing acrylic resin to be poured into the mould (Fig. 38.2).

The two halves of the flask are opened and modelling wax is melted into the impressions of the teeth, until their gingival margins are covered.

The flask is reassembled and a thin mix of self-curing acrylic is vibrated into the mould through one of the sprues until it is filled, as seen

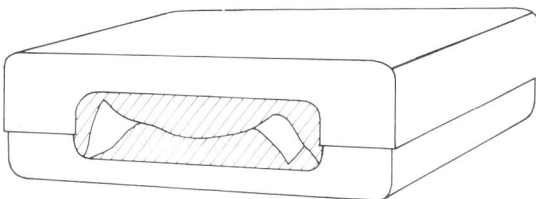

Fig. 38.2 The flask reassembled after removal of the denture and the forming of the sprue holes.

allowed to set while the patient maintains the mandible in the retruded contact position. As the mould of the teeth is preserved on the replica denture, it is only necessary to select the appropriate tooth shade at this stage.

Following suitable disinfection, the replicas which are now templates for the production of the new dentures, can then be conveyed to the laboratory. Instructions are given to pour casts in the impressions, then to mount the templates on an articulator, cut the pink wax teeth off the bases one or two at a time, and re-wax on stock teeth of the desired mould and shade.

Third visit

The waxed-up dentures are checked in a similar manner to that used for conventionally produced dentures:

1. Checking extension, retention and stability.
2. Checking aesthetics.
3. Checking the vertical component of jaw relationship.

4. Checking the horizontal component of jaw relationship.

Details of these procedures are described in Chapter 26.

The post-dam is carved to the optimum position and depth on the cast of the upper jaw, with due reference to the patient's mouth.

Fourth and fifth visits

The new dentures are fitted and reviewed as usual, using procedures as described in Chapters 27 and 28.

FURTHER READING

Basker RM, Chamberlain JD 1971 A method for duplicating dentures: some clinical applications. Br Dent J 131: 549

Heath JR, Davenport JC 1982 A modification of the copy denture technique. Br Dent J 153: 300

Heath JR, Johnson A 1981 The versatility of the copy denture technique. Br Dent J 150: 189

Scher EA 1964 A replacement denture technique. Dent Pract Dent Rec 14: 464

39. Overdentures

INTRODUCTION

An overdenture is a complete or partial denture which is supported by mucoperiosteum and prepared teeth or roots. In addition to the application of the principles of prosthodontics described throughout this book, a good understanding of the practice of general restorative techniques, including periodontal and endodontic treatment, is essential to the provision of overdenture treatment. This chapter will be confined to a consideration of the principles relating to overdentures. For further information concerning their application and details of clinical methods used in overdenture treatment, the literature should be consulted.

ADVANTAGES OF OVERDENTURES

These largely relate to advantages which accrue from the retention of tooth substance:

1. Retained roots provide a stimulus for the retention of alveolar bone. The loss of a tooth is invariably followed by alveolar bone loss and, to date, all attempts to prevent this have failed.

2. Sensory feedback is maintained. periodontal proprioception is retained, and this is equally true for endodontically treated teeth as for vital teeth. In addition, where the overdenture contacts the abutment teeth, tactile sensitivity is maintained so that, compared to those with complete dentures, overdenture wearers are better able to discriminate fine particles. They also retain the ability to perceive variation in the hardness of objects placed between the teeth.

3. Enhanced retention over that obtainable by conventional complete dentures is possible.

4. Denture stability and support are enhanced over those of complete dentures. The larger area of support of the retained periodontal ligament is brought into function. This also has the effect of diluting forces applied to the denture-bearing mucosa.

5. Overdenture treatment does not preclude the provision of conventional complete dentures at a later stage, should this prove to be necessary. In addition, as the form of an overdenture is similar to that of a complete denture, the potential of the patient for effective management of complete dentures may be enhanced.

6. Retention of overdenture abutments is said to reduce the disturbing experience suffered by many patients contingent upon loss of all the natural teeth.

DISADVANTAGES OF OVERDENTURES

1. The susceptibility of the overlaid teeth to caries is high and meticulous home care is required. Thus, there is a need for frequent recall for examination of the patient.

2. Periodontal disease of the retained teeth may continue or even be stimulated by the presence of an overdenture. Normal stimulation of the gingival tissues by the tongue and cheeks is absent and plaque accumulation is enhanced. The possibility of a transient bacteraemia after endodontic treatment and the development of periodontal infection may have unfortunate sequelae where certain medical conditions exist, such as a patient suffering from mitral stenosis.

3. Bony undercuts of the alveolar ridge are often found adjacent to retained teeth, especially where

isolated teeth are present. Such undercuts are usually situated on the buccal and labial aspects of the arch. The possibility of varying the path of insertion of an overdenture is limited and, consequently, where an undercut is present, the cast must be blocked out during the processing of the denture or the flange must be foreshortened. See Chapter 26, (pp. 226–227) for further consideration of these approaches. When either blocking out or foreshortening of the flange is used, aesthetic implications exist, as the former may result in excessive bulkiness of the flange, and the latter may cause uneven lip support.

4. Encroachment beyond the denture space. The presence of a prepared tooth, particularly where a precision attachment is to be used to aid retention, may produce excessively bulky contours. These may encroach on the tongue space and cause possible speech difficulties, or in some cases may even encroach on the available freeway space.

INDICATIONS FOR OVERDENTURES

Overdenture treatment should be considered whenever the decision is made to extract teeth and provide a denture. Even in those circumstances where the prognosis for the remaining teeth is such that long term use of the denture is unlikely, the advantages outlined above are such that the overdenture may be considered as a transitional appliance.

There are also several clinical situations where overdentures may be particularly indicated. These include:

1. The single complete denture. Where the extraction of the remaining teeth in one jaw would result in a complete denture being opposed by a natural dentition in the other, substantial difficulties may occur. The forces of mastication which develop may load excessively the mucosa underlying the complete denture, causing soft tissue damage and accelerated bone resorption. In such circumstances, balanced articulation is often difficult to achieve and obtaining a satisfactory aesthetic result may also present problems.

2. Gross attrition. Where gross loss of natural tooth substance has occurred, an overdenture may be a very practical solution to the problem of restoring the face height and appearance of the teeth, while providing maximal occlusal efficiency.

3. Where a patient suffers from hypodontia.

4. Where natural or acquired defects of the jaws are present, e.g. in cleft palate and post-surgical patients. The tissue remaining in the mouth may be so limited in extent and quality that the provision of a satisfactory functional prosthesis can present extreme difficulties. Suitable overdenture abutments can play a vitally important role for such patients.

CONTRAINDICATIONS TO OVERDENTURE TREATMENT

While overdenture treatment has potential advantages to all those patients who require tooth extractions and the provision of dentures, there are a number of conditions where it may be inappropriate:

1. Patients suffering from a severe debilitating condition which requires prolonged medical treatment. In such cases the essential high level of patient cooperation required for successful overdenture treatment may be wanting.

2. Any condition which contraindicates endodontic therapy where this is part of the planned treatment regime, e.g. where the prognosis for endodontic therapy is uncertain, as in a patient who is contemplating cardiac surgery.

3. Any handicap — physical or mental — which will prevent a patient from maintaining a satisfactory standard of oral hygiene.

4. The patient's attitude. Apart from periodontal, endodontic and other preliminary treatment (e.g. crowns and other restorations) stringent oral hygiene standards are required. When the extra clinical visits and the necessary home maintenance by the patient are productive of doubt as to the patient's willingness to provide complete cooperation, it may be unwise to proceed with overdenture therapy.

PRINCIPLES OF OVERDENTURE TREATMENT

The provision of an overdenture substantially alters the environment of the abutment teeth. The effect of this is the enhancement of the potential for plaque retention, accelerated caries and periodontal disease. As a consequence, a high standard of oral hygiene and plaque control is essential.

All the required restorative work is carried out and the unusable teeth are extracted. This leaves the teeth or roots which can be used for overdenture support. Where necessary, these teeth are then reduced in length in order to improve the crown/root ratio so that the potential for the effects of high laterally directed forces is substantially reduced. In most instances, reduction of the crown length to the extent required — some 2 mm above the gingival crest — will mean that endodontic treatment must be carried out first. In cases where gross attrition has occurred, further crown reduction may not be necessary, although some modification to the form of the remaining tooth substance will be required.

Support and retention for overdentures

The choice of supporting elements for overdentures is usually very limited. Whenever possible, support which is symmetrically distributed about the jaw should be sought. For example, a canine and molar on each side of the arch will be satisfactory. However, only two teeth, especially when present in the anterior part of the lower arch, may be usefully applied. Unilateral retention of teeth is less satisfactory, although such a situation still offers advantages over the conditions which may result from total tooth loss. Even teeth which exhibit clinically demonstrable mobility may be considered for use, as such movement will be found to diminish after decoronation of the tooth. The important point is that there must be at least

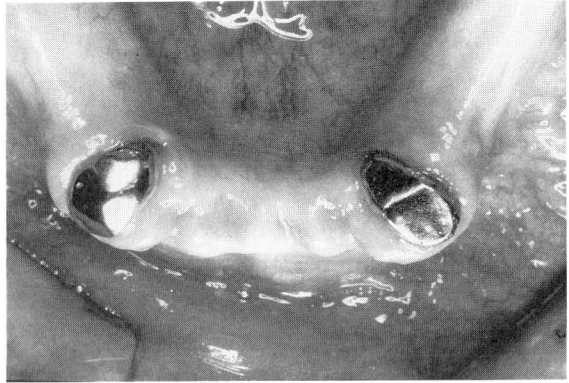

Fig. 39.2 Plan view of the lower arch with copings on 43 and 33 prepared for overdenture treatment.

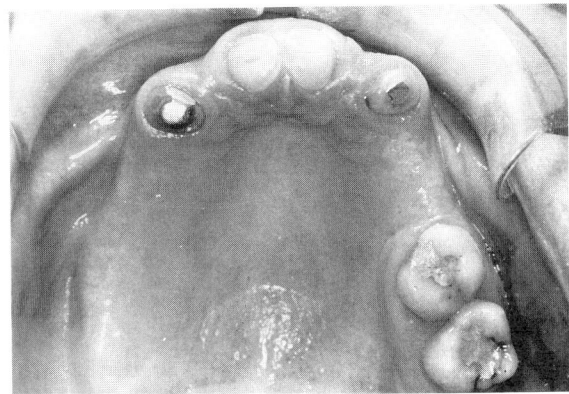

Fig. 39.3 Palatal view of the upper arch showing 13, 11, 21 and 23 prepared for overdenture treatment. Note that secondary dentine is visible on 11 and 21 and no exposure of the root canal has occurred.

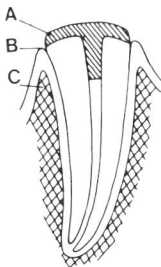

Fig. 39.1 Section through a tooth having a shallow dome form of casting cemented in position. A, casting; B, gingival margin; C, alveolar bone.

5–7 mm of bony support present, together with intact gingival tissues which can be brought to a healthy state.

Endodontic treatment is carried out and the crown of the tooth removed. For the simple type of overdenture, no additional retaining device is used beyond the normal forces utilised in the retention of complete dentures, along with any additional frictional forces generated by contact with the retained teeth. Where a cast coping is to be placed over the remaining root face(s) it is of a shallow dome form, retained in the root canal by means of a short post, and having margins slightly supragingivally placed (Fig. 39.1 and 39.2). If no casting is to be used, the exposed part of the root canal is sealed with amalgam, and the amalgam and dentine smoothed and polished to a rounded form (Fig. 39.3). Such a form is easy to clean and maintain by the patient.

Where an attachment device is to be used to provide positive retention and/or additional support, it may be of a type requiring cementation of a threaded post into the root canal, or one requiring the soldering of the patrix portion to the root face coping. Magnetic forces using cobalt–samarium magnets have also been successfully applied to assist overdenture retention. The splinting of roots together can also be undertaken using bar devices such as the Dolder bar, which will also provide positive retention.

Fabrication of the overdenture

In the cases of the simple overdenture, where no precision attachment devices are included in the denture design, conventional methods are used to construct the overdenture. The overdenture is mucosa supported at rest and becomes tooth and mucosa supported when loaded. A small space is present between the root face or coping and the denture, under resting conditions (Fig. 39.4). This may be provided by relieving the denture at a stage in denture processing as described in Chapter 26, for the provision of a relief area in a conventional denture. The gingival margin region must be relieved to prevent damage to these tissues as movement of the denture occurs during function. Excessive relief must be avoided as hypertrophy of

the tissues into the space created may occur.

Where precision attachments are to be used, the procedures to be followed for the impression stage and the location and incorporation of the attachments varies between the different devices and no attempt will be made to consider details of these. The major problem in the fabrication of such an overdenture is the incorporation of the retention device within the normal outline form of a complete denture. This may be found to be an impossible ideal and bulging of the denture in the region of the device is often necessary.

CARE OF OVERDENTURES

Whether the root facing is covered by a cast coping or not, the dangers of caries and periodontal disease are ever present. While the care of the gingival tissues is simplified by the loss of the crown of the tooth, the potential for plaque retention is considerably enhanced by the presence of the overdenture. Thus, meticulous oral hygiene procedures and denture cleansing must be impressed on the patient. Recall of the patient every 4 months is recommended so that any caries or deterioration of the gingival condition can be detected early and any necessary treatment and reinforcement of oral hygiene instruction undertaken.

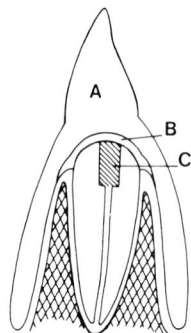

Fig. 39.4 Section through a simple overdenture resting in position over a prepared root. A, overdenture; B, space between root facing and the denture; C, amalgam plug in the root facing.

FURTHER READING

Basker R, Harrison A, Ralph JP 1988 Overdentures in general dental practice. British Dental Association, London
Crumm RJ, Rooney Jr GE 1978 Alveolar bone loss in overdentures: a 5-year study. J Prosthet Dent 40: 610
Fenton AH, Hahn N 1978 Tissue response to overdenture therapy. J Prosthet Dent 40: 492
Lioselle RJ, Crumm RJ, Rooney GE, Stuever CH 1972 The physiologic basis for the overlay denture. J Prosthet Dent 28: 4
McDermott IG, Rosenberg SW 1984 Overdentures for the irradiated patient. J Prosthet Dent 51: 314.
Preiskel HW 1985 Precision attachments in prosthodontics. Overdentures and telescopic prostheses. Quintessence, Chicago, vol 2
Smith GA, Laird WRE, Grant, AA 1983 Magnetic retention units for overdentures. J Oral Rehab 10: 481
Toolson LB, Smith DE, Phillips C 1978 A 2-year longitudinal study of overdenture patients. Part I. Incidence and control of caries on overdenture abutments. J Prosthet Dent 40: 486
Toolson LB, Smith DE, Phillips C 1982 A 2-year longitudinal study of overdenture patients. Part II. Assessment of the periodontal health of overdenture abutments. J Prosthet Dent 47: 4
Toolson LB, Taylor TD 1989 A 10-year report of a longitudinal recall of overdenture patients. J Prosthet Dent 62: 179.

40. Dental implants

INTRODUCTION

An implant is an object or substance which is implanted into the body for the purpose of restoration of function and/or the replacement of deficient tissues. A dental implant is implanted into or onto the tissues of the jaws with the object of providing anchorage for a tooth, bridge or denture, or for the augmentation of the resorbed residual alveolar ridge.

Some of the newer dental implant techniques have a wider application than replacement of deficient oral tissues, and are used for rehabilitation of patients requiring ear, ocular and other maxillo-facial prostheses.

TYPES OF DENTAL IMPLANTS

Dental implants may be designated as intramucosal, subperiosteal or endosseous, depending on whether they lie within the mucoperiosteum (intramucosal), beneath the mucoperiosteum and on the surface of the bone (subperiosteal) or actually enter the body of the bone (endosseous).

MATERIALS USED FOR IMPLANTATION

Stringent biological, chemical and mechanical properties are required of substances for implantation in the jaws. No single material has been identified as possessing ideal properties for all types of implants. It is, therefore, not surprising that a large number of different materials have been used in the production of implants for dental use.

Examples of materials which have been used for the production of dental implants include the following:

Implantable teeth and roots:
    Cobalt–chromium–molybdenum alloys
    Ceramics
    Vitreous carbon
    Titanium
Tissue augmentation:
    Hydroxyapatites
    Silicone rubbers
Subperiosteal implants:
    Cobalt–chromium–molybdenum alloys
Endosteal implants:
    Titanium
    Alumina
    Stainless steel
Intramucosal inserts:
    Titanium.

PARTIALLY BURIED IMPLANTS

Most dental implants may be described as partially buried, i.e. they are implanted into the body tissues and have part of the implant projecting through the soft tissues into the mouth. There are, however, several exceptions to this statement, including:

1. Intramucosal implants, in which stud-like projections (the mucosal insert) are processed into an upper denture base. These provide retention for the denture by engaging suitable receptor sites in the mucous membrane (Fig. 40.1).

2. Diodontic implants, which consist of a rod or pin which is implanted through the root canal of an existing natural tooth. This type is also known as an endodontic endosseous implant.

3. Materials used to augment deficient alveolar ridges. Hydroxyapatites are examples of such materials. These materials are placed subperiosteally,

Fig. 40.2 Subperiosteal implant framework. The polished vertical posts project through the mucoperiosteum into the mouth.

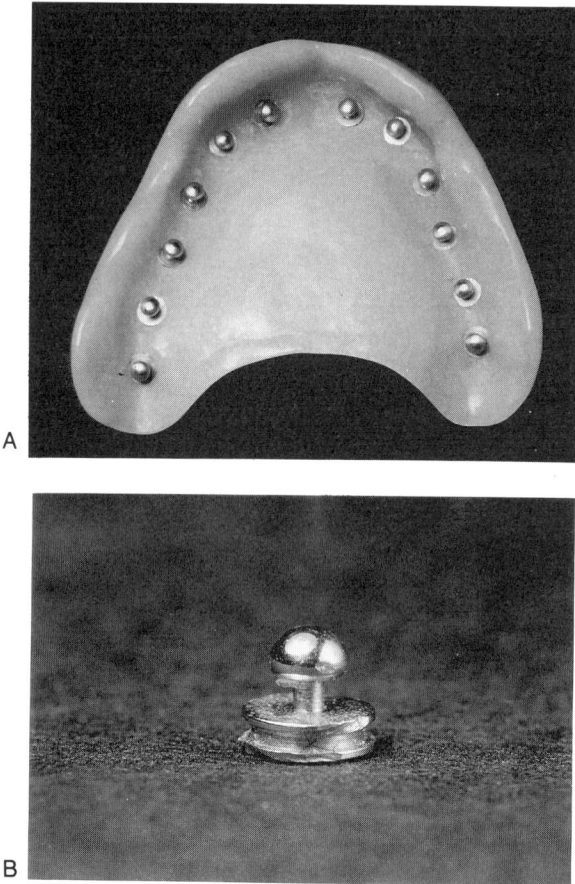

Fig. 40.1 **A** Intramucosal studs placed in an upper denture. **B** An intramucosal stud.

and may be used in particulate form, or as a porous block with the object of stimulating tissue ingrowth.

SUBPERIOSTEAL IMPLANTS WITH INTRA-ORAL PROJECTIONS

This type of implant has been in use for many years. These implants consist of a framework which fits against the surface of the bone of the jaw. In order to produce the framework, an operation is required in which the mucoperiosteum is reflected and an impression of the bone is obtained, after which the soft tissues are replaced.

The impression is used to make a model on which a cast metal framework (usually of cobalt–chromium alloy) is made (Fig. 40.2). This frame-

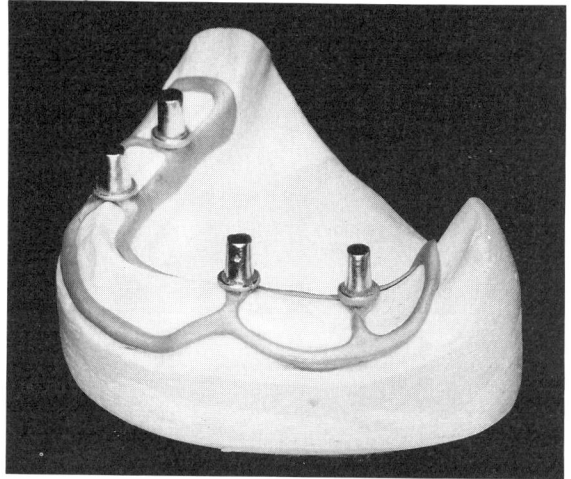

work includes the intra-oral projections of the implant and is inserted at a subsequent operation. The intra-oral projections act as abutments to retain and support a removable prosthesis.

When failure of this type of implant occurs, it is a result of breakdown at the soft tissue/implant interface associated with the intra-oral projections, and is commonly related to failure of effective plaque control.

ENDOSSEOUS IMPLANTS

There are many different types of endosseous implants having a wide variety of shapes and sizes. They are usually identified by the name of the clinician who introduced each type.

Each implant consists of a body which is a representation of a tooth or teeth, a neck portion which passes through the mucoperiosteum, and a post which projects into the mouth for the attachment of a prosthesis. The body of the implant may be solid or porous. Where pores are present, they should be some 100 µm or larger, if mineralization of the ingrowing tissue is to occur.

A variant of the endosseous implant is the transmandibular staple, in which a curved bar is fitted to the inferior border of the mandible in the anterior region by means of retentive pins. Two threaded transosteal pins penetrate through the bone into the mouth, where locking nuts are

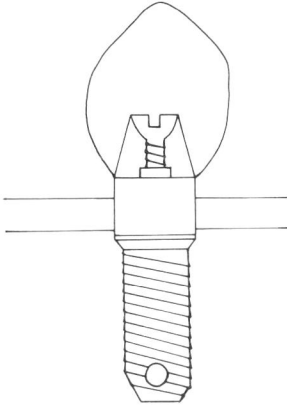

Fig. 40.3 Illustration of an implant of a type used in the osseointegration technique.

applied. An overdenture type of prosthesis utilises the transosteal pins as abutments.

Variable success has been reported for the different types of these implants and a substantial body of research has surrounded them. In particular, the tissue/implant interface has received most attention, since this is the region which is most prone to failure. Apart from the factors associated with the biocompatibility of the materials used, the shape and nature of the implant surface are important related factors, as is the extent of the loads applied

and the time of application following initial healing.

OSSEOINTEGRATED IMPLANTS

The basis of this type of implant is the formation of bone in immediate proximity to the intraosseous part of an implant. The term 'osseointegrated implant' is coined following the work of Branemark in which the artificial root portion of a pure titanium implant was implanted within the bone, and the soft tissue is then closed above it. After healing is complete, the tissues over the coronal end of the implant are reflected so that an abutment can be attached. A series of two or more abutments joined together can then be used to form the substructure for a fixed or removable prosthesis.

Using this system, no loads are applied to the body of the implant immediately following its placement, so that healing takes place without disturbing the tissues in proximity to the implant. Bone growth during the healing phase occurs to contact the oxide layer on the surface of the implant, without giant cell production or any intervening fibrous tissue. This principle has been applied to single-tooth implants as well as multiple-unit restorations. Results obtained using the osseointegrated system on carefully selected patients have shown a high rate of success (Fig. 40.3 and 40.4).

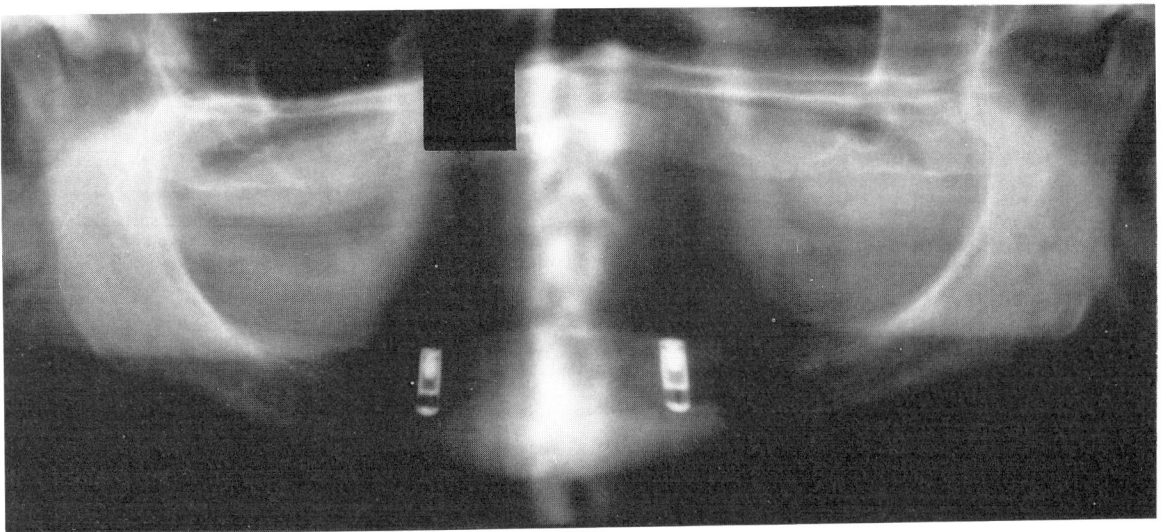

Fig. 40.4 An orthopantomogram radiograph showing osseointegrated implants in the 43 and 33 areas.

The contribution of the osseointegrated technique to dental implantation offers much promise for successful long-term rehabilitation of patients who have lost some or all of their natural teeth, and for whom this form of treatment can be applied.

FURTHER READING

Adell R, Lekhohn U, Rockler B, Brånemark PI 1981 A 15-year study of osseointegrated implants in the treatment of the edentulous jaw. Int J Oral Surg 10: 387

Babbush C, Kirsch A, Mentag PJ, Hill B 1987 Intramobile cylinder (IMZ) two-stage osseointegrated implant system with the intramobile element (IME). I, Its rationale and procedure for use. Int J Oral Maxillofac Implants 2(4): 203

Hoad-Reddick G, Grant AA 1989 Intramucosal inserts — time for a re-evaluation. Quintess Int 20: 879

McCord JF, Callis PD 1987 Localised alveolar ridge augmentation with dense hydroxyapatite: report of two restorative cases. Rest Dent 3: 112.

Quayle AA, Cawood JI, Smith GA, Eldridge D J, Howell RA 1989 The immediate or delayed replacement of teeth by permucosal intraosseous implants: the Tubingen implant system, part I: implant design, rationale for use and pre-operative assessment. Br Dent J 166: 365

Quayle AA, Cawood JI, Smith GA, Eldridge DJ, Howell RA 1989 The immediate or delayed replacement of teeth by permucosal intraosseous implants: the Tubingen implant system, part II: surgical and restorative techniques. Br Dent J 166: 403

Quayle AA, Marouf H, Holland I 1990 Alveolar ridge augmentation using a new design of inflatable tissue expander: surgical technique and preliminary results. Br. J Oral Maxfac Surg 28: 375

US Department of Health and Human Services 1980 Dental implants: benefit and risk. NIH — Harvard consensus development conference, Washinton DC

41. Obturators for maxillary defects

Intra-oral maxillofacial prosthodontics is that practice which is involved in the aesthetic and functional rehabilitation of patients requiring the replacement of deficiencies in the hard and/or soft tissues within the oral cavity.

Patients requiring such treatment may present with conditions in which direct intra-oral communication between the oral cavity and the maxillary sinus or the nasopharynx exists; or for whom essential treatment procedures will result in such communication.

The need for such treatment arises from:

1. Congenital abnormalities, such as cleft lip and palate.
2. Trauma from industrial, domestic, road traffic accidents or other penetrating injuries.
3. Surgery, especially that related to the treatment of oral and peri-oral malignancy.

Where congenital defects and the results of traumatic injury are concerned, the prosthodontist is faced with an existing set of circumstances from which to attempt to rehabilitate the patient. Such circumstances are often far from favourable in terms of the provision of a good end result of treatment.

On the other hand, where ablative surgery which will result in substantial tissue loss is contemplated, the prosthodontist should be involved in planning the overall treatment of the patient. The recording of the pre-surgical tissue relationships, the provision of splints and appliances used as an adjunct to surgery for the retention of postsurgical dressings, for example, as well as the definitive prosthodontic appliance, all form part of the treatment procedures.

OBTURATORS

An obturator is an object which closes an opening and, in dentistry, refers to a prosthesis used to functionally close a congenital or acquired opening in the palate. An obturator is sometimes referred to as a speech bulb, where it is an extension of a denture base which replaces a deficiency of the soft palate.

In general terms, the approach to the treatment of a patient in need of an obturator varies according to whether or not sufficient of the tissue, normally regarded as denture-bearing tissue, remains to enable accurate recording of jaw relations to be made. An example of conditions where adequate basal tissue might be present would be where the hard palate was perforated, or where a congenital cleft of the hard and soft palates existed. The results of ablative surgery, such as a maxillectomy for the treatment of oral cancer, would be representative of a lesion where insufficient normal denture-bearing tissue is present to permit stability of a denture base.

DENTURE RETENTION

The retention of dentures with obturators is one of the principal difficulties experienced by patients having deficiencies in the denture foundation tissues. Such difficulties are substantially reduced where natural teeth are present and can be utilised for the provision of direct retention, either by means of conventional clasping or by precision attachments.

In the absence of natural teeth, residual tissue undercuts may need to be engaged, and it may be necessary to consider the use of implants to assist in denture retention.

Patients with palatal defects who are not edentulous must have the importance of retaining their natural teeth stressed to them. Intensive oral hygiene instruction, and reinforcement of this, together with regular dental inspections and any necessary restorative treatment, must be carried out.

OBTURATOR PRODUCTION

Small defect

Where the palatal defect is relatively small, so that a stable denture base can be provided in order to secure an accurate record of jaw relations, treatment is commenced by producing a conventional type of denture. The obturator is subsequently added to the denture.

If the defect concerned involves a perforation of the hard palate only, the effect of sheeting over the defect with a denture base may provide adequate obturation (Fig. 41.1). During the impression stage, the space is covered with gauze impregnated with petroleum jelly, in order to prevent access of the impression material. The denture is then produced in the normal way.

Where a cleft of the hard and soft palates is present, the cleft is again protected from ingress of impression material using gauze impregnated with petroleum jelly at the impression stage. A denture having a base which extends posteriorly to the normal extension level is produced, but which has

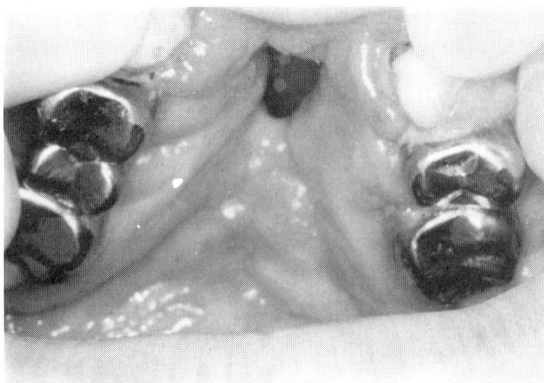

Fig. 41.1 Perforation of the hard palate which can be treated by sheeting over with a denture base.

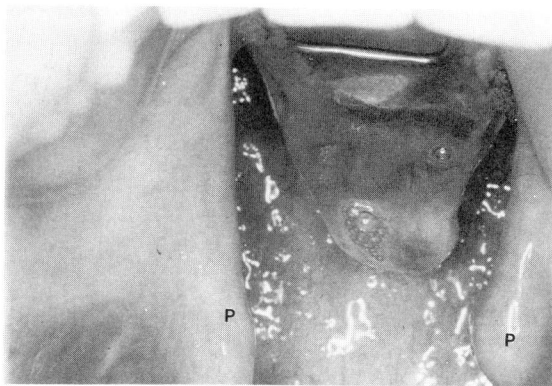

Fig. 41.2 Cleft of hard and soft palates. The pharyngeal extension of the obturator projects into the gap between the remnants of the soft palate (P,P). During functional activity the patient's soft palate remnants contacted the obturator to separate the oropharynx from the nasopharynx.

processed into it a loop of stainless steel wire. The loop of wire is positioned within the lateral remnants of the soft palate, and does not impinge on the posterior pharyngeal wall.

On the wire loop is moulded the pharyngeal extension of the obturator. The moulding process produces an obturator which, in functional activity during speech and deglutition, serves to separate the nasopharynx from the oropharynx (Fig. 41.2).

Large defects

Where insufficient tissue remains to enable a stable denture base to be produced, it is advantageous to obturate the cavity first. The obturator, together with the residual natural denture-supporting tissues, then provides a stable base on which to produce a denture.

The tissue cavity which remains following surgery may be very irregular in form, and a sectional impression will be required for its accurate reproduction. A sectional impression is one which is taken in several parts, which can then be separated for removal from the cavity and subsequently reassembled (Fig. 41.3). In this way, very irregularly shaped areas which may be severely undercut can be reproduced.

A hollow silicone obturator may be produced from the impression, which has advantages in

A

B

C

reducing the weight of the appliance. It can also be collapsed in order to insert the obturator into the mouth, and this can be very helpful, particularly where the oral opening is restricted.

The denture which is produced is attached to the obturator by means of undercut studs or by an undercut channel provided on the denture in the region where the denture bridges the oral defect at its narrowest level.

The above descriptions are illustrative only, and are representative of some of the many designs of obturator which may be used. The reader is referred to the literature for further details of these.

FURTHER READING

Benington IC 1989 Light cured hollow obturators. J Prosthet Dent 62: 322
Benington IC, Watson IB, Jenkins WMM, Allan GRJ 1979 Restorative treatment of the cleft palate patient. British Dental Association, London
Davenport JC 1983 Clinical and laboratory procedures for the production of a retentive silicone rubber obturator for the maxillectomy patient. Br J Oral Maxfac Surg 22: 378
Enderby P, Hathorn IS, Servant S 1984 The use of intra-oral appliances in the management of acquired velopharyngeal disorders. Br Dent J 157: 157
Schaaf NG 1977 Obturators on complete dentures. Dent Clin North Am 21: 395
Walter JD 1981 The design of prostheses used in the treatment of velopharyngeal insufficiency. Br Dent J 151: 338

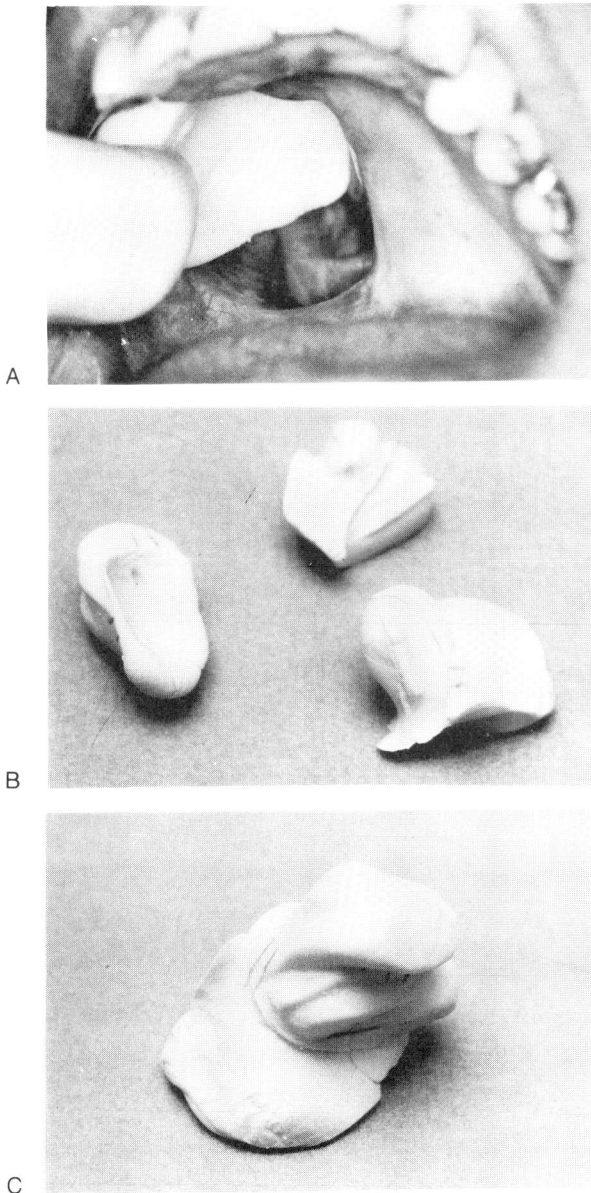

Fig. 41.3 **A** Silicone material being placed into the maxillectomy cavity by means of the operator's forefinger. This will form the first part of a three-part impression. **B** Three sections of the impression of the maxillectomy cavity. Each part is allowed to set and then coated with petroleum jelly before placement of the next part, so that separation of the sections is simplified to permit removal from the cavity. **C** The assembled impression.

General bibliography

Removable denture treatment cannot be undertaken successfully without acquaintance with related fields, and to this end the following textbooks are suggested as companions to the introductory study of clinical prosthetic dentistry:

CONSERVATIVE DENTISTRY
Kidd EAM, Smith BGN 1990 Pickard's manual of operative dentistry, 6th edn. Oxford University Press, Oxford

CROWN AND BRIDGEWORK
Shillingburg HT, Hobo S, Whitsett CD 1981 Fundamentals of fixed prosthodontics, 2nd Edn. Quintessence, Chicago

DENTAL MATERIALS SCIENCE
Combe EC 1986 Notes on dental materials, 5th edn. Churchill Livingstone, Edinburgh

DENTAL TECHNOLOGY
Wilson HJ, Mansfield MA, Heath JR, Spence D 1987 Dental Technology and Materials for Students, 8th edn. Blackwell, Oxford

ORAL MEDICINE
Jones JH, Mason DK 1990 Oral manifestations of systemic disease, 2nd edn. Baillière Tindall, London

ORAL SURGERY
Moore JR, Gillbe GV 1981 Principles of oral surgery, 3rd edn. Manchester University Press, Manchester

ORTHODONTICS
Foster TD 1990 A textbook of orthodontics. 3rd edn. Blackwell, Oxford

PERIODONTICS
Lindhe J 1990 Textbook of clinical periodontology, 2nd edn. Munksgaard, Copenhagen

Many excellent books on removable prostheses are referred to in the text.

Appendix

PERMANENT TEETH

Upper right   Upper left

18	17	16	15	14	13	12	11	21	22	23	24	25	26	27	28
48	47	46	45	44	43	42	41	31	32	33	34	35	36	37	38

Lower right   Lower left

DECIDUOUS TEETH

Upper right   Upper left

55	54	53	52	51	61	62	63	64	65
85	84	83	82	81	71	72	73	74	75

Lower right   Lower left

Index